THE PRINCIPLES
OF
HYPNOTHERAPY

MEDICAL HYPNOSIS

By

LEWIS R. WOLBERG, M.D.

*Chairman, Board of Trustees, Postgraduate
Center for Mental Health; Clinical Professor
of Psychiatry, New York Medical College*

Volume I

THE PRINCIPLES OF HYPNOTHERAPY

GRUNE & STRATTON

A Subsidiary of Harcourt Brace Jovanovich, Publishers

New York   San Francisco   London

Grune & Stratton, Inc.
111 Fifth Avenue
New York, New York 10003

Library of Congress Catalog Card Number 48-2929
International Standard Book Number 0-8089-0536-8

Printed in the United States of America

*To
My Wife*

CONTENTS

PREFACE

FEW THERAPIES in the history of medicine have enjoyed simultaneously such widespread acclaim and such universal condemnation as has hypnosis. To some extent these opposing attitudes still prevail. However, recent years have witnessed advances in experimental and therapeutic hypnosis which have tended to establish hypnotherapy firmly as a scientific treatment method.

The present volumes are a contribution to the growing literature on therapeutic hypnosis. They issue out of experimental work with hypnosis in the treatment of various emotional difficulties, and they attempt to delineate the utilities and limitations, as well as advantages and disadvantages, of hypnotherapy.

The teaching of any psychotherapeutic method is best achieved by personal observation and practical experience. For this reason, the manner of presentation in these volumes is somewhat unique. A considerable portion of Volume One is devoted to a step-by-step description of the induction process, illustrating various induction methods by excerpts from transcriptions of actual hypnotic sessions. There is a didactic discussion of the principles of psychotherapy, and of the psychopathologic factors in the different disease syndromes. Therapeutic methods applicable to the existing dynamics and the contributions hypnosis has to make to the treatment plan are elaborated on in some detail.

Volume Two contains three complete transcribed case histories which enable the reader to follow the various stages in treatment, and to observe the therapeutic management of the patient as if he were personally present at the sessions from the beginning to the end of therapy. In each instance, these illustrate a preceding discussion of the uses and limitations of the chief short-term psychotherapeutic methods.

Hypnosis adds speed and directness to psychotherapy, but it must not be regarded as a cure-all. A number of emotional problems fail to respond to hypnotherapy and require tra-

ditional long-term analytic approaches. However, where the
therapeutic goal does not demand an exhaustive rehabilitation of the character structure—and time itself is the essence
in the cure of obdurate interpersonal and habit patterns—a
short-term approach utilizing hypnosis may restore the
person to functional equilibrium. Furthermore, as will be
seen, the period of hypnotherapy may be utilized to create
an incentive in the patient to explore the deeper levels of
his neurosis and to prepare him to enter, at a later date,
should he need to do so, a more formal analytic type of
therapy.

The employment of psychotherapeutic technics calls for
certain personality qualifications and specialized skills in
the physician. Many indefinable elements enter into the
intense emotional experience that constitutes psychotherapy.
Among these are physical appearance, facial expression,
diction, forcefulness and mode of articulation of the therapist. These tend to structure, at the start at least, the type
of relationship the patient establishes with the physician.
They are qualities which are utilized by every physician in
what is euphemistically referred to as a "bedside manner."
However, a "bedside manner" alone is useless without addi-
tional personality qualities which make for a capacity to
empathize with the patient and to enter with him into a
therapeutic interpersonal relationship. Neurotic components
in the therapist which interfere with his ability to establish
and to maintain a relationship, or which cause him to act
hostile or to detach himself, will function as deterrents to
psychotherapeutic success.

Admittedly there are certain neurotic personality traits
in the physician to which the patient may respond in a
positive manner. A pompous, domineering and patronizing
attitude, for instance, may facilitate certain directive technics, and bring about symptomatic relief in dependent patients. However, serious neurotic traits in the physician will

interfere with the maintenance of that type of relationship which can succeed in bringing about deeper personality changes. The physician who desires to do any extensive type of psychotherapy must, consequently, be free from severe character difficulties, or at least aware of them sufficiently so that they are not projected into the therapeutic situation. A didactic psychoanalysis, accordingly, can be of inestimable value to the physician who desires to specialize in psychiatry.

Relative freedom from neurosis, nevertheless, will not suffice to make the physician a good therapist. What is essential is adequate training and experience, particularly supervised experience. Much as the surgeon requires postgraduate training, so the physician who seeks to treat emotional problems will need supplementary knowledge and training. While books such as this work are helpful, and constitute a convenient guide, they merely indicate the lines along which the physician may develop his therapeutic skills. Practical experience, particularly in some psychiatric training center, is indispensable in permitting of a full development and utilization of available therapeutic aptitudes.

Acknowledgment is made to Dr. Paul Hoch, editor, and to Grune and Stratton, publishers, for permission to reprint from the book, "Failures in Psychiatric Treatment," my article on "Therapeutic Failures with Hypnosis." I am deeply grateful to Dr. Milton H. Erickson who taught me, some years ago, the technic of induction of hypnosis by hand levitation which is included in this volume. Indebtedness is herewith expressed to the many patients and volunteer experimental subjects who shared with me the experiences which made this work possible.

LEWIS R. WOLBERG, M.D.

New York City
January, 1948

Part One

HISTORICAL, PHENOMENOLOGIC AND THEORETIC ASPECTS OF HYPNOSIS

I

THE HISTORY OF MEDICAL HYPNOSIS

Hypnosis is one of the oldest of the medical arts. Before discussing the principles of modern hypnotherapy it might be well to review briefly something of its history, the course of its development through a variety of rise and decline in favor, from the ancient concept of supernatural origin to the scientific theory and practice of today.

Medical hypnotism was practiced by the ancients who were convinced of the divine nature of the trance. The Persian Magi and Hindoo fakirs, inducing in themselves cataleptic states by strained fixation of the eyes, claimed supernormal powers of healing. The Egyptian "temple sleep" was probably a form of hypnosis during which curative utterances were suggested to the sufferer by the priest. These temples became so popular that they spread throughout Greece and Asia Minor.

With the development of Christianity, trance states were considered forms of witchcraft, and trance healing if employed at all was practiced secretly out of fear of ecclesiastic reprisal. It was not until the end of the eighteenth century that the phenomenon of hypnosis was recognized openly as a therapeutic agent.

In 1776, Franz Anton Mesmer wrote a thesis in which he

discussed the influence of planets on the human body. In his paper Mesmer postulated that this action occurred through the instrumentality of a universal fluid, a kind of impalpable invisible gas in which all bodies were immersed. The fluid had properties like those of a magnet and could be withdrawn by the human will from one point and concentrated on another. An inharmonious distribution of these fluids produced disease. Health could be attained by establishing harmony of magnetic fluids. The substance, which Mesmer called "animal magnetism," was said to flow from the hands of the operator directly into the patient. Animal magnetism could also be transferred to an animal or inanimate object which thereafter possessed mesmeric powers.

Mesmer was forced, by the hostile attitude of the medical profession, to leave Vienna and to take up residence in Paris where he founded with Deslon a clinic for the treatment of various diseases. Mesmerism became a fashionable fad, and throngs of wealthy followers filled his apartments to receive the magical nostrum. Mesmer's impressive manner and surroundings, his mystical passes and strokings, the slow music, and the expectation of benefit all contributed to the effect. Patients were placed in a large wooden tub filled with water, iron filings, bottles and iron rods which were applied to their various ailing parts. Mesmer, himself, appeared in a long silk robe with an iron wand with which he touched his patients. Several such treatments sufficed to cure a variety of disorders.

Mesmerism attracted a great many charlatans who as "magnetizers" made extravagant claims as to the efficacy of this treatment. Many of them professed supernatural powers which made it possible for them to detect lesions deep within the patient's body. Common expressions were as follows: "This patient's stomach is full of pimples. . . . I see a ball of hair blocking the bowel. . . . Your chest is all grazed inside, and you must not sing for several days; it looks as if it had been scraped with a knife, and your lungs are full of dust."[1]

A commission, appointed by the French Government in 1784, finally investigated the methods of Mesmer and pronounced him a fraud. Thereafter his popularity waned. But, while Mesmer was blinding himself with dazzling notoriety, one of his disciples, Marquis de Puységur, observed and described three cardinal features of hypnosis. He noted that the "magnetized" subject could hear only what the "magnetizer" said and was oblivious to all else, that he accepted suggestions without question, and that he could recall nothing of the events of the trance when restored to normal consciousness. This condition de Puységur called "artificial somnambulism." He explained that the subject was endowed with second sight, for he could accomplish incredible feats like reading sealed messages, suffering needles to be jabbed into his skin, and permitting, without flinching, the application of a red hot poker to his body.

Following the discreditment of Mesmer by the medical profession, few reputable physicians practiced mesmerism until the middle of the nineteenth century when James Braid, a Manchester surgeon, experimenting with the phenomenon, decided that it was not at all due to "animal magnetism" or to any other mysterious influence that passed from the subject to the patient. On the contrary, he contended that the mesmeric effect was entirely subjective. This finding was also arrived at independently by Bertrand and the Abbe Faria. In 1842, Braid offered to read a paper on the subject before the British Medical Association which was to meet in Manchester. The offer was rejected. In the same year Squire Ward presented before the Royal Medico-Chirurgical Society of London a paper on amputations performed painlessly on a hypnotized patient.[2] The paper was branded as ridiculous as were the reports of Braid to the effect that he had cured cases of contractures and disorders of sensibility such as deafness.

Braid renamed the phenomena of mesmerism *hypnotism*, and he stated that through the aid of hypnotism important physical and psychical effects might be obtained. Braid postulated the existence of an intelligent secondary consciousness, and he theorized that *rapport* was an artificial condition due to suggestion.

Several years later, the physician Elliotson was discharged from his position at the University College Hospital for choosing hypnosis as his subject for the Harveian Oration of 1846. Despite the fact that he was branded as a charlatan, Elliotson and his followers started the *Zoist*, a journal dealing with mesmerism and with cerebral physiology. Under the influence of Elliotson, Mesmeric Institutions were formed in various parts of the British Isles. At the Institution at Exeter, Parker claimed to have mesmerized twelve hundred persons and to have performed on them a total of two hundred painless operations.

Around the same time, James Esdaile, in India, reported to the Medical Board seventy-five operations performed under hypnosis, but his letter was never even acknowledged. When he had accumulated over one hundred hypnotic operations, he placed his results before the Government. A committee of investigation, appointed by the Deputy-Governor of Bengal, reported favorably on his experiments. Esdaile continued with his work, and before he left India he had to his credit thousands of minor operations and three hundred major surgical procedures done under the influence of hypnosis.

In 1882, a Society for Psychical Research was founded to investigate the therapeutic uses of hypnotism. Among the members were William James, Bernheim, Stanley Hall, Liebeault and Janet. The British Medical Association, in 1891, also appointed a committee to investigate the therapeutic value of hypnotism. The published report contained the opinion that "as a therapeutic agent hypnotism is frequently effective in relieving pain, procuring sleep and alleviating many functional ailments."[3]

In France, Charcot and his followers, at the Paris Hospital of Salpétrièr, tried diligently to devise scientific tests for hypnosis. Their contention was that hypnosis was a pathologic phenomenon akin to hysteria, the product of an abnormal nervous constitution. The methods and conclusions of Charcot were later exposed as unscientific by the Nancy School which proved hypnosis to be a normal manifestation.

Liebeault, who may be considered the real father of modern hypnotism, was one of the first physicians who experimented with the therapeutic value of hypnosis on a large scale. He treated thousands of patients suffering from a great assortment of physical symptoms. Hypnosis, he believed, could influence favorably not only functional, but also organic diseases. It could even, he imagined, cure cancer, and it might also act as an antidote to poisoning. He claimed cures for anemia, intermittent fever, pulmonary tuberculosis, menstrual difficulties, neuralgia and migraine. Liebeault published a book on hypnosis, but medical skepticism was so great that he was able to sell but one copy. Bernheim, a professor at the Nancy Medical School, incensed by the claims of Liebeault, decided to visit his clinic to expose him as a quack. He was instead so amazed at Liebeault's work that he undertook a study of hypnotism, and he soon became one of its most ardent devotees, publishing a book[4] in which he claimed cures for hysterical hemiplegia and aphonia, hysteroid crises, gastric difficulties, loss of appetite, "depression of the spirit," pains, tremors, "fixed ideas," sleepwalking and a number of other complaints associated with functional diseases. Bernheim ridiculed the idea of Charcot that hypnosis was a sign of weakness and of nervous indisposition.

Bernheim's work established hypnosis more firmly as a therapeutic method and inspired others to work with the hypnotic procedure. Charles Despine, Lasegue, Morel, Moll,[5] Quackenbos,[6] Hecker, de Jong, van Eeden, Gorodickze, Sturgis, Mavroukakis, Bourdon, Babinski and Heidenhain spoke enthusiastically of their cures, particularly with hysterical patients. Surgical operations under hypnosis were performed by Recamier, Cloque, Oudet, Ribaud and Tophan. Babinski treated cases of abasia associated with agoraphobia. Krafft-Ebing and Schrenck-Notzing reported good results in the treatment of satyriasis, nymphomania and homosexuality. Voisin, Berillon, Tanzi, Bauer, Marot, Fulda and Wetterstrand were successful in the handling of drug addiction, while Woods reported favorably on the treatment of epilepsy. Voisin, Brenaud and Burot claimed excellent results in depressive forms of insanity. Osgood, Stadelmann, Charpentier, Farez, Grossmann and Backman were convinced of the value ɔf hypnosis in skin diseases. Utilizing hypnosis as a means of moral pressure, Guyou, Delboeuf and Berillon treated such disorders in children as incontinence, untruthfulness and nail-biting. In Switzerland, Ladame claimed signal success with alcoholics. In Germany, Holland, Russia and other parts of Europe, hypnosis took on increasing significance as a form of treatment.

So many varied types of illness presumably were "cured" by hypnotism that one may justifiably suspect that the therapist's enthusiasm often overwhelmed his scientific judgment. For instance, Forel listed among diseases susceptible to hypnosis "spontaneous somnambulism, bodily pains, sleeplessness, functional paralysis and contractures, chlorosis, disturbances of menstruation, loss of appetite, nervous digestive disturbances, constipation, diarrhea, gastric and intestinal dyspepsia, psychical impotence, morphinism, chronic muscular and arthritic rheumatism, lumbago, neurasthenic disturbances, stammering, nervous disturbances of vision, blepharospasm, night terrors in children, seasickness, vomiting of pregnancy, enuresis, chorea, nervous attacks of coughing, hysterical disturbances and bad habits."[7]

One reason why unfounded claims were made for hypnosis during this period was that few follow-up studies were done on patients presumably cured. It must be remembered that at this time nothing was known of the defensive value of symptoms, and of their functional utility in the life adjustment of the individual. Hypnosis was used as a bludgeon to crush the patient's complaints. We therefore must suspect that failures were far more frequent than successes.

Around 1880, Breuer introduced an important innovation in hypnotic therapy which extended the application of hypnosis beyond the simple suggesting away of symptoms. While treating a hysterical patient, Anna O., whose illness was precipitated by the development on the part of her father of a peripleuritic abscess, he was confounded by the fact that in spite of all hypnotic efforts her symptoms became progressively worse. She was incapacitated by distressing physical symptoms and by alternating states of consciousness.

Breuer accidentally discovered that when Anna was induced to speak freely under hypnosis, she exhibited a profound emotional reaction and thereafter experienced a decided relief from her complaints. He learned from the utterances of Anna that the states of somnolence into which she lapsed each afternoon were repetitions of the vigils she held at her sick father's bedside while she nursed him in the early stages of his illness. Although Anna's general condition gradually improved, she continued to exhibit alternating states of consciousness, and she was indolent, moody, disobedient and at times actively hallucinated.

One afternoon, during a period of intense heat, Anna suffered from great thirst, but to her dismay she found that she was unable to swallow water. For six weeks thereafter she quenched her thirst exclusively by eating fruits and melons. During a hypnotic session she revealed, in a fit of anger, how, to her great disgust, a former governess had permitted a dog to drink water out of a glass in her presence. She had at the time refrained from protesting in order to be polite. Following this revelation she surprized Breuer by asking for a drink

which she imbibed without hesitation, awakening from hypnosis with the glass at her lips. There was no further recur-
rence of her refusal to drink. It was Breuer's belief that the
act of recalling the experience of the dog drinking from a glass
caused the symptom to vanish.

Breuer then attempted to associate all of the patient's peculiar habits with damaging or disgusting experiences in the
past. During the morning Anna was hypnotized and asked to
concentrate on her thoughts and memories concerning a particular symptom. As she talked her productions were jotted
down in rapid succession. In the evening, during a second
hypnotic session, she elaborated upon the events that had
been noted previously. There was in this way a gradual working back of situations to their primal causes. Only when the
basic cause was discovered did the symptom disappear. It
usually required a considerable amount of work to arrive at
the basic cause. For instance, in trying to understand why
Anna failed to hear a person entering the room, she detailed
one hundred and eight examples before she revealed the first,
in which her father was involved, which finally removed the
symptom.

Gradually Anna recalled under hypnosis all the events
associated with development of her hysteria. In July 1880
when her father had first become ill, she and her mother
shared the responsibility of nursing him. On one occasion during the absence of her mother, while awaiting a surgeon from
Vienna, she was awakened from her sleep by a sense of foreboding and great anxiety. She hurried to her father's sick
room and sat near his bed holding her right arm over the back
of the chair. As she started dozing, she fantasied a black
snake coming out of the wall toward her father as if to bite
him. She had an impulse to drive the snake away, but her
right arm seemed paralyzed and asleep. She gazed at her
fingers with dread and noticed that they had changed into
small snakes with skulls. She wished to pray, but her anxiety

was so great that the words refused to come, until she finally remembered an English nursery rhyme. In the English language alone could she get herself to think and pray. The blast of a locomotive however interrupted her reverie. On the following day, while outdoors, a bent twig evoked the snake hallucination which in turn automatically brought about a contracture of her right arm.

Anna's inability to eat was traced to the constant feeling of anxiety during her father's illness which had interfered with her appetite. Her deafness appeared first when she attempted to eliminate the sound of her father who was in a choking attack. Her visual disturbance, too, had originated in association with her father. Once as she sat near him tears filled her eyes. Her father asked her for the time, and because her vision was blurred, it was necessary to bring the watch close to her eyes. The face of the watch at short range appeared very large. Symptoms of makropsia and convergent strabismus symbolized this experience. A quarrel during which she had to suppress an answer caused her throat to contract, and this laryngeal symptom repeated itself later on. By discovering the experience associated with the first appearance of the symptom, Anna "related away" her anesthesia, cough, trembling, and other complaints, and finally her entire hysterical attack came to an end.

The importance of Breuer's work lies in the change of emphasis in hypnotic therapy, from the direct removal of symptoms to the dealing with the apparent causes of the symptoms. There is evidence that Janet simultaneously arrived at the technic of liberating "strangulated affects" associated with traumatic memories, although Breuer traditionally has been given credit for the discovery.

Breuer's method attracted a number of physicians, the most prominent being Sigmund Freud, who, with Breuer, in 1895, published a book, "Studien über Hysterie." "We found, at first to our greatest surprise, that the *individual hysterical symptoms immediately disappeared without returning if we succeeded in thoroughly awakening the memories of the causal process with its accompanying affect, and if the patient circumstantially discussed the process in the most detailed manner and gave verbal expression to the affect.*"[8] Breuer and Freud concluded that hysterical symptoms developed as a result of experiences so damaging to the individual that they had been repressed. The mental energy originally associated with the experience was blocked from reaching consciousness by the mechanism of repression. The energy was then converted into bodily innervations. Under hypnotic treatment, the discharge of strangulated affect ("abreaction") into normal channels of consciousness made it unnecessary to convert the energy into symptoms. Because this technic seemed to evacuate quantities of emotion from the unconscious, it was called the "cathartic method."

Another important modification in hypnotic technic was instituted by Freud. In attempting to hypnotize a young woman, Lucie R., who complained of depression and of subjective sensations of smell, he was unable to induce the somnambulistic trance essential for "cathartic" treatment. Remembering an experiment by Bernheim, who had caused a patient to remember in the waking state, by persistent urging, her experiences during a somnambulistic trance, Freud placed his hand on the patient's forehead and enjoined her to repeat everything that came to her mind. Recollections and fantasies which the patient thought too insignificant to mention were by this process of "free association" brought to the surface. Freud was thus able to recapture important pathogenic experiences without recourse to hypnosis.

Perhaps more significant was Freud's discovery of the motives and resistances decisive for the forgetting process. Because many memories were inaccessible to hypnotic recall even in the somnambulistic state, Freud concluded that there were forces that kept memories from invading consciousness, and he discovered that it was necessary to neutralize the repressing forces before recall was possible. An effective way to overcome the resistance was to permit the patient to relax and to talk freely about any idea or fantasy that entered his mind no matter how trivial or absurd. Freud could observe in this "free association" a sequential theme that was somehow related to the traumatic event. Other important ways of discovering traumatic episodes were the interpretation of the patient's dreams and of the irrational attitudes and fantasies the patient developed in relation to the physician, a phenomenon Freud called the "transference." He concluded that hypnosis was ineffective in the face of resistance, and he consequently abandoned the trance as a means of uprooting repressed memories.

Freud, in continuing his psychoanalytic work, laid less and less stress on the strangulated affects of early traumatic experiences as the chief cause of neurosis. More and more he became cognizant of the purposeful nature of the symptom, and, in 1926, he revised his theory of neurosis drastically, claiming that symptoms were not only manifestations of repressed instinctive strivings, but also represented defenses against these strivings.[9] Essentially they were technics to avert anxiety. By pointing out that symptoms served an economic function in the psychic life of the individual, Freud lent further emphasis to the irrationality of the use of hypnosis for removal of symptoms.

Freud's discoveries as well as current disappointment in hypnosis as a permanent cure of hysteria almost succeeded in dealing hypnosis a death blow. Whereas thousands of scientific articles and books on the subject had been published yearly, the number of publications dwindled to several dozen. A few authorities, nevertheless, proceded with hypnotic research, the most notable being Pierre Janet[10] in France, J. Milne Bramwell[11] in Great Britain, Morton Prince[12, 13] and Boris Sidis[14, 15] in the United States, all of whom published works on the subject. Rivers, Read, Southard, Ames, Hall, Salmon, Pavlov, Münsterberg, McDougall,[16] Brooks,[17] Baudouin[18] and Yellowlees[19] were also among those whose interest in hypnosis continued. However, the growth of the psychoanalytic movement and the development of other forms of psychotherapy reduced hypnosis to a place of relatively minor importance. Hypnotism became subject to the attack of the medical profession on the basis that it was allied to quackery and was a source of moral danger. Even Bernheim who did so much for hypnosis, no longer regarded it as having any real value.[20]

Janet, however, continued to believe in hypnosis as a most effective treatment for the neuroses. He warned that hypnotic suggestion could produce no action beyond the power of the normal will. Indeed, because neurotic persons suffered from "defects of the will," he contended that the physician should be satisfied if hypnosis produced actions no greater than those encompassed by the average will. He also felt that by exercising lost motor and sensory functions under hypnosis, these functions might be restored to normal activity involuntarily.

In the eyes of most physicians, nevertheless, hypnosis was a relic of the past. Although it was politely mentioned in textbooks of psychiatry, it was considered in the category of such ancient practices as cupping, leeching, and blood-letting.

During the first World War, the large number of victims suffering from functional contractures, paralytic and amnesic conditions, as well as other symptoms caused by the trauma of war, required, in view of the shortage of psychiatrists, an abbreviated form of therapy. Hypnotherapy was revived and was utilized both for direct symptom removal and for the restoration of repressed experiences. Excellent accounts of this historical phase are described by Thom,[21] Brown,[22] Wingfield,[23] and Hadfield.[24] Both Wingfield and Hadfield caused their patients during the trance to regress in time to the period of the damaging experience, and encouraged them to relive the event and to liberate the emotions relating to the experience during this regression. Hadfield originated the term "hypnoanalysis" which he applied to the latter procedure.

Success in the treatment of the war neuroses created a new wave of enthusiasm for hypnotherapy which has persisted to the present day. However, confusion as to methods and reasons for success and failures have made the application of hypnosis in medicine a hit and miss procedure.

Considerable controversy has existed as to the real value of hypnotherapy. The literature contains many reports of functional and even organic illnesses "cured" or ameliorated through the use of hypnosis. Thus hypnosis is said to have been used successfully in conversion hysteria,[25,26] in hysterical lethargy,[27] hysterical mutism and blindness,[28] amblyopia,[29] photophobia,[30] hysterical paralysis,[31,32] dissociation of the personality,[33] amnesia,[34-40] chorea,[41-43] speech disorders,[44-49] asthma,[50,51] enuresis,[52,53] various skin diseases,[54] including lichen planus,[55] eczema,[56-58] psoriasis,[59,60] warts,[61] arsphenamine dermatitis[62] and pruritis,[63] allergy,[64] sleep disturbances,[65,66] essential hypertension,[67] vomiting of pregnancy,[68] menstrual disorders,[69,70] anorexia nervosa,[71] various neuroses,[72-75] morbid fears,[76-78] kleptomania,[79] perverse sex practices,[80] alcoholism,[81-86] various mental diseases,[87] including depression and early schizophrenia.[88] It has been advocated in orthopedics,[89] in dentistry,[90-94] in diseases of the sympathetic nervous system,[95] for exhausting hemorrhages in hemorrhagic diathesis,[98] and in other organic diseases.[99]

With few exceptions these reports involve the use of hypnosis as a means of symptom removal through prestige suggestion. We may speculate that follow-up studies would reveal a considerable number of relapses, since the basic core of the emotional illness is not affected by suggestion. This is not to say that some symptomatic recoveries have not been permanent. Wells,[100] for instance, reported the cure of a patient suffering from hysterical headaches, contractures, paralyses, anesthesias, somnambulism and fugues. After several hypnotic treatment sessions the patient recovered and remained symptom-free during the intervening fourteen years.

While the treatment of symptoms by direct suggestion is occasionally successful, failures have, in the experience of most practitioners, been the rule rather than the exception. Attempts have consequently been made to see if methods other than direct symptom removal might be more effective. Following the technic advocated by Dubois,[101, 102] several physicians have claimed gratifying results from hypnosis by using it in a reassuring, persuasive manner to bolster up the self confidence of the individual. A number of the reports mentioned above employ this method. The dynamics of how hypnotic persuasion operates has not been satisfactorily described, but some years ago Hollander[103] made the challenging assertion that persuasive suggestions penetrated through the conscious layers of mind and reconstructed the personality by influencing the subconscious.

That hypnosis often exerts a healing influence without the patient's conscious participation has been observed by many other therapists. One way in which this influence is probably effected is the partial modification of the patient's values and standards, perhaps by virtue of the fact that the hypnotist becomes for the patient, temporarily at least, an omniscient authority.

In some instances the hypnotist, assuming the role of a new, more lenient authority, has attempted an alteration of misconceptions gleaned from past experiences with repressive and overdisciplinary authorities. Here, while under hypnosis, the patient has been reassured about his fears and guilt feelings, and an attempt has been made to re-educate him with the object of reducing the severity of his conscience.

While such attempts generally have been inconclusive, since the incorporated disciplines of past contacts with authority are not easily dissipated, success has been reported by some physicians. Morgan,[104] for example, treated a young woman with such strong guilt feelings about sex that suicide was a possibility. She was inaccessible to other approaches. Under hypnosis suggestions were made to her to the effect that sex was natural, and that irreparable wrong was not done when an individual yielded to sexual impulses. Depression vanished and the patient made an excellent adjustment to a more normal outlook on life.

The use of hypnosis to implant re-educational suggestions presupposes a precise knowledge of areas of psychobiologic malfunctioning. The understanding of the manner in which the individual fails in his relationships with life is mandatory. For instance, if a symptom is traced to certain powerful emotions that issue out of disturbed interpersonal relationships, suggestions directed at the causative emotion rather than at the symptom may bring success. This principle is illustrated by the early case of von Renterghen,[105] who, in treating a patient with torticollis, emphasized that it was essential to control his anger. From the case history it would seem that the hostility of the patient was associated with his symptom, and that the patient's acceptance of the injunction to repress hostility produced an alleviation of his complaint. Dealing with symptoms by tackling their emotional source has resulted in a more effective use of hypnosis. The work of Prince and Sidis has been principally in this direction.

In spite of certain published claims, the use of hypnosis along traditional persuasive and re-educational lines is only moderately more successful than persuasive and re-educational methods without hypnosis. Obdurate habit patterns and devaluated self esteem are not disposed of by appeals to reason. More and more physicians are arriving at the conclusion that before a real cure can be obtained through psychotherapy, it is essential to work through the dynamic sources of the patient's neurosis. Consequently we have witnessed an increasing emphasis in the direction of determining and removing the cause of the patient's conflicts, employing hypnosis to facilitate this process.

The fact that repressed traumatic experiences can act as foci of emotional difficulty has centered much attention on the hypnotic recall of buried memories. The war neuroses have provided the most dramatic examples of how effective hypnosis can be in the amelioration of symptoms through a reliving of the traumatic scene. Recent efforts have been extended toward encouraging recall during hypnosis, particularly through hypnotic regression and reorientation to the period of the traumatic event.

Utilizing this method, Erickson and Kubie[106] reported a case of a young woman who had been plunged into a depression by a proposal of marriage. Hypnosis with regression to ages between ten to thirteen revealed that she had, at that period, received many faulty ideas regarding sex from her mother. Misconceptions were clarified and the patient developed insight into her condition. She recovered completely and shortly afterward married the man whose proposal had initiated her depression. The treatment of an acquired food intolerance by a similar technic was also reported by Erickson.[107]

The most detailed published work in this field is that of Lindner,[108] who hypnoanalyzed a criminal psychopath and enucleated memories of traumatic events that had occurred prior to the age of one. A microphone, concealed in the room, transmitted the productions of the patient to a stenographer who recorded and later transcribed the proceedings in detail. Lindner contends that hypnoanalysis is equivalent to a surgical removal of barriers and hazards, that it pierces the psychic substrata and raises the repressed to the level of awareness.

A variety of technics other than regression and revivification have been employed during the trance state to help recapture forgotten traumatic experiences. Among these are dream induction, drawing, automatic writing, mirror gazing, play therapy and free association.[109-115] Although therapeutic effectiveness has been increased to some extent by these hypnoanalytic methods, there are definite limitations, as has been shown,[116] to what can be achieved through technics which depend exclusively on the restoration of repressed memories. While some neurotic conditions, like hysterical and traumatic neuroses are influenced by this procedure, most emotional difficulties are not particularly responsive.

In an effort to expand the application of hypnosis, studies have been made and reported, most notably by the Menninger group[117,118] and Wolberg,[119] on the hypnotic handling of transference and resistance. Evidence exists that hypnosis can catalyze the working through of both transference resistances as well as resistances to recall. As more is learned about the dynamics of hypnotherapy, and as more analysts utilize hypnosis as a therapeutic adjunct, further data will be available on which to judge the value of hypnosis in the psychoanalytic process.

One hypnoanalytic technic which is of particular interest to some physicians is that of the experimental conflict. No other method can approach the spectacular directness with which the basic problems of the individual can be brought to his attention and his ego resources mobilized to help him overcome certain difficulties. Luria[120] originally worked with this technic in investigating various aspects of human behavior, and he undoubtedly inspired such workers as Erickson[121] who have utilized and perfected the procedure.

In treating a man suffering from premature ejaculation, Erickson,[122] suggested a fictitious incident which involved the man's placing a lighted cigarette in a painted glass ash tray, the heat of the cigarette cracking the tray. Guilt at having destroyed the article was successfully induced. Following hypnosis, the subject's spontaneous conversation was filled with references to vases, broken glassware, bric-a-brac and art treasures, and his mental stream was frequently interrupted by stammering, blocking and repetition of ideas. Furthermore, the man could not get himself to use a nearby ash tray, and he showed extraordinary caution in putting out cigarette butts and matches. The subject was then rehypnotized and instructed to recall the entire incident upon awakening. In so doing he seemed to recognize a similarity between the experimental conflict and his own emotional problem, and several days later he was able to perform his first successful act of sexual intercourse.

Eisenbud[123] utilized the experimental conflict to induce hostility in a patient with migraine and amnesia in order to demonstrate to him how his headaches were the result of repressed hostility. Although many incidents of the amnesic period were finally recalled, a gap of six weeks remained that could not be bridged. Prior to the onset of the patient's illness, his father was hospitalized with diabetic gangrene which necessitated a foot amputation. During this period the patient had pawned his father's clothes in order to redeem some worthless checks. No great amount of work was required to reveal repressed hostility toward the father even though the patient's conscious attitude was one of dutiful concern. Wishes for the father's injury or death were revealed by dreams. Headaches followed such dreams as a psychosomatic sequel.

During hypnosis the patient recovered several memories of events that had occurred at puberty when, in a fit of rage, he had tried to poison his father by putting Lysol in the latter's whiskey and rat poison in one of his medicinal powders. The gradual removal of the six week amnesic gap brought out open hostility and aggression directed at the father. Headaches disappeared, but anxiety resulted that distressed the patient greatly. After twenty-five days the amnesia was re-induced through hypnotic suggestion, and the patient's anxiety suddenly disappeared, but a return of headaches was the consequence.

In order to test the hypothesis that the repression of hostile aggressive attitudes gave rise to headaches, Eisenbud decided to implant in the patient's mind an experimental conflict. In deep hypnosis, a fictitious story was related to the patient involving a quarrel between a male nurse and himself during which he was falsely accused of breaking into the nurse's office. Although he was angry at this unjust accusation, he was told that he had to hide his true feelings. The next morning the patient woke up feeling grouchy, complaining of a severe generalized headache. The following day under hypnosis the incident was repeated and the next morning he had an even more severe headache. That noon he was again hypnotized, and he was informed that the event had never really occurred. He immediately showed a happy-go-lucky attitude and complete freedom from headaches. Other complexes were induced under hypnosis involving situations in which the patient had to repress his aggression either out of fear or out of politeness. The consequence of this repression was always an attack of migraine.

The most interesting phase of this experiment was that desensitization gradually developed. Hypnotically induced conflicts became less and less capable of invoking attacks, and, along with this, spontaneous headaches also disappeared. Finally, the reinduction of the original amnesia which had been associated with migraine failed to produce headaches, and its removal produced no anxiety. Some months after the experiment, the patient was subjected to harsh criticism by his employer and had to repress his hostility in order to retain his job. No headaches resulted. Finally his father was admitted to a hospital with a severe heart attack, and the patient was able to weather this without the development of symptoms.

The ability of the individual to master neurotic symptoms through the medium of experimental conflicts contributes to self confidence and helps to strengthen the weakened ego. Another means of achieving this goal is by demonstrating to the patient under hypnosis that he is capable of establishing control over his functions. Kardiner and Spiegel[124] illustrate the latter use of hypnosis by the case of a patient with a persistent tic who, through suggestion, was convinced that it was possible to increase and diminish the intensity of his tic, that it could be transferred from one side of the body to the other, and finally that he himself could control it. He thus became convinced that he was not the helpless victim of his symptoms, but could actually master them through his own resources.

What the future holds for hypnosis cannot be foreseen. A number of new books have appeared, most notably those of Brenman and Gill[125] and Le Cron and Bordeaux,[126] which review the historical phases of hypnosis and outline existing treatment procedures. Such efforts are commendable because they present the experiences of workers in the field of therapeutic hypnosis. They are of help in permitting hypnosis to emerge from its past mysticism and oversimplification. Unfortunately these efforts are constantly being sabotaged by the fantastic claims of untrained people whose enthusiasm with a few rapid hypnotic successes causes them to voice judgments about the method that are essentially untrue. The history of hypnosis demonstrates conclusively that it is no miracle worker, but that, shorn of extravagant claims made for it by some of its adherents, it is an important and useful therapeutic tool.

REFERENCES

1 HERMES: 1826, p. 216.
2 YELLOWLEES, H.: A manual of Psychotherapy, London, A. & C. Black, 1923, p. 82.

3 BRAMWELL, J. M.: Hypnotism. London, Rider, 1930.

4 BERNHEIM, H.: Suggestive Therapeutics. New York, Putnam's, 1900.

5 MOLL, A.: Hypnotism (translated by A. F. Hopkirk). London, Walter Scott Publishers, 1909.

6 QUACKENBOS, J. D.: Hypnotic Therapeutics in Theory and Practice. New York, Harper, 1908.

7 FOREL, A.: Hypnotism: or suggestion and psychotherapy (translated by H. W. Armit). New York, Rebman, 1907.

8 BREUER, J. AND FREUD, S.: Studies in Hysteria (translated by A. A. Brill). New York & Washington, Nervous & Mental Disease Publishing Co., 1936, pp. 3, 4.

9 FREUD, S.: The Problem of Anxiety. New York, W. W. Norton, 1936.

10 JANET, P.: Psychological Healing. New York, Macmillan, 1925.

11 BRAMWELL, J. M.: op. cit., reference 3.

12 PRINCE, M.: The Unconscious. New York, Macmillan, 1921.

13 ———: Clinical and Experimental Studies in Personality. Cambridge, Sci-Art, 1929.

14 SIDIS, B.: Psychopathological Researches. New York, G. E. Stechert, 1902.

15 ———: Foundations of Normal and Abnormal Psychology. Boston, Badger, 1914.

16 McDOUGALL, W.: Outline of Abnormal Psychology. New York, Scribners, 1926.

17 BROOKS, C. H.: The Practice of Autosuggestion by the Method of Emile Coue. New York, Dodd Mead, 1922.

18 BAUDOUIN, C.: Suggestion and Autosuggestion. London, Allen & Unwin, 1920.

19 YELLOWLEES, H.: op. cit., reference 2.

20 JANET, P.: op cit., reference 10, vol. I, p. 324.

21 THOM, D. A.: Suggestive therapy. Am. J. Insan. 76: 437, 1920.

22 BROWN, W.: Psychology and Psychotherapy, ed. 3. Baltimore, Wm. Wood, 1934.

23 WINGFIELD, H. E.: An Introduction to the Study of Hypnotism, ed. 2. London Vailliere, Tindall & Cox, 1920.

24 HADFIELD, J. A.: Functional Nerve Disease. London, H. Frowde, 1920.

25 SIMONSON, E.: Successful therapy of severe multiple conversion hysteria by catharsis; case. Internat. Ztschr. f. Psychoanal. 20: 531–542, 1934.

26 RAEDER, O. J.: Hypnosis and allied forms of suggestion in practical psychotherapy. Am. J. Psychiat. 13: 67–76, 1933.

27 ANGULO, L. MUNIZ: Hysterical lethargy cured by hypnotism. Rev. med. cubana 46: 875–882, August 1935.

28 ———: Hysteric mutism and blindness cured by psychoanalysis and hypnotism; case. Rev. med. cubana 48: 675–678, July 1937.

29 EBERT, E. C.: Hypnosis in psychogenic amblyopia. U. S. Nav. M. Bull. 29: 248–463, July 1931.

30 RAEDER, O. J.: op. cit., reference 26.

31 CABALLERO, C. PEREZ: Facial paralysis of hysterical origin cured by hypnosis and high frequency therapy: case. Siglo med. 87: 413–415, April 18, 1931.

32 WAGNER, F.: Functional paralysis cured by hypnosis and suggestion. Ugesk. f. laeger. 106: 258, March 15, 1944.

33 COPELAND, C. L. AND KITCHING, E. H.: A case of profound dissociation of the personality. J. Ment. Sc. 83: 719–726, 1937.

[34] STERN, R.: Ztschr. f. d. ges. Neurol. u. Psychiat. *108:* 601–624, 1927.

[35] EVPLOVA, N. N. AND FAKTOROVITCH.: Klin. J. Saratov. Univ. *5:* 145–154, February 1928.

[36] VINER, N.: Amnesia: dual personality with special reference to case recalled by hypnotism. Canad. M. A. J. *25:* 147–152, August 1931.

[37] ERICKSON, M. H.: Development of apparent unconsciousness during hypnotic reliving of a traumatic experience. Arch. Neurol. & Psychiat. *38:* 1282–1288, 1937.

[38] BECK, L. F.: Hypnotic identification of an amnesia victim. Brit. J. M. Psychol. *16:* 36–42, 1936.

[39] COPELAND, C. L. AND KITCHING, E. H.: Hypnosis in mental hospital practice. J. Ment. Sc. *83:* 316–329, 1937.

[40] HART, H. H.: Hypnosis in psychiatric clinics. J. Nerv. & Ment. Dis. *74:* 598–609, 1931.

[41] PODYAPOLSKY, P. P.: Successful treatment of chorea in children. Klin. J. saratov. univ. *6:* 51–56, June 1928.

[42] ESZENYI, M.: Hypnosis in chorea minor. München med. Wchnschr. *81:* 1340–1342, August 31, 1934.

[43] ——: Hypnosis—effect in choreatic movement disorders. Psychiat. neurol. Wchnschr. *37:* 499–504, Oct. 19, 1935.

[44] DONATH, J.: Hypnosis for stammering. Med. Welt. *2:* 1532–1533, Oct. 13, 1928.

[45] SCHULZE, H.: Hypnosis of stuttering. Therap. d. Gegenw. *73:* 521–522, November 1932.

[46] DONATH, J.: Hypnosis in stuttering. Therap. d. Gegenw. *73:* 456–457, October 1932.

[47] VOLGYESI, F.: Hypnosis in speech disorders. Monatschr. f. Ohrenh. *69:* 339–349, March 1935.

[48] LEVBARG, J. J.: Hypnosis—potent therapy for certain disorders of voice and speech. Arch. Otolaryng. *30:* 206–211, August 1939.

[49] MOORE, W. E.: Hypnosis in a system of therapy for stutterers. J. Speech Disorders. *11:* 117–122, 1946.

[50] JACOBI, E.: Treatment of asthma by hypnosis. Deutsche med. Wchnschr. *52:* 452, 1926.

[51] TAPLIN, A. B.: Hypnotism and Treatment by Suggestion. Liverpool, 1928.

[52] NARATH, U.: Causal treatment of enuresis. Klin. Wchnschr. *5:* 1446, 1926.

[53] BILLSTROM, J.: Hypnosis in enuresis nocturna. Acta Paediat. *26:* 62–65, 1939.

[54] ESTRIP, J.: Hypnosis as supportive symptomatic treatment in skin diseases; cases. Urol. & Cutan. Rev. *45:* 337–338, May 1941.

[55] KARTAMISCHEW, A. J.: Hypnosis for lichen ruber planus; cases. Dermat. Wchnschr. *96:* 788–791, June 10, 1933.

[56] DUBNIKOV, E. I.: Hypnosis of eczema of nervous origin. Vrach. delo. *15:* 634–636, 1932.

[57] BUNNEMANN, O.: Successful use of hypnosis in psychogenic eczema. Med. Welt. *8:* 87–88, Jan. 20, 1934.

[58] KARTAMISCHEW, A. J.: Hypnosis in eczema. Dermat. Wchnschr. *102:* 711–714, May 30, 1936.

[59] WISCH, J. M.: Hypnosis in psoriasis. Dermat. Wchnschr. *100*: 234–236, Feb. 23, 1935.

[60] KARTAMISCHEW, A. J.: Hypnosis in psoriasis. Dermat. Wchnschr. *102*: 260–263, Feb. 29, 1936.

[61] BONJOUR, J.: La guerison des condylomes par la suggestion. Schweiz. med. Wchnschr. *57*: 980, 1927.

[62] KARTAMISCHEW, A. J.: Arsphenamine dermatitis and its cure: case. Arch. f. Dermat. u. Syph. *174*: 36–37, 1936.

[63] BEZYUK, N. G.: Hypnosis in cutaneous pruritus. Vrach. delo. *21*: 397–400, 1939.

[64] MARCUS, H. AND SAHLGREN, E.: Hypnosis and allergy. Acta psychiat. et neurol. *11*: 119–126, 1936.

[65] TUCKEY, C. L.: Treatment by hypnotism and suggestion or psychotherapeutics. London, Baillière, Tindall & Cox, 1921.

[66] KOGERER, H.: Psychotherapy. Vienna, Wilhelm Mandrick, 1934.

[67] STOKVIS, B.: Hypnosis as psychotherapy in essential hypertension. Nederl. tidschr. v. geneesk. *81*: 5676–5682, Nov. 27, 1937.

[68] ANGULO, L. Muniz: Incoercible vomiting of pregnancy cured by hypnotism; case. Rev. san. mil., Habana *6*: 65–70, January–March 1942.

[69] KROGER, W. S. AND FREED, S. C.: Psychosomatic treatment of functional dysmenorrhea by hypnosis. Am. J. Obst. & Gynec. *46*: 817, 1943.

[70] ERICKSON, M. H.: Am. J. Obst. & Gynec., *42*: 817, 1943.

[71] BIRNIE, C. R.: Anorexia nervosa treated by hypnosis in out-patient practice. Lancet *2*: 1331–1332, Dec. 5, 1936.

[72] KOSTER, S.: Hypnosis for neuroses. Nederl. tijdschr. v. geneesk. *1*: 2600–2606, June 1, 1929.

[73] VOLGYESI, F.: Hypnosis in anxiety neurosis. Gyógyászat *70*: 640; 665; 682, 1930.

[74] ANGULO, MUNIZ, L.: Anxiety neuroses cured by hypnotism; case. Rev. med. cubana *47*: 135–142, February 1936.

[75] REISTRUP, H.: Historical development of hypnotherapy and its present status illustrated by three cases of psychoneuroses treated by hypnosis. Ugesk. f. laeger. *100*: 29–36, Jan. 13, 1938.

[76] SMITH, G. M.: A phobia originating before the age of three cured with the aid of hypnotic recall. Char. & Pers. *5*: 331–337, 1936–1937.

[77] ERICKSON, M. H.: op. cit. reference 37.

[78] COPELAND, C. L. AND KITCHING, E. H.: op. cit., reference 33.

[79] BYCHOWSKI, G.: Kleptomania after encephalitis; successful hypnosis. Nervenarzt *5*: 82–84, Feb. 15, 1932.

[80] FREY, E.: Hypnotic possibility of curing homosexuality. Schweiz. Arch. f. Neurol. u. Psychiat. *28*: 100–125, 1931.

[81] FAYBUSCHEVICH, V.: Hypnosis in alcoholism. Vrach. gaz. *32*: 587–592, 1928.

[82] WOLFFENBUTTEL, E.: Hypnotic method in case of alcoholism with cure lasting 8 years. Brasil-med. *49*: 447–448, May 18, 1935.

[83] GOLDSTEINAS, L.: Hypnosis in alcoholism. Medicina, Kaunas *19*: 12–30, Jan. 1938.

[84] COTLIER, I.: Chronic alcoholism treated by hypnotic suggestion and psychic reeducation of personality. Rev. argent. de neurol. y psiquiat. *3*: 102–109, Mar. 1938.

[85] KALLENBERG, K.: Emotional hypnosis in therapy of alcoholism. Svenska lak-tidning *35:* 2149–2152, Dec. 30, 1938.

[86] MEYERS, T. S.: Hypnosis in the treatment of chronic alcoholism. J. Am. Osteop. A. *44:* 172–174, 1944.

[87] WAGNEROVA, H. AND PROKOP, J.: Hypnosis in mental diseases. Bratisl. lepar. listy. *10:* 226–243, April 1930.

[88] RAEDER, O. J.: op. cit., reference 26.

[89] MAYER, E.: Hypnosis in orthopedics. Verhandl. a. deutsch. orthop. gesellsch., Kong. *21:* 387–392, 1927.

[90] DORLAND, J. W. Hypnotic therapeutics and modern dentistry. Dent. Cosmos. *63:* 810–813, 1921.

[91] STEIN, M. R.: Anesthesia by mental dissociation. Dent. Items *52:* 941–947, 1930.

[92] HOLLANDER, B.: Hypnosis and anesthesia. Dent. Surg. *29:* 239–244, 253–257, 1932.

[93] HAWKES, L. A.: Hypnotism and anesthesia. Oral Hyg. *19:* 1948–1950, 1929.

[94] WOOKEY, E. E.: Uses and limitations of hypnosis in dental treatment. Brit. Dent. J. *65:* 562–568, 1938.

[95] KOSTER, S.: Hypnosis in diseases of sympathetic nervous system. Nederl. Tijdschr. v. geneesk. *2:* 2689–2694, 1926.

[96] MILBRADT, W. AND KOHLER, A.: Hypno-analytic therapy of alleged sciatica. Med. Welt *8:* 408, March 24, 1934.

[97] KZENDZOVSKEY, M.: Hirschsprung's disease in boy 8 years old cured by sugges-tion; case. Sovet. vrach. Zhur. *41:* 917–922, June 30, 1937.

[98] KLEMPERER, G.: Hypnosis for exhausting hemorrhages in hemorrhagic diathesis. Therap. d. Gegenw. *72:* 21–24, Jan. 1931.

[99] KOSTER, S.: Hypnosis in organic diseases. Psychiat. en neurol. bl. *41:* 138–165, Jan.–Feb. 1937.

[100] WELLS, W. R.: The hypnotic treatment of the major symptoms of hysteria: a case study. J. Psychol. *17:* 269–297; 1944.

[101] DU BOIS, P.: The Psychic Treatment of Nervous Disorders. New York, Funk & Wagnalls, 1909.

[102] ——: Education of Self. New York, Funk & Wagnalls, 1911.

[103] HOLLANDER, B.: Methods and Uses of Hypnosis and Self-hypnosis. London, Allen & Unwin, 1928.

[104] MORGAN, J. J. B.: Hypnosis with direct psychoanalytic statement and sugges-tion in the treatment of a psychoneurotic of low intelligence. J. Abnorm. & Social Psychol. *19:* 160–164, 1924.

[105] RENTERGHEN, A. W. VON: Ein Fall von Muskelkramph (tic rotatoire). Ztschr. f. Hypnotismus *4:* 259–265, 1897.

[106] ERICKSON, M. H. AND KUBIE, L. S.: The successful treatment of a case of acute hysterical depression by a return under hypnosis to a critical phase of child-hood. Psychoanal. Quart. *10:* 583–609, 1941.

[107] ——: Hypnotic investigation of psychosomatic phenomena. A controlled experi-mental use of hypnotic regression in the therapy of an acquired food intoler-ance. Psychosom. Med. *5:* 67–70, 1943.

[108] LINDNER, R. A.: Rebel Without a Cause: the hypnoanalysis of a criminal psycho-path. New York, Grune & Stratton, 1944.

[109] ERICKSON, M. H.: The investigation of a specific amnesia. Brit. J. M. Psychol. *13:* 143–150, 1933.

[110] ——, AND HILL, L.: Unconscious mental activity in hypnosis, psychoanalytic implications. Psychoanal. Quart. *13:* 60–78, 1944.

[111] ——, AND KUBIE, L. S.: The permanent relief of an obsessional phobia by means of communications with an unsuspected dual personality. Psychoanal. Quart. *8:* 471–509, 1939.

[112] ——: The use of automatic drawing in the interpretation and relief of a state of acute obsessional depression. Psychoanal. Quart. *7:* 443–466, 1938.

[113] KUBIE, L. S.: The use of hypnagogic reveries in the recovery of repressed amnesic data. Bull. Menninger Clin. *7:* 172–82, 1943.

[114] WOLBERG, L. R.: Hypnoanalysis. New York, Grune & Stratton, 1945.

[115] ——: The mechanism of a hysterical anaesthesia revealed during hypnoanalysis. Psychoanal. Quart. *14:* 1945.

[116] ——: op. cit., reference 114, pp. 224–256.

[117] BRENMAN, M. AND KNIGHT, R. P.: Hypnotherapy for mental illness in the aged: case report of hysterical psychosis in a 71 year old woman. Bull. Menninger Clin. *7:* 5–6, 188–198, 1943.

[118] GILL, M. M. AND BRENMAN, M.: Treatment of a case of anxiety hysteria by a hypnotic technique employing psychoanalytic principles. Bull. Menninger Clin. *7:* 5–6, 163–171, 1943.

[119] WOLBERG, L. R.: op. cit., reference 114, pp. 257–312.

[120] LURIA, A. R.: The Nature of Human Conflict. New York, Liveright, 1932.

[121] ERICKSON, M. H.: The method employed to formulate a complex story for the induction of an experimental neurosis in a hypnotic subject. J. Gen. Psychol. *31:* 67–84, 1944.

[122] ——: A study of an experimental neurosis hypnotically induced in a case of ejaculation praecox. Brit. J. M. Psychol. *15:* 34–50, 1935.

[123] EISENBUD, J.: Psychology of headache. Psychiat. Quart. *11:* 592–619, 1937.

[124] KARDINER, A., AND SPIEGEL, H. S.: War Stress and Neurotic Illness. New York, Paul B. Hoeber, 1947, pp. 830–850.

[125] BRENMAN, M., AND GILL, M. H.: Hypnotherapy: A survey of the literature. New York, Int. Univ. Press, 1947.

[126] LECRON, L. M., AND BORDEAUX, J.: Hypnotism Today. New York, Grune & Stratton, 1947.

II

THE PHENOMENA OF HYPNOSIS

IN RECENT years many of the objective phenomena of hypnosis, originally described by Bernheim,[1] have been exposed to experiment and re-evaluated in the light of newer discoveries. It is the aim of this chapter to elucidate some of these findings.

The study of human behavior, and particularly so complex a form of behavior as hypnosis, involves many variables not present in work with animals or inanimate objects. Unfortunately a large number of workers in the field of experimental psychology have neglected to take this into account. As a consequence sundry contributions to hypnotic literature are outmoded and misleading. Erickson has appropriately pointed out that much of the work in the field of experimental hypnosis is a comprehensive demonstration of how hypnotic experiment should not be performed. Contradictory findings in the trance state are largely the result of inadequate experimental methods and controls. As more clinically trained workers enter the field of hypnotic experiment, contributions will be less dogmatic and more scientific.

For purposes of convenience hypnotic phenomena may be divided into those of the induction phase, those which occur during the trance state itself, and those of the posthypnotic period.

PHENOMENA DURING THE INDUCTION PHASE

Important psychologic changes are present during the induction phase. With standard induction technics, immobilization and monotonous repetition of the hypnotist's commands produces a gradual narrowing of sensory avenues until the hypnotist becomes the sole channel of communication with the world.[2] A state develops akin to early stages of sleep. It is difficult to say how much the apparent resemblance to sleep is actually assumed because of suggestion, and how much is due to the spontaneous development of a sleeplike tendency. Professor W. R. Wells has performed what he calls "waking hypnosis" in which there is no mention of sleep. The subject at all times appears to be in complete contact with his surroundings. In certain subjects I have been able to induce catalepsy and analgesia by direct suggestion without any prior sleep suggestions. It is likely, therefore, that feelings of relaxation and of drowsiness are, at least to some extent, the result of specific suggestions that are accepted by the subject.

Spontaneous thoughts and feelings during induction are especially prominent during the first few trance sessions. Later on, the subject passes through the induction stage so rapidly that he may not be conscious of his emotions or thought processes. Even at first, the fleeting images and fantasies may be recalled only with difficulty, and one may get the erroneous impression that there has been a cessation of cognitive activities. This is not at all true, for the mental functions continue to operate, sometimes in an intensely vivid manner.

The nature of the ideational processes depends upon the subject's attitudes toward the hypnotist and toward hypnosis itself. If he interprets hypnosis as an invasion of his privacy or as a potentially dangerous adventure, he will have fearful or hostile thoughts. If he feels contempt toward or animosity for the hypnotist, he may inwardly defy him and depreciate his suggestions. If he has great expectations concerning the benefits he will derive from hypnosis and from the hypnotist, he may symbolize these by appropriate ideas or fantasies.

With an induction technic utilizing a fixation object, some subjects experience various visual illusions and even hallucinations. Streaks of light, kaleidoscopic patterns, fantastic shapes or abstract forms apparently symbolize the monotony and rhythm of the induction process. One patient described himself as an egg-shaped disk over which I was suspended in the form of an embracing luminous crescent. The sound of the hypnotizer's voice may be symbolized as a drum or orchestral instrument. Feelings of relaxation and sleepiness are occasionally represented as "descending into a shaft" or "rising up in an elevator." A hysterical patient visualized himself on a magic carpet soaring up into the clouds. There may be illusions of the room widening or shrinking, of the furniture warping, of the physiognomy of the hypnotist changing. An art student described her surroundings as a surrealistic painting. Skin warmth or coldness, and paresthesias, like tingling and feelings of electricity, are occasionally experienced. Brenman and Gill[3] credit these experiences to a change in the ego which leads to a minimization of the importance of external reality, and to alteration in bodily sensation and body image.

As the induction gets deeper, some subjects become aware of their helplessness and inability to resist the commands of the hypnotist. In fearful subjects anxiety may become so intense as to make hypnosis impossible. Other subjects may respond to the trance with a feeling of not wanting to resist suggestions.

Sensations of strangeness are common and the individual may develop ideas that his body or identity has changed. One subject saw himself as a mechanical man whose limbs moved without his participation. Other reports are: "My mind and body were disjointed." "I'm separated into fragments." "I felt like I couldn't recognize myself apart from you." "My body seemed strange as if it didn't belong to me." "I felt like several different people all at the same time." "My body seemed to be made out of rubber." "I seemed to be standing in a corner of the room looking at myself on the couch." Not a few subjects have ideas of death or rebirth.

Feelings of depersonality and unreality, and inability to distinguish the self from others, resemble closely the fantasies in schizophrenia as well as the subjective experiences during the onset of normal sleep or upon awakening. They are probably the psychologic components of regression with beginning dissolution of ego boundaries.

Ego dissolution is apparently a temporary phenomenon, as Kubie and Margolin[4] have noted, for as soon as the subject enters into a real state of trance, and upon the command of the hypnotist, he emerges partially from his regression and re-enters into better contact with the world.

During the induction phase, the subject may feel intense emotions which in part are due to an automatic release of inhibitions with liberation of repressed affects, and in part are the product of the patient's own interpretation of the trance experience. The quality of mood varies from joy to fear. In most cases the experience is a pleasurable one associated with feelings of lightness and relaxation, but in instances where the image of authority is destructive or fearful, the emotion may be of great terror. One patient remarked: "As you were talking to me, I felt as if you were a black priest sneaking up to strangle me with your bony fingers." In other instances, the patient may regard the experience as a seduction and may have vivid sexual fantasies concerning the hypnotist. This fact has been recognized by many hypnotists, and some have advocated the presence of a third person where the subject is a female in order to avoid legal entanglements.

Objective phenomena during the induction phase depend upon the character of the induction technic. If a fixation object is used, there will be immobilization of the head, neck and skeletal system. Strained fixation causes a fatigue of the eye muscles, a watering of the eyes and blinking of the lids. Relaxation suggestions produce general muscle atonicity. The manifestations with other induction technics depend upon the specific suggestions made.

Phenomena during the Trance State

Spontaneous Phenomena. In some subjects, for no apparent reason, the mere assumption of a state of trance suffices to produce phenomena spontaneously such as ordinarily would be invoked by suggestion. One might try to explain this on the basis that hypnosis dissolves resistance and makes possible the conscious expression of subconscious impulses. To some extent this is correct because hypnosis tends to nullify the inhibitory mechanism of the ego. Spontaneous manifestations are also the result of a desire on the part of the subject to comply with the hypnotist by demonstrating those responses which, according to his experience or intuition, he believes will be expected of him.

A common spontaneous manifestation is the recall of memories that were, in the waking state, forgotten. There appears to be an easier access in the trance to repressed memories and conflicts. Another spontaneous occurrence is the development of certain psychosomatic symptoms. In producing such phenomena as deafness, blindness, amnesia, analgesia, anesthesia and age regression, Erickson[5] discovered a number of apparently unrelated spontaneous psychosomatic and ideational manifestations. For instance, induced hypnotic deafness caused visual and motor disorders in one subject, while another subject with induced color blindness showed a spontaneous loss of meaning for the word "three." It is a common observation that suggested amnesia may cause spontaneous headaches until the memories which were forgotten have been recalled. These developments are probably not fortuitous, but have an associated symbolic meaning to the subject. In the case of an alcoholic treated by myself, all hypnotically induced dreams with a traumatic implication produced a spontaneous glove anesthesia; these were related to fantasies of destruction, aggression and masturbation.[6]

In hysterical individuals, hypnosis may spontaneously produce uncontrollable fits of laughter or crying, screaming rages and even convulsive seizures. Paresthesias, anesthesias, hyperesthesias, tics, tremors, choreiform movements, spasms, twitchings, paralysis, aphonia, blindness, deafness, amnesia, hallucinations and "trance speaking" are occasionally demonstrated. Profound alterations of personality may develop with mood changes and even reorganized attitudes and values. Repressed drives for superiority, domination, ambition, power and masochism may come to the surface with amazing force. Spontaneous regression may suddenly release a somnambulistic reliving of an emotionally surcharged period in the past life. On the other hand, hypnosis may, without further suggestion, suffice to remove temporarily hysterical paralysis, amnesia, anesthesia or multiple personality.

Other spontaneous phenomena during hypnosis are sudden awakening and a progression of the trance into actual sleep. Awakening is often the product of resistance, or the result of an anxiety-provoking suggestion that interferes with the motivation for hypnosis. Because of strong affects, escape from the trance situation may be sought in a manner similar to awakening from sleep during a nightmare. The transference of hypnosis into real sleep may occur without provocation, or may follow a posthypnotic suggestion of a conflictual nature which the subject does not desire to carry through, yet feels powerless to resist. If sleep occurs, it lasts for a short period, although Schilder and Kauders[7] reported cases in which sleep continued for several days.

Hypersuggestibility. Perhaps the most characteristic phenomenon of hypnosis is a state of exaggerated suggestibility. The degree of suggestibility varies in different persons. It is dependent upon the training of the subject as well as on the depth of trance. It goes without saying that somnambules are most suggestible.

In some persons suggestibility is so great that the mere induction of hypnosis brings on, without further command, phenomena that have been induced in previous trance states. Often the subject shows a remarkable plasticity with an unqualified acceptance of the hypnotist's injunctions. However, there are definite limits to suggestibility and the subject will emphatically resist, and resist successfully, any suggestion that arouses too much anxiety. In spite of his apparent lack of volition, the subject can refuse to do anything he feels is against his best interests. So long as suggestions do not involve a fundamental issue, the subject will conform without hesitation. But when a basic conflict is touched on, resistance is the rule. For example, a woman with a mouse phobia may develop anesthesia on suggestion and will permit her arm to be burned by a cigarette without flinching; but when it is suggested that she no longer fears mice, and when she is threatened with real exposure to a mouse, she will in all probability awaken.

Rapport. For a long time *rapport* was considered a basic characteristic of hypnosis, occurring spontaneously in each subject. Some observers, including Hull[8] and Young,[9,10] believe that *rapport* is not a spontaneous phenomenon, but develops only when the subject has a conviction during hypnosis that he must respond solely to the hypnotist. Nevertheless, under average conditions, *rapport* seems to be part of the hypnotic state, although, it may not, in some persons, be exclusively directed toward the hypnotist. *Rapport* is not as real as it seems because the subject is quite aware of the presence of others. He merely acts as if they do not exist.

"Types" of Trance. Various "types" of response to the hypnotic situation have been reported[11-12] In the main there are two types, active or alert, and passive or lethargic. The "active" type, according to White,[13] exhibits no delay in executing movements, enjoys submission, is deferential and affiliative in his behavior, and his mind throughout hypnosis remains alert. The "passive" type resists any disturbance in his repose, is more inclined to anxiety, and his mind is

relatively blank. This attempt to split up reaction types is quite arbitrary, as Friedlander and Sarbin[14] have pointed out. The conduct of the patient in the trance state is related to how he believes he is expected to behave, and what he wants to get out of the trance. Initial reactions based on these factors can be altered by training.

Muscular Phenomena. Among the muscular manifestations that can be induced during hypnosis are alterations in tonicity, paralysis of muscle groups, spasms, contractions, tremors, choreiform movements, catalepsy, stereotypy, automatic movements, and interference with such special functions as talking and writing. Any voluntary muscular activity can be increased, decreased, or inhibited. Good subjects may be trained to produce hysteric-like gait disorders, astasia-abasia and convulsive seizures.

Suggestions of muscle relaxation, hypotonicity and paralysis usually cause the subject to feel a lazy disinclination for active movements or an inability to make up his mind as to whether or not to move his limbs. There is actually no loss of motor power; merely a temporary suspension of tonicity and motion. Paralysis may involve small groups of muscles, such as the eyelids, or larger groups, as the limbs or trunk. It may be of a flaccid or spastic nature. The paralysis does not follow the distribution of the motor nerves and is based entirely on the subject's conception of how a paralyzed person behaves. Some subjects make no effort to struggle against suggestions of paralysis, while others vigorously attempt to move the extremity in spite of the hypnotist's command. In such struggles the subject usually fails, and as he contracts the muscles of the paralyzed part, one may observe antagonistic muscles opposing the action. Some persons will attempt to overcome inhibition by a ruse which may or may not be successful. They usually sense their helplessness and this realization in some subjects can precipitate panic.

Rigid catalepsies may be produced in various parts of the

body. The common stage phenomenon of supporting a subject by a chair placed under the head and another beneath the low extremities is the result of catalepsy of the muscles of the trunk. *Cerea flexibilitas* may often be induced making it possible to mold the extremities into awkward positions which can be maintained for extraordinarily long periods. Automatic movements, such as hand levitation and inability to stop the hands from rotating around each other, may also be suggested. Muscle tremors and spasms can be produced directly or may develop spontaneously with suggested rigid catalepsies.

The successful performance in hypnosis of muscular feats of supernormal strength and power has been reported by some observers. Such increased power is largely the result of an inability to feel fatigue. Williams[15,16] and Nicholson[17] claim that in hypnosis the subject can maintain uncomfortable postures longer and can perform work with less tremor and fatiguability than in the waking state. This overexertion is undoubtedly carried out at the expense of the physical reserve of the body.

Sensory Phenomena. Hypnotic paresthesias, hyperesthesias and anesthesias are distinguished from organic disturbances by their variability, the ease of change on suggestion, and by their failure to follow any anatomic distribution. Paresthesias in various areas are relatively easy to suggest. Among these are numbness, tingling, itching, prickling, burning, sensations of coldness, and increased sensitivity to stimuli of pain, pressure, temperature and touch. On suggestion a subject may be made to exhibit acute sensitivity to stimuli, and may be able to distinguish variations in texture and temperature that could not be differentiated in the waking state. Young[18] asserts that this excessive responsiveness to sensory stimuli is illusory, based not upon a real hypersensitivity, but upon the subject's belief that he is more sensitive. There is reason for feeling, however, that the sensory threshold is actually lowered in an organic manner as a result of suggestion.

Hypnotic anesthesias, like hysterical disorders of sensation, conform to popular notions of function rather than to anatomic areas. In suitable subjects, suggestion will produce a loss of the sense of touch (anesthesia), of pain (analgesia), and of temperature (thermoanesthesia). Often this loss is relative, and the subject will attest to a diminished rather than to a total absence of sensation. In trained subjects, however, sensory loss can be complete. Dental work, obstetric procedures, minor and even major surgery may be possible here.

Whether anesthesia is real or whether the subject is playing a role and merely acting as if he did not feel pain is a question about which different opinions have been expressed. Sears[19] has reported that in hypnotic anesthesia, physiologic reactions to painful stimuli, as registered by changes in respiration, pulse and galvanic skin reflexes, are definitely diminished. This would indicate that the anesthesia is genuine. Dynes[20] also reported that respiratory and cardiac reflex changes are abolished. Thus, it is probable that an actual though reversible organic change is involved.

In suitable subjects there may be induced an impairment, perversion or increase of deep sensations involving muscle, tendon and joint senses. Disturbances of the sense of position, movement, resistance, weight and vibration may be suggested, producing syndromes of ataxia and astereognosis.

Phenomena of the Special Senses. Paresthesias of the special senses include those of vision, in the form of flashes of light and color (photomata), of hearing, such as buzzing or roaring in the ears, of perverted taste sensations (paraguesia), and smell (parosmia). Presented with a blotter and instructed that he is partaking of a tenderloin steak, the subject will proceed to eat and swallow the blotter with satisfaction as if he were actually eating a tenderloin. A deeply hypnotized person, exposed to spirits of ammonia presented to him as perfume, will inhale the fumes with obvious enjoyment and without the physical reactions characteristic of smelling ammonia.

In deep somnambulistic states the eyes may be opened without awakening. Visual hallucinations may often be induced here, and they evoke the same kind of behavior one might expect were the perception produced by a real stimulus. The subject will flee from imaginary lions in great terror or, upon suggestion, he will pick up and pet tenderly a hallucinated kitten. If it is suggested that he go into a restaurant to appease his hunger, he will enter a fantasied restaurant, seat himself and go through the procedure of scanning the menu, of inquiring about the various dishes, of imbibing the ordered courses from cocktail to dessert, even wiping his mouth with a napkin and leaving an imaginary tip for the waiter. Stage performers depend upon such hallucinations for their effects.

"Crystal gazing" or mirror gazing, are forms of visual hallucination. Upon suggestion the subject will gaze intently into the crystal or mirror, and he will see scenes that are the product of his own ideational processes. This technic is used in hypnoanalysis. Gustatory, olfactory and auditory hallucinations, both pleasant and unpleasant, may also be induced. Thus the subject will listen intently to an orchestra or to a speech with appropriate facial gestures and other reactions. "Shell hearing," in which communications from a sea shell or a teacup held over the ear are received on suggestion, is a type of auditory hallucination.

In hypnosis, a degree of keenness in vision, hearing, touch and smell may be obtained which is not possible in the waking state. The subject may perceive stimuli that would escape ordinary observation. A favorite trick of stage hypnotists is to show the subject a blank card, then ask him to select it from a shuffled pack of apparently similar blank cards.

Telepathic abilities and powers of second sight are held responsible for a successful performance. What actually happens is that the subject observes creases or imperfections on the card that will enable him to distinguish it from others later on. These flaws are so slight as to evade scrutiny unless attention is specifically focused on the most minute details. Increased sensitivity to noises, tastes and odors can also be obtained.

Negative hallucinations are possible only in deepest somnambulism, and, as Erickson[21] has shown, require a careful formulation of commands. In the visual area one may produce an elimination of specific objects in the environment, blindness of half the visual field (hemianopsia), the development of various blind spots (scotomata), color blindness (achromatopsia), concentric narrowing of vision, such as one finds in hysteria, and total blindness (amaurosis). Suggested deafness may involve one or both ears, may be partial or complete with loss of varying portions of the tonal range. The complete absence of taste (aguesia) and of smell (anosmia), or the obliteration of specific taste sensations or odors may also be produced.

The nature of these sensory changes has been debated. There are some observers who believe that they are merely the result of a changed attitude, and that all phenomena can be explained on the basis of playing a role. Pattie,[22] Lundholm[23] and Dorcus[24] are of this opinion. The majority of workers, however, believe that an organic change of some kind is involved.[25] Doupe, Miller and Keller,[26] for instance, contend that stimulation of an anesthetic limb produces much less vaso-constriction than would be possible if painful impulses were perceived. Loomis, Harvey, and Hobart[27] fastened the lids of their subjects with adhesive so that it was impossible to close the eyes. They then measured the brain potentials with an electroencephalographic apparatus. Every alternate fifteen seconds they suggested first that the subject was totally blind, and then that he could see. In every case, upon suggestion that the subject could not see, brain waves appeared of the character found in a totally blind person, or in a person whose eyes were shut. Brain waves ceased upon suggestion that the subject could see. Lemere[28] and Lundholm and Löwenbach[29] disagree with this work, not having been able to duplicate it.

Contradictory opinions have also been expressed about pupillary reactions to hallucinations of light. Hypnotic blindness is usually associated with a normal pupillary response to light stimuli, and hallucinations of light produce no contraction of the pupil. However, in very deeply hypnotized subjects who have been conditioned properly, pupillary contractions can be obtained. Erickson and Erickson[30] suggested hallucinatory color vision in a group of subjects and discovered the interesting fact that these were followed by after-images of complementary colors even in cases where preliminary word tests showed no correct associations of the various colors. Furthermore, Erickson[31] reported that hypnotically induced deafness was not distinguishable from neurologic deafness by any of the ordinary tests.

The contradictory findings which have been reported can possibly be explained on the basis that some subjects in the trance will play a role and simulate a suggested situation, while others will respond with organic reaction patterns. A definite aptitude seems to be required for positive psychosomatic responses.

Ideational Processes. Although the subject appears to be in a state of suspended animation, his thought processes always continue to function. In asking one man to recall his hypnotic experiences, he reported: "My eyelids become extremely heavy, and I am contented to close them though I feel with some effort I could keep them open. It seems that I am not asleep, for I am aware of things. I can hear the sound of a voice, though things seem a bit jumbled. Things pass through my mind, not exactly like logical thinking, but perhaps like day dreams." Subjects are usually aware of environmental stimuli even though they do not concentrate on them. In later trance states they can recover a surprising number of details that occurred in early hypnosis, of which, at the time, they seemed unaware. There may be a peculiar slowness and some difficulty in thinking. Occasionally one finds incoherence and blocking of thought.

Spontaneous fantasy and imagery may be increased in some persons even to flight of ideas. The fantasies depend upon the meaning of hypnosis to the subject and upon his aptitudes in symbolizing his experiences. There may be present fantasies of rebirth, of being fed, sexually stimulated, injured or destroyed. Sensations of lightness may be represented by such ideas as being converted into a bird who flies, or into a sponge full of air. Heaviness may be conceived of as being in chains or wearing lead boots. Space perception may be so distorted that the room appears boundless, approaching infinity. This type of imagery is more related to sleep than to waking life, and mechanisms of condensation, substitution and symbolization are often utilized as in dreams.

Both abstract and conceptual thinking may remain facile even in the deepest hypnosis. Creative imagination, organization and proper relation of memory images, and the ability to formulate ideas and to relate them to familiar ideas and experiences are relatively unimpaired. The associative functions continue, as do processes of reasoning and the capacity for analytic and logical discrimination. Nevertheless, upon suggestion, these functions can be eliminated or distorted with resulting disorders of association and apperception, and disturbances of symbolic functions, such as aphasia, alexia, asymbolia, amusia and agraphia. Disturbances of attention can be induced, such as the inability to concentrate on specified activities in the environment (aprosexia), or a morbid focusing of attention on a restricted area (hyperprosexia).

During hypnosis, archaic thinking and associations may be brought to the surface. This occurs especially during induced regressive states or upon attaining deeper unconscious levels through dream induction and automatic writing. Unconscious mentation differs in character from conscious thinking in utilizing such mechanisms as condensation, displacement, chronological running together, plural identification, representation by opposites or by small details. Phallic symbolism is frequently encountered in the representation of ideas and attitudes. Erickson[32] and Erickson and Kubie[33,34] have contributed excellent papers on unconscious thinking processes that prevail during automatic writing and drawing. Farber and Fisher[35] have shown that individuals under hypnosis are capable of interpreting, with astonishing accuracy, the unconscious productions of other persons. They have commented on a prevailing sexual preoccupation.

Among hypnotic procedures utilized during hypnoanalysis are free association, dream induction, automatic writing, dramatics, play therapy, drawing, mirror gazing and the induction of experimental conflicts. These involve complicated ideational processes and will be considered in detail in a later chapter.

At first glance the weird outcroppings from the unconscious appear senseless, and one might suspect that the levels of mind reached through hypnosis are disorganized and absurd. This is by no means the case, for as Freud[36] has shown, unconscious thinking can have a definite purpose and function.

In subjects capable of deep hypnotic states, it is possible to produce obsessive ideas, compulsions, phobias, ideas of reference, persecutory trends, grandiose ideas, depressive and nihilistic delusions, ideas of unreality, hypochondriacal ideas and delusions of influence. These disorders of mental content resemble very closely those found in actual neuroses and psychoses, and the subject's spontaneous reactions may be the same as in these disorders. Once an obsession or delusion is induced, the individual may defend it vigorously with fabrications and rationalizations. Even ideas of an absurd nature may seem real to the subject by suggesting to him that he will remember them as true facts after he awakens from the trance.

Demonstrating this phenomenon before a group of medical students, I once suggested to a volunteer subject that several days previously he had attended the Kentucky Derby and that he would remember this upon awakening. In talking about his experiences, the subject skillfully wove in the fact that he had recently won a sizeable sum of money in the Kentucky Derby, but that he had lost it at the track. It was pointed out to him that he could not possibly have attended the Kentucky Derby because the race was scheduled several months in advance of the day he claimed having attended it. He quickly manufactured the story that, because of unusual conditions, several races were being run that year. Several of his colleagues testified that he had been in New York City on the day he claimed he was away, and they reminded him that they had attended several classes with him. The subject then asserted that he actually was in New York in the morning, but that afternoon had boarded an airplane, returning by plane after the race. No amount of argument or logic could dissuade him from this idea.

Situations created during hypnosis may seem as real to the subject as if they actually existed. During a play therapy session with a patient who had been regressed to a ten year level, the latter got into an imaginary fight with another boy over disputed occupancy of a swing. The fight got so extreme and the rage of the patient became so intense that the fight had to be stopped.

Learning Process. A number of studies have appeared which allege a facilitation of the learning process in hypnosis. Scott[37] found that defensive movements of the finger were easier to establish in the trance than in the waking state. Mishchenko[38] similarly demonstrated that conditioned responses were more easily developed in hypnosis. Stalnaker and Riddle,[39] experimenting with the recall of one year old material, reported a gain of 38.5 per cent in hypnosis over the waking state. White, Fox and Harris[40] also demonstrated hypermnesia for recently learned material, while Rosenthal[41] found that while there was no blanket hypermnesia, there was a tendency toward increased recall of disparaged or failed items to which the subjects had been exposed. In a subject tested by myself, an eight digit series, repeated during hypnosis, was recalled in a trance two years later.

That memories which have been forgotten can be recalled during hypnosis is a well known fact. This hypermnesia may be demonstrated by hypnotizing an individual and testing his memory of recent events. Often he will be aware of situations that had not seemed to register themselves on him because his attention had apparently been directed elsewhere.

Recovery of incidents that have occurred during childhood and even infancy may sometimes be obtained by inducing hypnotic regression. Hypnosis can remove some inhibitions and repressions that keep memories from awareness. The availability of forgotten memories to recall depends to a large extent on the amount of nascent anxiety associated with the memory. It depends also upon the degree to which the process of forgetting is a purposeful defensive mechanism shielding the individual from conflict.

On the other hand, the learning process may be impaired or blocked by suitable suggestions. In deep hypnosis, induced amnesia may produce a forgetting of entire segments of experience. Paramnesia may also be invoked with acceptance of falsified memories as factual. The latter phenomenon is often used in experimental conflicts and in provoking dreams and fantasies which give clues to unconscious conflictual situations.

Regression. It is possible to create a state of disorientation during hypnosis in spheres of place, person and time. In hypnoanalysis this phenomenon is utilized, the patient being regressed to an earlier age level and encouraged to recall experiences that may be etiologically related to his emotional disorder.

Considerable disagreement exists as to whether hypnotic regression is actual in the sense that it is a recapitulation of a previous stage of development, or whether the subject re-enacts and dramatizes an earlier developmental stage on the basis of his present-day concepts of what a person at the suggested age level is supposed to do. Without question hypnotic subjects are capable of simulating behavior at a suggested regressed age much better than conscious subjects. They are similarly able to remember things at regressed age levels that are not available to them at adult levels.

On the basis of intelligence tests, Hakebush, Blinkovski and Foundillere[42] claim to have regressed patients to infancy, and they believe that it is possible to secure regression to a neonatal state. They report that intelligence tests at regressed ages correspond precisely with performances at actual chronological levels. By a similar method Platonow[43] attempted to show that the transformation in the subject during regression was a real reproduction of an earlier developmental period. Platonow subjected his subjects to intelligence tests after regressing them to age levels of four, six and ten. Each of the subjects at the suggested age was able to pass only those tests which did not go beyond the corresponding age as established by the Binet-Simon method. Furthermore, the behavior of the subject during regression was in all details similar to what one might find in children at those ages. For instance, at four and six year levels, the subjects were very fidgety, easily distracted and fatigued. When given complicated tests, they faltered and refused to go on. At the regressed age of ten, their behavior changed completely, and they worked quietly and attentively. Handwriting also corresponded to the various age levels. In the waking state, the subject easily passed all tests including those at the adult level. Platonow is convinced that his results definitely disproved any kind of simulation or role-playing. He explains the phenomenon of regression on the basis that conditioned reactions once developed do not disappear completely, but leave organic traces in the nervous system. This makes possible an actual reproduction of previous developmental stages later on. Word stimuli in hypnosis reanimate earlier conditioned reflexes. Thus, suggestion brings forth an organic reproduction of engrams, the formation of which occurred in earlier periods of the individual's life. Dolin[44] is of a similar opinion.

Young,[45] on the other hand, has criticized the work of Dolin, Hakebush and Platonow on the basis that they utilized too few cases to warrant such sweeping generalizations. Regressing fourteen trance subjects to the third birthday, he found that intelligence tests revealed an average mental age of six. Although their speech and grammar as well as their mannerisms were very childish, the subjects did not enter into activities so circumscribed as those of a three year old child. Seven unhypnotizable control subjects who were asked to simulate a three year old child approached more closely a three year level of performance than did the hypnotized subjects. Young concludes that hypnosis is playing a role and that regression as obtained in hypnosis is an artifact.

The consensus at the present time is that regression actually does reproduce early behavior in a way that obviates all possibility of simulation. This is the opinion of such authorities as Erickson, Estabrooks,[46] Lindner,[47] and Spiegel, Shor and Fishman.[48] My own studies[49] have convinced me of this fact, although the regression is never stationary, constantly being altered by the intrusion of mental functioning at other age levels. These shifts are probably the result of dynamic forces. They are responsible for a fluctuating age-level picture during regression, so that intelligence tests and handwriting usually show items of greater maturity than one would expect at the age to which the subject has been regressed.

Two types of regressive phenomena are generally obtained as indicated by Erickson and Kubie.[50] In the first type, there is an actual return to a developmentally earlier stage of development with a total amnesia for events subsequent to that period. For example, if a subject is regressed to a five year level, he will remember experiences at that level and will have forgotten completely all of the events subsequent to that period. He will even fail to recognize the hypnotist and may get out of rapport with him. Art productions at a regressed age level are so typically childish that they could scarcely be simulated. Even an accomplished artist will draw grotesque figures common to the age level suggested. Motor behavior patterns also correspond with the regressed age level, and a revivification of past experiences may occur. On the other hand, in some subjects, suggested regression brings about not an actual reproduction of an earlier childhood level, but a simulated copy of what this level must have been. The fact that these two types of phenomena occur may explain why observers have differed in opinion as to the actual significance of hypnotic regression. Where it can be obtained, the first type of regression is, I believe, a definite organic reproduction of a developmentally earlier period.

To what earliest period a subject can be successfully regressed is difficult to say with certainty. On one occasion I attempted to regress a somnambulistic subject to the first year of life. The subject was unable to speak, and he exhibited definite sucking and grasping movements. He was instructed to remember his experiences when brought back to an adult level. He revealed the following details: "I was very small. I didn't understand anything. Everything was new. I didn't know what things meant. I was trying to get hold of things, reaching for things. I didn't know what it was, what I was doing. I didn't know the meaning of things. Somebody was leaning over me, mother. She picked me up and held me tight. She was fixing things up around me. She was fixing up my body, the clothes where I was lying. I had all kinds of sensations. I didn't know what anything meant. I saw different kinds of things. I saw mother, the different things, the walls. There were spots of light in the walls. I didn't know the names of anything. I took hold of things that came toward me, the covers. They dropped to the floor. I didn't know what made them drop. I didn't know what became of them when they dropped. I didn't know why mother was there. I took hold of her. I played with everything. I was reaching out, grabbing things, clothes, feet, everything." Lindner[51] reports regression and revivification in a psychopath to a period between six months and one year.

Time Sense. There is conflicting evidence as to whether or not hypnosis gives the individual a better capacity to judge the passage of time than in the waking state. If a subject under hypnosis is asked to perform a task after passage of a certain number of minutes, he will usually do so with considerable accuracy. Similarly, upon appropriate suggestion, a subject may go through a posthypnotic act or series of acts after a prescribed time.

Perhaps the most intensive work in this field has been done by Bramwell,[52] whose subjects under hypnosis have shown an uncanny time sense. Bramwell's work, however, has never been duplicated by others. In a controlled experiment, Stalnaker and Richardson[53] have reported that the ability to judge time is no more increased during hypnosis than in the ordinary waking state provided the individual concentrates on the task.

It is probably dangerous to generalize, but the varying results obtained may depend upon differences in the aptitudes of the subjects under test. It is quite possible to train a hypnotic subject to judge time with extraordinary accuracy. On the other hand, there are persons who are capable of estimating time in the waking state with a remarkable degree of precision. Appropriate suggestions cause the subject to concentrate more intensively on the passage of time during hypnosis. Were he to devote himself to the problem as keenly in the waking state, he might possibly be able to obtain as good results as in the trance.

Personality Changes. Distinct changes in personality can be provoked during hypnosis, the subject acting the role of various suggested characters. Multiple personalities can be produced experimentally in this way. Multiple personalities may also be created spontaneously while teaching the subject such technics as automatic writing or crystal gazing.[54,55]

In order to test how fundamental personality changes were under hypnosis, Sarbin[56] first obtained a Rorschach record of each of his subjects in the waking state and also while under hypnosis. He then created two new personalities in each subject, the first being Madame Curie, the second, Mae West. Rorschach tests were taken of the different personalities. Under hypnosis, the "organizing energy" was increased, and the externally imposed "aufgaben" circumscribed the response pattern to a greater extent than the self-imposed "aufgaben." The respective psychograms showed the W/D was significant in differentiation. For instance, in the waking state the values were 11/24 or .46. In hypnosis with the normal personality they were 14/15 or .93; with the "Madame Curie" personality they were 21/15 or 1.40; with the Mae West personality, 19/12 or 1.58. Levine, Grassi and Garson[57] and Bergman, Graham and Leavitt[58] similarly have reported significant Rorschach changes with hypnotically induced moods and during regression. Unpublished studies of Rorschach records taken during hypnosis on a number of my subjects demonstrates no remarkable alteration in personality during hypnosis, but do show marked alterations in the responses when anxiety develops or when the subject is regressed. The regressed Rorschachs are not identical with corresponding age levels in the waking state, but are sufficiently similar to eliminate any suspicion that regression is "play acting."

Emotional Changes. Spontaneous emotional changes have already been considered in the form of feelings and attitudes that are related to the hypnotic state and to the hypnotist. If the hypnotic situation fulfills satisfactorily certain needs, the subject may experience sensations of ecstasy, joy and pleasure. On the other hand, with suggestions that stir up anxiety, he may experience emotions of fear, rage or scorn. Various moods can be artifically induced under hypnosis by suggesting a situation that automatically arouses that mood. For instance, requested to hallucinate an approaching lion, the subject, if he accepts the suggestion, will probably react with terror.

Fisher and Marrow[59] have reported that hypnotic mood changes can materially influence cognitive and conative processes. Emotions of rage, panic, depression and elation may be stimulated, and the subject's associations and thought content will correspond to the prevailing mood.

By removing inhibitions, repressed emotions may be liberated. This is a most common observation during the trance. Keir[60] has reported a case that demonstrates this phenomenon most vividly.

Psychosomatic Phenomena. Hypnosis can produce a number of effects beyond the bounds of normal volition. Among the most spectacular of these is an increased control over the autonomic nervous system. Some of the phenomena which have been reported seem so incredible that the possibility of fraud must always be kept in mind. Knowing that the hypnotist expects certain things of him, the subject may contrive to please with remarkable ingenuity. He may later develop an amnesia for his connivance. For instance, I once suggested to a subject that he would develop hives over the forearms posthypnotically, and that he would report to me as soon as hives appeared. Several days later he demonstrated a markedly irritated skin, but no evidence of hives. He denied that he had in any way irritated the skin, insisting that when he awoke from sleep that morning he found the skin scratched and inflamed. Under hypnosis, however, he confided that he had, following the trance, taken a walk through the woods. Here he picked poison ivy leaves and rubbed them vigorously on the inner surfaces of his arms. Later, he developed a complete loss of memory for this, probably to convince me that he had spontaneously complied with my request.

The old hypnotists reported such rare phenomena as bleeding from the mucous membranes, local redness of the skin, blisters,[61,62] and changes in milk secretion induced by suggestion. Such reports must reasonably be accepted with caution because of the element of unconscious deception that might have been involved. Ullman[62a] has described producing herpes and a second degree burn by hypnotic suggestion.

Almost as spectacular are studies on the influence of hypnosis on metabolic processes. Glaser[63] noted that the calcium content of blood could be brought down by hypnotic command. Povorinskij and Finne[64] suggested to their subjects that they were partaking of large amounts of honey and then discovered a marked increase in the blood sugar. On the other hand, when suggestions were made that there was an absence of sugar and sweetness in food eaten, the blood sugar rise is said to have been inhibited even though sugar was imbibed. Langheinrich[65] suggested to his subjects that they were first drinking bouillon and then eating butter. He had the contents of the duodenum examined, and, following the first suggestion, found these to be thin and yellow, while after the second suggestion, they were dark, viscous and increased in quantity similar to what would have occurred were the suggested substances actually incorporated. Delhougne and Hansen[66] also fed fictitious meals to a subject, consisting, first, of protein, second, of fats, and third, of carbohydrates. During the first suggested meal, he reports an increase in pepsin and trypsin in the stomach contents, during the second, an increase of lipase, and during the third, an increase of diastase. Heilig and Hoff[67] administered meals to a group of subjects, some being told that they relished the food, and the rest that the food was repulsive to them. Analysis of the contents of the stomach is said to have shown a greater acid content than normal in the first group, and in the second group a very much reduced acid content. Heyer[68] suggested to his subjects the ingestion of an imaginary meal and claimed to have produced gastric secretions, the amount and content of which corresponded with what one might expect were the foods actually eaten. In another experiment, he gave a subject a constipating dose of opium under the guise of castor oil and observed that the results were cathartic. Marx,[69] suggesting to a subject that he was drinking large quantities of water from an empty glass, noted that the urinary output was markedly increased, with a loss of bodily fluids. Platonow and Matskevich[70] report that they were able to cause symptoms of acute alcoholic intoxication to disappear by hypnotic command. Both elevation of temperature and altered basal metabolism are claimed to have been brought about by hypnotic suggestion.

Suggestions of hunger may stimulate gastric motility and secretion, and Bramwell[71] reports having seen subjects made hungry after they had just finished eating a hearty meal. Gastrointestinal symptoms which may be invoked hypnotically are vomiting, disturbed digestion, increased or diminished intestinal peristalsis, diarrhea or constipation.

Increased pulse rate and blood pressure, and local ischemias and hyperemias may also be produced by direct suggestion. However, evidence points strongly to the fact that cardiovascular symptoms are the consequence of stimulated emotions. Suggestions of relaxation spontaneously lower the blood pressure and pulse rate as in sleep. Suggestions of excitement and other strong emotions will elevate the pulse rate and blood pressure. That direct verbal suggestions under hypnosis have no power to increase the heart rate without the intermediary action of emotion is claimed by Jenness and Wible.[72] Doupe, Miller and Keller[73] allege that the lumen of cutaneous blood vessels cannot be altered by hypnotic suggestion except when these suggestions induce emotional states. Nevertheless it is essential to consider that cardiac and vascular responses can be conditioned to verbal cues once they have been obtained through emotional stimulation. Responses originally produced by emotional reactions can in this way be elicited in trained subjects by mere verbal suggestions. This fact holds true not only for cardiovascular responses, but for all other vasomotor activities which may, through the process of conditioning, be provoked by verbal command.

Emotional states can influence other somatic reactions during hypnosis. The emotion of excitement, for example, may produce an increase in the number of red blood corpuscles, probably through contraction of the spleen. Tear production may be caused by appropriate depressive moods. Heilig and Hoff[74] have reported producing cold sores in a subject by recounting unpleasant experiences while stroking the lower lip and suggesting itchiness as in a cold sore. A swelling of the lip developed followed by a real cold sore. The same authors[75] reported producing diuresis in subjects by creating an emotional upset in the trance. Contraction and dilatation of the pupils can also be emotionally incited. Allergic phenomena, menstrual changes, hydrosis of the face,[76] angioneurotic edema,[77] asthmatic attacks,[78] and migraine[79] have been reported in the literature.

POSTHYPNOTIC PHENOMENA

Spontaneous Phenomena. Immediately upon awakening, the subject probably undergoes an ego synthesis, with restoration of ego boundaries, a general reorientation in time and place, and a re-establishment of volitional control. This reintegrative process is sometimes delayed for a short period, and the subject may be dazed or confused for some time after the trance.

Psychosomatic symptoms as headache, nausea, tremors and shivering may appear spontaneously in some individuals. These symptoms are usually of very short duration, unless they are reactions to a posthypnotic suggestion the subject wishes to resist. In the latter instance, symptoms can continue for an extended period, until the individual follows the posthypnotic command or until the compulsive influence of the hypnotist's suggestions have worn off. There may be associated with these symptoms an intense dislike for the hypnotist.

A similar lingering hostility may develop following therapeutic hypnotic suggestions. In treating an alcoholic patient, I suggested to him while in trance that he would develop an increasing distaste for alcohol because he would gradually realize how much it undermined him and was against his best interests. Immediately upon awakening the patient began to talk excitedly about how doctors often overcharged their patients. He speculated that probably ninety per cent of physicians did this and he remarked that this was the reason why so few patients had confidence in their doctors. Further associations revealed that this trend of thought had been stimulated by a resentment over the suggestion I had given him to abstain from alcoholic beverages.

Where the subject during hypnosis has been forced to act in a manner opposed to his usual nature, he may harbor antagonism and rage posthypnotically. Estabrooks[80] cites an amusing incident while personally witnessing a demonstration by a stage hypnotist. The latter found a good subject in a dignified member of the community who was the deacon of his church. Under hypnosis he made the deacon, among other things, stand on his head, bark like a dog and crawl around on all fours. Upon awakening the deacon promptly knocked the hypnotist down for forcing him into such a shameful exhibition.

In certain individuals, induced hypnotic phenomena spontaneously continue in the waking state. Paralysis, analgesia, and other symptoms may persist to the great astonishment of the subject. Usually this occurs when the hypnotist fails to give the subject a posthypnotic command to the effect that all of his functions will be restored to normal. Upon analyzing the meaning of the persistence of hypnotic phenomena in the waking state, one usually discovers an unconscious desire to please the hypnotist by continuing to fulfill his implied wishes. Sometimes hysteric-like phenomena follow repeated inductions. These occur in hysterically inclined persons who are motivated toward the development of specific symptoms. This is not a casual happening, but follows dynamic laws that govern unconscious wishes.

A very common reaction following the first trance induction is disappointment in hypnosis due to the excessive expectations on the part of the subject, or because of distorted notions concerning the uniqueness or exotic nature of the hypnotic trance. Another common reaction is a denial by the subject that he has been hypnotized because he was conscious of everything that went on. This denial may persist after subsequent trances, and only upon demonstrating to the subject during hypnosis that he cannot voluntarily open his eyes or resist automatic movements may he actually concede the fact that he has entered the hypnotic state. Even then he will usually assert that he could easily have resisted the hypnotist's commands had he so desired. Theoretically this is true, but what the subject overlooks is the fact that the motivation for hypnosis usually robs him of this desire.

In some instaces the hypnotic experience may be followed by emotional instability, depression or anxiety, especially where posthypnotic suggestions have been given the subject which are opposed to his common sense, habits and interests. Occasionally, emotional instability is the product of a realization in a compulsively independent individual that he has yielded his control, and that, in spite of his resolutions to defy the hypnotist, he has finally succumbed. In other cases, great elation, ecstasy and joy may develop as a result of the experience. These emotions are most pronounced in persons whose sole motivation for hypnosis is to find a godlike figure who will magically fulfill their wishes and demands.

Feelings related to hypnosis may be carried over into waking life for a considerable period affecting it in a manner similar to dreams with a strong emotional tone.

Posthypnotic Amnesia. Deep hypnosis is usually associated with the loss of memory on awakening which increases with the depth of the trance. The subject may remember all details of the trance state upon awakening, and then gradually forget some or all of his experiences. He may remember nothing, and then later recover some or all of the events. Although some authorities like Bramwell[81] deny that lost memories can ever be recalled through association of ideas, experience does not corroborate this.

It is probable that posthypnotic amnesia is due to a direct or implied suggestion to forget what has occurred. The fact that sleep has been suggested, automatically means to many persons that they must not remember the events during the trance. Complete posthypnotic amnesia is found only in the deepest hypnotic states. In certain instances, the subject's character structure demands that he maintain control, and, even though he succumbs to a deep trance, he will recall all of his experiences or a sufficient number of them to satisfy his personality needs. Trance events, shielded from consciousness by amnesia, are usually remembered in subsequent trances, unless there are specific directions to the contrary. On the other hand, if the individual during hypnosis is directed to remember events that have occurred, he will in all likelihood have no amnesia. In somnambulistic subjects, posthypnotic amnesia may be induced for certain aspects of waking life. The amnesia may even involve the individual's own identity much as in hysterical amnesia.

The phenomenon of posthypnotic amnesia raises an important question in therapy. How much does the amnesia nullify curative, persuasive and re-educative suggestions given during hypnosis, and will it cause the repression of forgotten memories recalled in the trance? There is considerable evidence that even a so-called complete posthypnotic amnesia is not perfect. Often subjects will remember hypnotic incidents, but will consider them a product of their own fantasies or conclusions. Sometimes they will confuse events during hypnosis with actual happenings. I have repeatedly confirmed the fact that patients, through free association or slips of speech, will bring up material of the trance state without being fully aware of the origin. Suggestions given the patient during hypnosis, even though not remembered, can be effective, operating from subconscious layers of the mind.

Experimentally it has been shown that posthypnotic amnesia is artificial. Strickler[82] and Patten[83] contend that hypnotic events leave indelible impressions on the mind so that relearning of the supposedly forgotten material occurs with relative ease. Scott[84] experimented with conditioned reflexes established during hypnosis to see whether they could be abolished by posthypnotic amnesia. Hypnotized subjects exposed to an apparatus that imparted to the skin a mild electric shock were conditioned to the sound of a buzzer, which sufficed to produce the customary hand withdrawal from the electrode. The changes within the subject resulting from the shock were recorded in differences in breathing, heart action and galvanic skin reaction. Scott discovered that the conditioned reflex continued in the waking state even though the subject had no recollection of the experiment. Bitterman and Marcuse[85] found that differential automatic responses occurred to test words posthypnotically, even though the words themselves were not remembered. In hypnotherapy suggestions given the patient in the trance will influence him even though he has an apparent amnesia for his hypnotic experiences.

Posthypnotic Suggestions. Any phenomenon induced during hypnosis may also be executed posthypnotically upon suggestion. In some cases, posthypnotic suggestions will be carried out even if the trance has been relatively light, and in spite of the fact that the subject remembers the suggestions. Such subjects are probably extremely suggestible and would be easily influenced in the waking state also. In most cases, however, posthypnotic suggestions are effective only after the subject has developed a deep trance which has been followed by amnesia.

To illustrate how sincerely the subject believes in the authenticity of his posthypnotic experiences, I may cite an example of a posthypnotic negative hallucination induced in a man in the presence of one of my colleagues, Dr. S. The latter physician, skeptical about hypnosis, entered my office unexpectedly at a time when an experimental subject, known to both of us, was in a hypnotic trance. I suggested to the subject that when he woke up he would neither be able to see nor hear Dr. S. Upon awakening, the subject engaged me in a conversation regarding the pennant possibilities of the Dodgers, in the middle of which he casually asked if I had seen Dr. S. recently. I rejoined by asking him the same question. During this conversation, Dr. S. was leaning up against a window. I informed the subject that I was expecting Dr. S. and asked him to look out of the window to see whether he was in sight. The subject looked directly at Dr. S. and said, "No, he isn't." Inquiring as to what he saw, he remarked that he noticed the usual trees, grass, and buildings. At this point, Dr. S. addressed the subject directly.

The latter interrupted him in the middle of a sentence with a remark pointed at myself. Dr. S. continued talking, but the subject paid absolutely no attention to him as if he were not in the room. At this point, I held an inkwell in the air and asked him if he saw it. Perplexed, he admitted that he could and wondered why I had asked him so silly a question. I then handed the inkwell to Dr. S. and asked the subject again if he could see the inkwell. He looked intently at the inkwell and exclaimed, "My God, you will think I am crazy, but the inkwell is floating around in space." He appeared to be genuinely alarmed. I took the inkwell from Dr. S. and he said, "You have the inkwell now." Even though I insisted that Dr. S. was in the room and pointed him out, the subject continued to believe that I was joking. He remarked that fortunately he had not yet lost his mind. He was certain that there was no other person in the room until I rehypnotized him and removed the suggestion.

The compulsive nature of the posthypnotic act is one of its most characteristic features. This is not to say that the suggestion cannot be resisted. Usually, however, resistance takes a tremendous effort. Bleuler[86] underwent hypnosis to test this point. He describes his experience in attempting to resist a posthypnotic suggestion as follows: "I was able to resist the carrying out of a posthypnotic suggestion. However, this cost me considerable trouble, and if I forgot for an instant during talking my resolve not to take any notice of the plate, which I was supposed to place somewhere else, I suddenly found myself fixing this object with my eyes. The thought of what I had been ordered to do worried me until I went to sleep, and when I was in bed I nearly got up again to carry it out, merely to ease my mind. However, I soon fell asleep and the action of the suggestion was then lost."

Commands that are reasonable and are in keeping with the individual's personality are usually carried out. Unreasonable suggestions, those that are ridiculous or not in keeping with the individual's personality, may not be carried out even though the subject is a somnambule. I once gave a patient a posthypnotic suggestion to reach for a cigarette and light it as soon as I returned to my chair. He did not follow the command. When I inquired whether he had remembered my giving him any posthypnotic suggestion, he declared that he did not. At the next hypnotic session, he confided that a private physician had advised him against cigarettes because of a heart condition, and he insisted that his refusal to comply with my suggestion was based upon a feeling that it might do him harm.

In certain cases, suggestions that are incompatible with the subject's customary behavior or outlook may be carried out with great resistance. Schilder and Kauders[87] state that in general posthypnotic suggestions of an unreasonable type will be accepted by those persons who are fundamentally very suggestible. Often a tremendous struggle results against compliance, with resulting psychosomatic phenomena, anxiety or emotional disturbance that may assume psychotic proportions. Brickner and Kubie[88] ascribe this struggle to a conflict between the commands given the subject by the hypnotist and the unconscious commands of his own superego which would be violated by the posthypnotic act. The compulsive quality of posthypnotic suggestions may be so intense that anxiety will force the person into compliance.

The way a posthypnotic suggestion is phrased also influences whether or not it will be followed. If the subject detects from the expression of the hypnotist that obedience is not mandatory, he will better be able to resist the command. If, however, he believes that he is expected to obey, he will feel more obliged to comply.

Frequently the enactment of a posthypnotic suggestion is defended by numerous rationalizations. The subject may refuse to believe that the act had been suggested by the hypnotist and he may justify it as his own impulse. A physician friend of mine, skilled in hypnosis, often used his wife, who was a good subject, to demonstrate the induction of trance. On one occasion, his wife decided to defy him. Upon awakening from the trance, she suddenly experienced great thirst. She assumed from the compulsive nature of the impulse to drink that her husband had given her this suggestion, which was, of course, correct. In spite of her resolve she felt herself being lifted out of her chair and pulled toward the kitchen. However, she clutched her chair and was for a while able to resist the compulsion. But she soon started to experience a dryness of the throat that became so extreme that she felt that it was foolish to torture herself. She then went into the kitchen, quenched her thirst and explained that the only reason she had done this was because she really was thirsty and had intended to get a drink anyway.

An experimental neurosis unwittingly produced in a medical student by myself[89] illustrates the compulsive character of posthypnotic suggestion. In order to illustrate the induction of hypnosis, a student volunteer was hypnotized in front of the class. A suggestion was given to him that upon awakening he would return to his seat and listen attentively to the lecture. As soon as I went to the blackboard and wrote the word "psychiatry," he would write his name, but in the process would misspell it. Before awakening he was instructed to sleep for three minutes, following which I would arouse him by rapping three times on the table top. After three minutes, the prescribed rappings failed to arouse the subject who was still deeply in a trance. Five more minutes passed without my being able to awaken him, and his only response was violent shaking and tremors. Finally, I told him that the posthypnotic suggestion might have aroused some resistance in himself and that he did not have to comply if he did not wish to.

He then aroused himself, opened his eyes, but his shaking became even more violent. He took his seat, but his tremors became so bad that he could hardly sit. I rehypnotized him and attempted to remove the tremors by direct suggestion. Although his tremors were diminished somewhat in intensity, they were still present, and he was obviously uncomfortable. He complained of nausea and feelings of tenseness and anxiety. He remembered the posthypnotic suggestion I had given him, and he recalled also the instruction that he did not have to carry it out.

I then went over to the blackboard and wrote the word "psychiatry." As soon as he saw the word, he reached for his pencil, but he paused in midair and forcefully brought his hand back. His tremors and anxiety became much more intense. I then advised him that it would probably be best for him to write his name in spite of his resistance. He grasped the pencil, but his fingers would not move. When he started writing, his hand shook violently and he was unable to form letters. He tried to steady his right hand with his left, but his pencil moved so slowly that it took him almost five minutes to write his first name. His hand stopped, and he seemed to exhibit a superhuman effort to force himself to write. Upon reaching the last two letters, his hand refused to go further. Finally, after a pause of several minutes, he finished his name. To his amazement he had misspelled it. His anxiety and tremors vanished immediately, and he became extremely cheerful. He was able to write his name then without any difficulty.

He confided spontaneously that he resented deeply any misspelling of his name. People frequently misspelled it, and he often wondered why they could not write accurately so simple a name as his. In commenting on the experiment, he said that he did not want to write his name wrong, yet he found himself forced to do so for reasons he could not understand.

It seemed obvious that his sleeping beyond the signal to awaken was a mechanism to avert the conflict. The release from the obligation to write his name inaccurately was sufficient to arouse him, but he felt compelled, nevertheless, to react to the command. The phenomenon acted as an excellent demonstration to the class of the dynamics of neurosis.

A letter written to me by the subject is interesting in detailing his subjective reactions:

"When the experiment started, I found it very easy to concentrate. When you told me I was asleep, I truthfully didn't believe it because I could still hear you talking and was still conscious of the fact that I was being hypnotized. I believe I remember everything you told me to do since I do not feel that I lost consciousness during the hypnosis. I simply felt more or less drowsy. The best comparison that I can make is this: I felt that I just ingested some alcoholic beverage (which I very rarely do because I never got into the habit) and was just about to doze off. When you told me that my right arm felt very light, it really did feel that way, and the same held true when you told me that my left arm felt heavy. And yet throughout all of this, I kept being amazed at it all, because I didn't see how it could be possible. When you gave me the command to write my name incorrectly spelled, I was not conscious of the fact that such a task would be distasteful, nor that it would create an experimental neurosis. When you asked me to dream, I did not dream but felt very relaxed and saw a soothing red or pink color in front of my eyes. When you tried to waken me, I felt very much as I do when I wake up in the morning, i.e., I hated to awaken. I know I trembled while still under hypnosis and even after I came out (I'm not sure that I did come out when you told me to) I could not stop trembling no matter how much self control I tried to exert.

"When I sat down in the chair, I wanted to write my name on the paper largely because of curiosity, especially since you began to analyze the situation at the time, referring to experimental neurosis created, etc. When I tried to write, I could hardly hold the pencil, since I was shaking so violently. As you well know, it turned out to be a child's scrawl. I had difficulty in getting out every single letter. I just could not get it out. All through this performance, I kept murmuring to myself that the whole thing was ridiculous, especially the tremors and trembling which affected my entire body. Finally, in exasperation, I murmured: 'What the hell,' and ended my name wrong against my will. When I did this, the trembling immediately ceased, and I felt kind of relieved. Someone then asked me to misspell my name again, and I could do it with no trouble.

"After this I felt tired because of the strain of concentration and trembling. But sure enough, on my way home from school on the train, I felt very gay and lively, in spite of the fact that I was up late the night before and would ordinarily be tired. I was with some friends. I kept joking with them, inviting them to come out with me that night to 'tear the town apart' and felt very contented as one does in the early stages of alcohol intoxication. When I got out of the subway, for some strange reason I ran all the way home and did not feel at all tired when I got there (and I'm hardly in good athletic form at this time). That evening I felt very well, not at all tired as I usually am (from a full day at school), and studied very efficiently. When I turned in, I was not tired, and I think that I could have worked efficiently the entire evening. (We'll have to try this again before finals.)"

The nature of posthypnotic behavior has been subjected to an intensive analysis by Erickson and Erickson.[90] These authors believe, as Bramwell[91] had contended previously, that posthypnotic suggestions are not carried out in a normal condition, but in a state that resembles hypnosis. During the performance of a posthypnotic act, a spontaneous self-limited posthypnotic trance develops. One frequently observes that some subjects do act dazed during the execution of a posthypnotic act, as if they were following it automatically. This is especially true where the subject is forced to interrupt one form of behavior to execute an act that differs markedly from what the individual was doing at the time. Amnesia for the posthypnotic act occurs particularly where the action is unusual or ridiculous, or conflicts with the customary behavior of the subject and may serve the purpose of averting embarrassment or anxiety.

In other cases, where the act is harmonious with the personality of the subject and with his surroundings, he may appear fully conscious during its execution. He will then remember his behavior, often rationalizing it as a product of his own doing. This occurs most often where the suggestions are so phrased that he can perform the act at his own timing. Unconsciously he will wait for an opportune moment to inject the act into the course of his behavior in such a way that it does not conflict with his standards or with what other people are doing at the time. This is not to say that during the actual execution of the posthypnotic act the subject may not be in a special form of trance. However, it is usually impossible to differentiate this behavior from the ordinary waking state.

Another problem is the actual extent and duration of posthypnotic suggestions. Do the suggestions themselves fade eventually or can they be made to persist indefinitely? Many observers have corroborated the fact that when a posthypnotic suggestion is to be executed after a long period of time, the passing of time does not obliterate the intensity of the compulsion. For example, a subject was told by myself that exactly two years and two days from the date of trance he would read one of Tennyson's poems. He complied with this suggestion on that date, having a week before developed a yearning to read poetry. Perusal of the book shelves of a library caused him to finger through one of

Tennyson's volumes which interested him so that he borrowed it. He then placed it on his own desk until the prescribed day when he suddenly found an opportunity to read the poem. He was positive that his interest in Tennyson was caused by a personal whim.

Estabrooks[92] mentions the case of a person in whom a posthypnotic suggestion was strong after twenty years, and he believes that with occasional reinforcement the posthypnotic suggestion can last indefinitely. Without reinforcement, a posthypnotic suggestion often persists for many days. In one subject, I induced hypnotically a craving for vinegar. This led to a desire for vinegar so intense that for several days the subject doused all of his food with that substance to the disgust of his roommates.

Wells[93] urged three subjects in a hypnotic trance to memorize a series of nonsense syllables. Posthypnotic amnesia was suggested for one year, and an appointed hour was set for remembering the syllables. This suggestion was carried out precisely. Further experiments proved that hypnotically induced suggestions were not necessarily obliterated by time, a fact that may have great therapeutic significance.

REFERENCES

[1] BERNHEIM, H.: Suggestive Therapeutics: a Treatise on the Nature and Uses of Hypnotism (Translated by C. A. Herter). New York, Putnams, 1900.

[2] KUBIE, L. S., AND MARGOLIN, S.: The process of hypnotism and the nature of the hypnotic state. Am. J. Psychiat. *100:* 611–622, 1944.

[3] BRENMAN, M., GILL, M. M., AND HACKER, F. J.: Alterations in the state of the ego in hypnosis. Bull. Menninger Clin. *11:* 60–66, 1947.

[4] KUBIE, L. S., AND MARGOLIN, S.: op. cit., reference 2.

[5] ERICKSON, M. H.: Hypnotic induction of psychosomatic phenomena. Psychosomatic interrelationships studied by experimental neurosis. Psychosom. Med. *5:* 51–58, 1943.

[6] WOLBERG, L. R.: A mechanism of hysteria elucidated during hypnosis. Psychoanal. Quart. *14:* 1945.

[7] SCHILDER, P., AND KAUDERS, O.: Hypnosis (Translated by S. Rothenberg). New York, Nervous & Mental Disease Publ. Co., 1927.

[8] HULL, C. L. Hypnosis and Suggestibility. New York, Appleton-Century 1933, p. 388.

[9] YOUNG, P. C.: Hypnotism. Psychol Bull. *23:* 504-523, 1926.

[10] ———: Is rapport an essential characteristic of hypnosis? J. Abnorm. & Social Psychol. *22:* 130-139, 1927.

[11] ———: An experimental study of mental and physical functions in the normal and hypnotic states. Am. J. Psychol. *36:* 214-232, 1925.

[12] DAVIS, R. C., AND KANTOR, J. R.: Skin resistance during hypnotic states. J. Gen. Psychol. *13:* 62-81, 1935.

[13] WHITE, R. W.: Two types of hypnotic trance and their personality correlates. J. Psychol. *3:* 279-289, 1937.

[14] FRIEDLANDER, S. W., AND SARBIN, T. R.: The depth of hypnosis. J. Abnorm. & Social Psychol. *33:* 453-475, 1938.

[15] WILLIAMS, G. W.: The effect of hypnosis on muscular fatigue. J. Abnorm. & Social Psychol. *24:* 83-95, 1930.

[16] ———: A comparative study of voluntary and hypnotic catalepsy. Am. J. Psychol. *42:* 83-95, 1930.

[17] NICHOLSON, N. C.: Notes on muscular work during hypnosis. Johns Hopkins Hospital Bull. *31:* 89, 1920.

[18] YOUNG, P. C.: An experimental study of mental and physical functions in the normal and hypnotic states. Am. J. Psychol. *36:* 214-232, 1925.

[19] SEARS, R. R.: An experimental study of hypnotic anesthesia. J. Exper. Psychol. *15:* 1-22, 1932.

[20] DYNES, J. B.: An experimental study in hypnotic anesthesia. J. Abnorm. & Social Psychol. *27:* 79-88, 1932.

[21] ERICKSON, M. H.: The induction of color blindness by a technique of hypnotic suggestion. J. Gen. Psychol. *20:* 61-89, 1939.

[22] PATTIE, F. A.: The genuineness of hypnotically produced anesthesia of the skin. Am. J. Psychol. *49:* 435-443, 1937.

[23] LUNDHOLM, H.: An experimental study of functional anesthesias as induced by suggestion in hypnosis. J. Abnorm. & Social Psychol. *23:* 337-355, 1928.

[24] DORCUS, R. M.: Modification by suggestion of some vestibular and visual responses. Am. J. Psychol. *49:* 82-87, 1937.

[25] YOUNG, P. C.: Experimental hypnotism: a review. Psychol. Bull. *38:* 98, 1941.

[26] DOUPE, J., MILLER, W. R., AND KELLAR, W. K.: Vasomotor reactions in the hypnotic state. J. Neurol. Psychiat. *2:* 97-106, 1939.

[27] LOOMIS, A. L., HARVEY, E. N., AND HOBART, G.: Brain potentials during hypnosis. Science *83:* 239-241, 1936.

[28] LEMERE, F.: Electroencephalography as a method of distinguishing true from false blindness. J.A.M.A. 118-884, 1942.

[29] LUNDHOLM, H., AND LÖWENBACH, H.: Hypnosis and the alpha activity of the encephalogram. Char. & Pers. *11:* 145-149, 1942-1943.

[30] ERICKSON, M. H., AND ERICKSON, E. M.: The hypnotic induction of hallucinatory color vision followed by pseudo-negative after-images. J. Exper. Psychol. *22:* 581-588, 1938.

[31] ———: A study of clinical and experimental findings on hypnotic deafness. J. Gen. Psychol. *19:* 127-167, 1938.

[32] ——: The experimental demonstration of unconscious mentation by automatic writing. Psychoanal. Quart. *6:* 513, 1937.

[33] ——, AND KUBIE, L. S.: The use of automatic drawing in the interpretation and relief of a state of acute obsessional depression. Psychoanal. Quart. *8:* 443–446, 1938.

[34] ——, AND ——: The permanent relief of an obsessional phobia by means of communications with an unsuspected dual personality. Psychoanal. Quart. *8:* 471–509, 1939.

[35] FARBER, L. H., AND FISHER, C.: An experimental approach to dream psychology through the use of hypnosis. Psychoanal. Quart. *12:* No. 2, 1943.

[36] FREUD, S.: The Psychopathology of Everyday Life. In The Basic Writings of Sigmund Freud. New York, Modern Library, 1938.

[37] SCOTT, H. D.: Hypnosis and the conditioned reflex. J. Gen. Psychol. *4:* 113–130, 1930.

[38] MISHCHENKO, M. N.: The rate of formation of conditioned reflexes in the hypnotic state. Eksp. med, Kharkov, No. 3, 33–40, 1935.

[39] STALNAKER, J. M., AND RIDDLE, E. E.: The effect of hypnosis on long delayed recall. J. Gen. Psychol. *6:* 429–440, 1932.

[40] WHITE, R. W., FOX, G. F., AND HARRIS, W. W.: Hypnotic hypermnesia for recently learned material. J. Abnorm. & Social Psychol. *35:* 88–103, 1940.

[41] ROSENTHAL, B. C.: Hypnotic recall of material learned under anxiety and non-anxiety producing conditions. J. Exper. Psychol. *34:* 369–389, 1944.

[42] HAKEBUSH, BLINKOVSKI AND FOUNDILLERE: An attempt at a study of development of personality with the aid of hypnosis. Trud. Inst. Psikhonevr. Kiev, *2:* 236–272, 1930.

[43] PLATONOW, K. I.: On the objective proof of the experimental personality age regression. J. Gen. Psychol. *9:* 190–209, 1933.

[44] DOLIN, A. O.: Objective investigation of the elements of individual experience by means of the method of experimental hypnosis. Arkh. biol. Nauk. *36:* 28–52, 1934.

[45] YOUNG, P. C.: Hypnotic regression—fact or artifact. J. Abnorm. & Social Psychol. *35:* 273–278, 1940.

[46] ESTABROOKS, G. H.: Hypnotism. New York, Dutton, 1943, p. 65.

[47] LINDNER, R. M.: Rebel Without a Cause: The hypnoanalysis of a criminal psychopath. New York, Grune & Stratton, 1944.

[48] SPIEGEL, H., SHOR, J., AND FISHMAN, S.: An hypnotic obeation technique for the study of personality development. Psychosom. Med. *7:* 273–278, 1945.

[49] WOLBERG, L. R.: Hypnoanalysis. New York, Grune & Stratton, 1945, pp. 208–214.

[50] ERICKSON, M. H., AND KUBIE, L. S.: The successful treatment of a case of acute hysterical depression by a return under hypnosis to a critical phase of childhood. Psychoanal. Quart. *10:* 592, 1941.

[51] LINDNER, R. M.: op. cit., reference 47.

[52] BRAMWELL, J. M.: Hypnotism; Its History, Theory and Practice, ed. 3. London, Rider, 1921, pp. 114–139.

[53] STALNAKER, J. M., AND RICHARDSON, M. W.: Time estimation in a hypnotic trance. J. Gen. Psychol. *4:* 362–366, 1930.

[54] HARRIMAN, P. L.: The experimental production of some phenomena related to the multiple personality. J. Abnorm. & Social Psychol. *37:* 244–255, 1942.

[55] WOLBERG, L. R.: op. cit., reference 49.

[56] SARBIN, T. R.: Rorschach patterns under hypnosis. Am. J. Orthopsychiat. *9:* 315–318, 1939.

[57] LEVINE, K. N., GRASSI, J. R., AND GARSON, M. J.: Hypnotically induced mood changes in the verbal and graphic Rorschach; a case study. Rorschach Res. Exch. *7:* 130–144, 1943.

[58] BERGMAN, J. S., GRAHAM, H., AND LEAVITT, H. C.: Rorschach exploration of consecutive hypnotic age level regressions. Psychosom. Med., Jan.–Feb. pp. 20–28, 1947.

[59] FISHER, V. E., AND MARROW, A. J.: Experimental study of moods. Char. & Pers., *2:* 201–208, 1934.

[60] KEIR, G.: An experiment in mental testing under hypnosis. J. Ment. Sci. *91:* 346–352, 1945.

[61] DOSWALD, D. C., AND KREIBICH, K.: Monotshefts f. prakt. Dermat. *43:* 634–640, 1906.

[62] HELLER, F., AND SCHULTZ, J. H.: München med. Wchnschr. *56:* 212, 1909.

[62a] ULLMAN, MONTAGUE: Herpes simplex and second degree burn induced under hypnosis. Am. J. Psychiat. *103:* 828–830, 1947.

[63] GLASER, F.: Med. Klin. *20:* 535–537, 1924.

[64] POVORINSIJ, J. A., AND FINNE, W. N.: Ztschr. f.d. ges. neurol. u. Psychiat. *129:* 135–146, 1930.

[65] LANGHEINRICH, O.: Psychische einflusse auf die Sekretionstatigkeit des Magens und des Diodenume. München Med. Wchnschr. *69:* 1527–1529, 1922.

[66] DELHOUGNE, F., AND HANSEN, K.: Die suggestive Beeinflussbarkeit der Magen und Pankreassekretion in der Hypnose. Deutsches Archiv. f. Klinische Medizin *157:* 20–35, 1927.

[67] HEILIG, R., AND HOFF, H.: Beitrage zur hypnotischen Beeinflussung der Magenfunktion. Med. Klin. *21:* 162–163, 1925.

[68] HEYER, G. R.: Das korperlich-seelische Zusammenwirken in dem Lebensvorgangen. Munchen, 1925.

[69] MARX, H.: Untersuchungen über den Wasserhaushalt. II. Mitteilung. Die psychische Beeinflussing des Wasserhaushaltes. Klin. Wchnschr. *5:* 92–94 1926.

[70] PLATONOW, K. I., AND MATSKEVICH, A. N.: Hypnosis and the nervous system under the influence of alcohol. Trudi ukr. psikhonevr. Inst. *15:* 93–106, 1931.

[71] BRAMWELL, J. M.: op. cit., reference 52, p. 92.

[72] JENNESS, A., AND WIBLE, C. L.: Respiration and heart action in sleep and hypnosis. J. Gen. Psychol. *16:* 197–222, 1937.

[73] DOUPE, J., MILLER, W. R., AND KELLER, W. K.: Vasomotor reactions in the hypnotic state. J. Neurol. & Psychiat. *2:* 106, 1939.

[74] HEILIG, R., AND HOFF, H.: Psychische Beeinflussing von Organfunktionen, Insbesondere in der Hypnose. Sammelreferat. Allgem. arztl. Zeitschrift f. Psychotherapie u. Psychische Hygiene, vol. 1, no. 4, Verlag von S. Hirzel, in Leipzig C. I Konigstrasse 2.

[75] ——, AND ——: Über hypnotische Beeinflussing der Nurenfunktion. Deutsche Med. Wchnschr. *51:* 1615–1616, 1925.

[76] BENEDEK, L.: Influence upon the vegetative nervous system of hypnosis. Gyógyászat *14:* 1–2, 1933.

[77] DOSWALD, C. D., AND KREIBLICH, K.: Zur Frage der post-hypnotischen Hauptphaenomene. Monatschr. f. prakt. Dermat. *43:* 634–640, 1906.

[78] LAUDENHEIMER, R.: Therap. d. Gegnw. *67:* 339–344, 1926.

[79] EISENBUD, J.: Psychology of headache. Psychiat. Quart. *11:* 592–619, 1937.

[80] ESTABROOKS, G. H.: op. cit., reference 46, p. 42.

[81] BRAMWELL, J. M.: op. cit., reference 52, p. 105.

[82] STRICKLER, C. B.: A quantitative study of post-hypnotic amnesia. J. Abnorm. & Social Psychol. *24:* 108–119, 1929.

[83] PATTEN, E. F.: Does post-hypnotic amnesia apply to practice effects? J. Gen. Psychol. *7:* 196–201, 1932.

[84] SCOTT, H D.: Hypnosis and the conditioned reflex. J. Gen. Psychol. *4:* 113–130, 1930.

[85] BITTERMAN, M. E., AND MARCUSE, F. L.: Autonomic response in post-hypnotic amnesia. Bull. Canad. Psychol. Assoc. *5:* 31–32, 1945.

[86] BLEULER, E.: Psychology of Hypnosis. Munich Med. Wchnschr., 1889, No. 5.

[87] SCHILDER, P., AND KAUDERS, O.: op. cit., reference 7, p. 5.

[88] BRICKNER, R. M., AND KUBIE, L. S.: A miniature psychotic storm produced by superego conflict over a simple post-hypnotic suggestion. Psychoanal. Quart. *5:* 467–487, 1936.

[89] WOLBERG, L. R.: Hypnotic experiments in psychosomatic medicine. Psychosomatic Medicine. *9:* 337–342, 1947.

[90] ERICKSON, M. H., AND ERICKSON, E. M.: Concerning the nature and character of post-hypnotic behavior. J. Gen. Psychol. *24:* 95–133, 1941.

[91] BRAMWELL, J. M.: op. cit., reference 52, p. 111.

[92] ESTABROOKS, G. H.: op. cit, reference 46, p. 81.

[93] WELLS, W. R.: The extent and duration of post-hypnotic amnesia. J. Psychol. *9:* 137–151, 1940.

III

THE NATURE OF HYPNOSIS

SINCE the time of James Braid[1] who demonstrated conclusively that hypnosis was purely a subjective experience, there have been three main lines of inquiry into the nature of hypnosis: pathologic, physiologic and psychologic.

PATHOLOGIC THEORIES

Charcot and his students, Binet and Féré, conducted a series of experiments at Salpétrière which convinced them that hypnosis was a pathologic phenomenon. The trance to them was merely a symptom of hysteria, principally because it could most easily be induced in hysterical patients.

Although this notion was rejected by Bernheim who exposed the fallacies of Charcot's experiments, Charcot's theory gained a number of supporters. Even today there are those like Brown[2] who believe in the hysterical character of hypnosis. Little evidence exists to support this theory as Eysenck[3] has pointed out. Indeed nonhysterical persons are often as hypnotizable and even more so than many patients suffering from hysteria.

PHYSIOLOGIC THEORIES

Physiologic theories contend that the process of hypnosis s accompanied by a physical change within the cerebral cortex. Bennett, for instance, advanced the idea that there was a suspension of activity in the white substance of the cerebral lobes with an overactivity of the remaining parts. Heidenhain[4] speculated that the trance resulted from an inhibition of the ganglion cells of the brain. Vincent similarly suggested an inhibition of one set of mental functions and an acceleration of another. Sidis believed hypnosis to be due to a functional dissociation between the nerve cells. Ernest Hart suggested cerebral anemia as a cause of hypnosis, reviving ideas held formerly by Carpenter and Hack Tuke. More recently attempts have been made, with little or no evidence, to classify hypnosis as an obscure function of the autonomic nervous system.[5] Eysenck,[6] leaning toward an ideomotor hypothesis, believes that hypnosis can be explained by referring to the properties of the synaptic nerve junctions. Hypnosis, he claims, directs the whole force of nervous energy into a smaller number of nervous channels, thereby reducing the synaptic resistance and facillitating the passage of nervous energy. This contention is somewhat similar to the belief of McDougall[7] who accounted for the somatic manifestations of hypnosis on the basis that voluntary attention withdrawn from the outer world could be concentrated in force upon the vasomotor system, producing changes not possible in normal consciousness.

Evidence that hypnosis is a physiologic phenomenon is usually pointed out because of the similarity of hypnosis to animal hypnosis, to sleep, to dissociative states and to conditioned reflexes.

Hypnosis and Animal Hypnosis. It is known that birds, frogs, alligators, crayfish, opossums, rabbits, guinea pigs, and some insects enter a state resembling hypnosis when subjected to certain stimuli. Thus alligators, frogs, and toads when turned over on their backs and stroked rhythmically on their undersides lose their muscle tonus and become unconscious. Other animals when placed in strange or unaccustomed positions develop catalepsy. During the mating season, female spiders become limp and nonresistant when males imbed their jaws into a sensitive spot in the abdomen. In many animals, these trancelike conditions are produced by fear and appear to be a mechanism of simulated death which serves a defensive purpose. Verworn has demonstrated that such reactions are tonic recumbency reflexes. Ablation of the cerebrum apparently does not destroy the reaction, and Spiegel and Goldblom believe that the red nucleus is the governing center for these responses.

The question that arises is whether such manifestations are really hypnotic in nature. There is serious doubt that catalepsy in animals is similar to a trance in human beings. Even though humans do show signs of catalepsy during hypnosis, these are among the more minor phenomena of the trance state.

Hypnosis as a State of Sleep. A common theory of hypnosis purports it to be a modified type of sleep. Pavlov[8] insisted that hypnosis and sleep were identical in that they both were dependent upon areas of inhibition spreading over the cerebral hemispheres. Rabinovich,[9] subscribing to the ideas of Pavlov, believed that eye fixation during hypnotic induction exhausted and finally inhibited a specific area in the cortex. Absence of disturbing stimuli encouraged the spread of inhibitions over adjacent areas until hypnosis ensued.

More recently Kubie and Margolin[10] have elaborated on this mechanism. According to these authors the basic physiologic prerequisite for hypnotic induction is the creation of a focus of central excitation with surrounding areas of inhibition. This condition is insured by immobilization and by a monotonous stimulus of low intensity. Fixation of the eyes on a single spot immobilizes the individual. A reduction of excitation occurs in the segmental oculo-motor apparatus, the suprasegmental levels, and in the entire sensori-motor system that adjusts the person to exploratory activities of the eye. At the same time sensory stimuli are decreased and those that remain are monotonously repeated. Repetition of rhythmic stimuli induces relaxation. The sensory adaptation that results has a hypnogogic effect. The onset of hypnosis thus appears to correspond to a partial sleep.

Other authorities believe that the resemblance of hypnosis to sleep is wholly superficial. They point out that eye fixation is not essential to the induction process and that subjects can pass into the trance state by mere suggestion that they do so.

Physiologic tests prove that the hypnotic state itself is not at all similar to sleep. For instance, a person asleep does not react to stimuli of average intensity, whereas a hypnotized person will respond to even subliminal stimuli. Reflexes which are diminished or abolished in sleep are not affected by hypnosis. Bass,[11] for example, found that the patellar reflex in hypnosis is more like that in the waking state. Wible and Jenness[12] reported that electrocardiographic and respiratory studies during hypnosis approximated the findings of normal consciousness rather than of sleep. Loomis, Harvey and Hobart[13] discovered that the brain potentials of subjects in a trance were characteristic of the waking state. The work of Nygard[14] on cerebral circulation, of Goldwyn[15] on blood pressure, blood count and chemical analysis, and of Beck,[16] Dorcus[17] and Pattie[18] on mental activity all fail to correlate hypnosis with sleep.

It is true that rapport can sometimes be established with a sleeping person and that suggestions may be given him to which he will respond. This does not necessarily prove that sleep is a type of hypnosis or vice versa. More probable, as Hull[19] has pointed out, the individual may pass from the sleep state to the hypnotic state in the same way that he can during somnambulism fall into a deep sleep from which he cannot be aroused.

The consensus is that although the phenomena occurring during the induction of hypnosis with a fixation object resemble early stages of sleep, the actual state of hypnosis is in no way related to sleep. Hypnosis as a form of sleep fails to explain the myriad manifestations of the trance as well as its dynamic function.

Hypnosis as a Dissociative Process. In hysterical somnambulism and fugue states, an unconscious group of memories

and activities temporarily appropriate the stream of consciousness and function autonomously. These are usually
repressed in the normal waking state. Janet[20] attributed this
phenomenon to a splitting off of an important group of
memories and ideas from the main stream of cognition. He
recognized that dissociated strivings, even though subconscious, were able to influence behavior. Because it was possible to induce, under hypnosis, phenomena which resembled
the symptoms of hysteria, and, because the individual could
perform complicated mental feats involving thinking and
judgment without resorting to customary symbolic processes, Janet looked upon hypnosis as a species of somnambulism analogous to hysteria. Operative were the workings
of a secondary dissociated consciousness which Janet called
the "co-conscious." Prince,[21] Burnett[22] and Sidis[23] supported
Janet's contention that in hypnosis intellectual processes
could function simultaneously and independently.

The theory of dissociation was, for many years, regarded
as the key to hypnosis. Depth of hypnosis was presumably
related to the degree of dissociation. Both hysteria and hypnotic susceptibility were considered dependent upon an aptitude to dissociate. In hypnosis, it was believed, the various
functions governed by the brain were, by suggestion, split off
from each other.

The dissociation hypothesis particularly was suited to the
idea of hypnosis as a form of automatism. This notion had
its origin in the early theory that there were two distinct
levels of behavior, the one a level of purposeful, volitional
striving, the other a level of reflex activity. Since hypnosis
appeared to abolish volition, a reflex kind of behavior would
automatically come into being. The latter was dissociated
from consciousness, particularly in the posthypnotic state.

Although posthypnotic amnesia would seem to bear out
the fact of dissociation of a complex group of memories, investigation has revealed that the amnesia is an artificial one,

being more apparent than real. The work of Patten,[24] Life,[25] Scott,[26] and Mitchell[27] leads them to conclude that there is no real barrier between two apparently isolated and dissociated groups of mental activity. Dorcus,[28] Pattie,[29] and Lund-holm[30] contend that instead of dissociation there is actually a very high degree of coordination in hypnosis. Barry, Mac-Kinnon, and Murray[31] and White and Shevach[32] have approached the problem of dissociation from another viewpoint, attempting to determine whether a correlation exists between hypnotizability and the aptitude of the individual in the waking state to perform simultaneously two mental activities. These observers found no such correlation.

Dissociation, while explaining some phenomena of hypnosis, does not account for many others. It fails to explain the arbitrary and changeable nature of the systems allegedly dissociated. It also fails to account for the active participation of supposedly dissociated elements in the total behavior of the subject.

Prince originally emphasized that dissociation was a function of the normal brain mechanism and, like association, existed for the purpose of adapting an individual to his environment. Freud[33] demonstrated that a large part, perhaps the greatest part, of mental life was unconscious, and that precise thinking and reasoning could occur outside the range of awareness. He demonstrated, too, that under certain conditions, as when anxiety was associated with the execution of a certain act or impulse, repressive influences excluded the act or impulse from consciousness. Repression did not reduce the dynamic activity of the excluded group of strivings, which utilized slips of speech, dreams, symbolic acts and symptoms of neuroses to gain expression, thereby circumventing excitation of the ego to anxiety. Another example is in hysteria, where purposeful complicated behavior patterns result during fugue states, somnambulism and operation of a multiple personality.

Dissociation thus can serve an important function and it may be looked upon as a form of motivated behavior. The dissociative tendency can be enhanced through suggestion, particularly during the hypnotic state. This, however, does not prove that hypnosis is basically a state of dissociation, nor does it imply that a person in a trance can always carry out two independent activities better than in the waking state.[34] White [35] has pointed out that the hypnotized person acts in a dissociated manner because the suggestions given him make him feel that he is required to carry out separate activities. While there is much question as to White's contention that the subject is really always playing a role, since organic changes can occur which are beyond the range of mere volitional control, his pointing out the purposeful nature of activity in hypnosis is more rational than attributing it to a mechanical dissociative process.

Hypnosis as a Conditioned Response. The fact that a mere verbal stimulus can, during hypnosis, induce changes of an organic nature has directed attention to the possibility that hypnotic phenomena are types of conditioned reflexes. In 1922, Cason,[36] utilizing the technic of Pavlov, was able to condition the constriction and dilatation of the pupil of the eye to the ringing of a bell. This work was continued by Hudgins[37] who conditioned pupillary contraction to the sound of a bell and later permitted the subject to operate the bell and the light circuits himself while uttering the word "contract." The word "contract," after some time, produced a reaction of the pupil. Pupillary contraction was then successfully conditioned to the subject's own whispered utterance, and finally to the mere thought of the word. Menzies[38] reported conditioning peripheral vascular constriction and dilatation to verbal stimuli. For example, when some of his subjects spoke and even thought of the word "cold" or "snow," the blood vessels constricted. On the other hand thinking of words with warm or hot connotations produced a vasodilatation. Jacobson[39] measured the action currents in muscles and discovered that a thought related to muscular activities could stimulate action currents in the appropriate muscles. Thus when his subjects visualized themselves as flexing their arms, action currents immediately were generated in the arm muscles which lasted until the person stopped thinking of this activity.

Both Pavlov[40] and Bechterev pointed out that words can become conditioned to both internal and external stimuli, and that they may in themselves produce even organic reactions. Platonow[41] presents the hypothesis that in hypnosis the word becomes the stimulus that sets up conditioned reflexes of a physiologic nature. Such reflexes, he states, are copies of organic inherited unconditioned reflexes. Suggestion, he continues, is a typical simple conditioned reflex, and, for this reason, there is no function which, under certain conditions, cannot be facilitated, inhibited or changed to its opposite by means of a verbal cue.

These studies seem to lend some scientific credence to the time-worn ideomotor theory of William James who postulated that any idea, unless inhibited, tended to express itself automatically in behavior. There is, as has been pointed out, evidence that thoughts are associated with corresponding muscular activities. Eysenck[42] attempted to test the theory that every motor idea tends to be carried out in action. In his experiments he utilized the body-sway test, and he reported that in those persons who reacted positively, there was first the idea of falling forward which was either acted on or inhibited. The idea of swaying could be implanted into the subject by another person, by listening to a phonograph record which contained appropriate suggestions, or by seeing another person sway. The idea of falling created the urge to fall forward, and this actually occurred if it was not countered by inhibition. Eysenck concludes that suggestibility is a resultant of two forces, ideomotor action and inhibition. Young[43] similarly favors this revised ideomotor hypothesis.

While the conditioned reflex theory is an intensely interesting one, and while it undoubtedly accounts for physical reactions and even for certain complex psychologic reactions during hypnosis, it does not seem to explain many important and complex phenomena of the hypnotic state. In itself, it is not a complete answer to the problem of the nature of hypnosis.

Psychologic Theories

Hypnosis as a Form of Suggestion. Most authorities feel that hypnosis is a state of exaggerated suggestibility.[44] Hull[45] asserts that all phenomena seen in hypnosis can be induced to a lesser degree by suggestion in the waking state. Increased suggestibility expresses itself both as ideomotor action in that an idea tends to induce automatic behavior, and as a response to social stimuli, particularly to a prestige relationship.

The average individual is relatively more susceptible to suggestions uttered by a person who is impressive in terms of strength, stature, clothes, mien, gestures, eloquence, age, education, experience and "magnetic personality." There is considerable evidence that the powers of the hypnotist are based to a large degree upon the mantle of prestige with which the subject cloaks the hypnotist. Some investigators[46] claim that the successful practice of suggestive hypnosis is dependent on the establishing and maintenance of an atmosphere of faith in the hypnotist. Anything that lowers the intensity of faith decreases the strength of suggestion. Where the subject doubts the skill and power of the hypnotist, there develops a powerful deterrent to hypnosis. Where he accepts on faith the strength of the hypnotist, he will respond to suggestions for which there are no logical grounds.

Knowledge that prestige suggestion may induce a trance actually tells us little about the nature of hypnosis. It is necessary to understand the meaning of the subject's willingness to respond to illogical suggestions. Furthermore, it is essential to explain why under certain circumstances the individual can be hypnotized without recourse to prestige suggestion, as for instance, by means of a phonograph record, and, under certain circumstances, by self suggestions in the technic of autohypnosis.

Psychoanalytic Theories. The emphasis by Bernheim and his contemporaries on the suggestive nature of hypnosis gradually focused attention on the fact that hypnosis was a special kind of relationship in which the hypnotist attempted to wrest from the subject control over his volition and action. The peculiar susceptibility of the subject to these designs on him by the hypnotist were regarded by Freud as due to an unconscious desire for libidinal gratification on the part of the subject.

Ferenczi[46] expanded this idea explaining that hypnosis was a reactivation of the subject's infantile attitude of blind faith and implicit obedience based on both love and fear of his parents. The curious authority with which the hypnotist was endowed was thus a projection of repressed infantile impulses which made the subject regard the hypnotizer as the authoritative parent. The capacity to be hypnotized, Ferenczi[47] alleged, depended upon the extent of transference. The hypnotist with an imposing exterior was often successful because he resembled the stern all-powerful father who expected the child to obey and to imitate him. A situation in which the mother-child relationship was repeated might also be conducive to hypnosis. Soft monotonous words spoken to the subject during the process of induction simulated those of the tender mother lulling the child to sleep. Although the feeling of awe for the parents and the compulsive need to obey them implicitly disappeared as the individual matured, Ferenczi explained that there persisted within each person a need to worship someone. This need was reactivated in the hypnotic state, and the subject actually regarded the hypnotist as if he were a revived image of the parent.

The hypnotic situation thus reanimated unconscious desires and fantasies that existed during the early stages of the child's development. Jones[48] emphasized that infantile incestuous thoughts embodied in the Oedipus complex were projected outward toward the hypnotist as a parental substitute. In a later study, Freud[49] pointed out the similarity between the state of being in love and hypnosis. He also stressed the fact that feelings of helplessness in the face of a superior power might be aroused provoking a passive-masochistic yielding to the hypnotic trance.

The most exhaustive analysis of the psychoanalytic theory has been made by Schilder and Kauders.[50] These authors stress the fact that both hypnosis and suggestibility are essentially of an erotic nature. They point out that sexual accusations are frequently made against the hypnotist. Even though the sexual nature of hypnosis is not at first always apparent to the subject, the trance is in essence an erotic state with inhibited goals. The first goal of hypnosis is a desire for erotic gratification. Another goal, which is also seen normally during the evolution of the Oedipus complex, is that of unconditional subjection. Hypnosis becomes a medium for the expression of self subordination. This masochistic attitude is not to suffer pain, but to subject oneself completely and unconditionally. A study of the psychology of masochism reveals that the masochist identifies himself with his ruler, and that he vicariously shares the latter's greatness and power by means of his subjection. To the hypnotized person the hypnotizer is omnipotent, a magician. The subject projects his own desire for magical power on to the hypnotist, and he participates, through the path of identification, in power he could not attain through his own efforts. The desire for omnipotence normally exists in each child in early stages of his development and is encompassed in the wish to control the world by thought alone. The hypnotizer arouses this infantile wish by inducing, during hypnosis, regression to a stage where the child shares the magical qualities of the parents by identifying himself with them. The hypnotizer on the other hand feels omnipotence more or less unconsciously, and he demands the unconditional masochistic subjection on the part of his subject as well as the latter's sexual subordination.

Two papers by Speyer and Stokvis[51] and Lorand[52] have attempted to confirm the psychoanalytic theory. Speyer and Stokvis studied the difference in the fantasies produced in a male physician, first by a female and then by a male hypnotist. Sensations and ideas during the trance state were recorded by a concealed auditor. Later, as a check, the subject, himself, wrote down his experiences. With the female hypnotist ideas of coitus, of being sexually vanquished and subjected to pain were prominent. With the male hypnotist there were fantasies concerning the latter's penis, and fears of his own castration at the hands of the hypnotist. There were hallucinations of having intercourse with his mother, of being converted into a phallus and entering the vagina and womb of a woman. From this evidence, Speyer and Stokvis conclude that the erotic attitude of the person hypnotized towards the hypnotizer plays an important part in hypnosis. They feel that during hypnosis a regression takes place to the stage of the Oedipus situation with a reactivation of the castration complex.

Lorand attempted to prove Ferenczi's idea that the entire phenomenon of hypnosis was based on the latent child-parent attachment with its attendant neurotic coloring. Through a coincidence he was able to psychoanalyze both a patient who had received hypnotic treatments, and the physician who had administered them. The patient suffered from severe anxiety attacks which came upon her in certain situations, such as when walking on the street, while attending the theater or during lunch with her friends. Under suggestive hypnosis she became symptom-free, but after four months she developed a new symptom — a compulsion to look at every man who passed her on the street. There were also obsessions that men would approach her and that she would not know what to do. She would then rush home for safety and she would experience relief only after she had resorted to masturbation. Her condition grew so aggravating that she finally applied for psychoanalysis.

During psychoanalytic therapy, she described hypnosis as a deep sleep from which she awoke elated, but without recollection of what was told her. As her analysis progressed, an increased amount of material, in dreams and free associations, threw light on her unconscious feelings about hypnosis. Hypnosis represented to her a means of being irresponsible and dependent upon the therapist for support, guidance and love. She revealed an unconscious desire for seduction by the hypnotist. She had abandoned hypnosis because she felt her emotional attachment had been unreciprocated and because she experienced too much anxiety. Lorand concludes that hypnotizability is correlated with "masochist yielding."

Hypnosis as a Psychosomatic Phenomenon

The psychoanalytic school has lent emphasis to the fact that hypnosis is a form of relationship between two people: the hypnotist and the subject. Without question the dynamic core of the hypnotic experience lies in this interpersonal relationship. However, the trance explained solely as an interpersonal experience does not account for the remarkable physiologic manifestations which are engendered by hypnosis. Furthermore, the hypnotic state under some circumstances may develop in the absence of a second person as when the subject listens to sleep suggestions from a phonograph record, or gives appropriate suggestions to himself (autohypnosis), or focuses his attention in solitude on a rhythmic monotonous verbal or visual stimulus.

My own work with hypnosis has convinced me that the

trance state connot be explained exclusively on either a psychologic or physiologic basis. Rather it is a complex psychosomatic reaction which embraces both physiologic and psychologic factors.

Before considering the psychologic aspects of the trance, it may be helpful to attempt an explanation of the physiologic manifestations.

Some observers have been so intrigued by the unique transference situation between subject and hypnotist, and by the motivational factors that lead the subject to act like a hypnotized person, that they regard physiologic phenomena as play-acting. One of the chief characteristics of hypnosis is hypersuggestibility. The subject, responding to an impulse to conform with and even to anticipate the demands made on him by the hypnotist, will therefore play a role, acting as if he experiences the phenomena suggested to him. For example, his reaction to suggestions that he regress to an earlier age level will, with appropriate tests, be shown to be not an organic reproduction of this level, but an intellectualized version of how a person of this age must react. Or, if anesthesia or blunting of the higher senses is suggested, examination will disclose that he is maintaining conscious control and merely acting as if his sensitivities were actually impaired.

These are not true physiologic reactions, but are the product of the subject's desire to conform. Such play-acting does not vitiate the fact that reversible organic reactions do occur in hypnosis, particularly in the deeper trance states.

Physiologic reactions are most common in those induction technics where sleep suggestions are utilized or where there is fixation on rhythmic stimuli. An inhibitory process seems to spread over the higher cortical centers. As in narcosis or sleep, there occurs a diminution of the reality sense, and alterations in awareness of body sensation and body image. A removal of repressive controls releases emotions and motor actions which have hitherto been held in check. The individual may become overwhelmed by powerful affects which are acted out in random or in purposeful behavior. Recall of painful memories or traumatic experiences may flood the attention. Frequently a regressive type of thinking develops, with primitive language forms and imagery of an oral, anal or sexual nature. In part the sexual fantasies are the result of the universal concern with sexual problems; in part they are the product of a symbolic form of unconscious thinking in which the phallus is conceived of as an instrument of power, aggressiveness and intactness. The content of thought is furthermore influenced less by reality factors than by inner strivings and conflicts.

The suspension of activity of the higher brain centers is associated with the capacity on the part of the individual to exercise an extraordinary influence over his somatic apparatus. The ego in hypnosis is, by virtue of release of higher controls, apparently in closer contact with subcortical systems. The subject may therefore, in response to suggestions from the hypnotist, be capable of controlling various organs and somatic functions. In self hypnosis this is also possible, as illustrated by the remarkable control over organic functions effected by adherents of the Yoga system.

The question of what is responsible for the phenomenon of cortical inhibition, and the mechanism of its development, has given rise to interesting theories by Pavlov[53] and Kubie and Margolin.[54] The process involves alterations in brain physiology produced by a gradual circumscription of sensori-motor channels, such as occurs in sleep. It is possible that hypnosis removes barriers between the cortical and subcortical areas analagous to the situation that exists in the infant prior to the myelinization of the higher neurones. Thus, during the trance a type of regression develops which brings into play areas of the subject's central nervous system that are not ordinarily available to him in normal waking life. This may explain the readiness with which vasomotor conditioned reflexes may be established during the trance. It perhaps accounts for the somatic reactions to verbal suggestions which have caused such observers as Pavlov, Bechterov and Platonow to regard phenomena of hypnosis as forms of conditioned reflexes.

The state of inhibition of the higher centers is temporary, and on suggestion is superseded by an alertness which is as great or greater than in waking life. The individual, nevertheless, with proper conditioning and training, may continue to influence his somatic system.

The psychologic components of the hypnotic state are more difficult to explain than the physiological manifestations. An interesting question is what makes the individual susceptible to the induction of hypnosis. Why does he allow himself to enter into a relationship with the hypnotist in which he yields up control of his various functions?

In recent years there has been a tendency to regard all behavior as dynamically motivated toward specific goals. In line with this many observers have emphasized that hypnosis does not occur as a fortuitous experience, but rather develops as a response to goal-directed strivings which are intensely meaningful to the individual.[55-58] R. H. White[59] contends that the driving force in hypnosis is the motive to behave like a hypnotized person as defined by the operator and understood by the subject. What produces the motive to behave like a hypnotized person, what needs are actually satisfied by the assumption of the trance state, is, of course, a crucial question, and it is in explaining this point that the various schools of psychology differ.

McDougall[60] contended some years ago that the subject succumbed to hypnosis to satisfy a "submissive instinct" and that those with a greater quantity of this "instinct" were most hypnotizable. Many psychoanalysts believe that hypnosis satisfies infantile attitudes rooted in the Oedipus complex, and gratifies a goal-inhibited erotism, a masochistic yielding and a striving for omnipotence through identification with the hypnotist. Other observers have postulated various other kinds of needs which are propitiated through entering a trance state.

During the past few years I have been interested in this problem and have attempted to study both conscious motives for hypnosis and those that emerge in fantasy, free association and dreams during the trance. The impression gained has been that hypnosis does not gratify any one or even several motives or needs exclusively. Rather the person utilizes hypnosis as an individual experience fitting it into the framework of his own personal values and goals.

The needs which hypnosis fulfills keep shifting with the individual. For instance, at the beginning many patients desire hypnosis because of a wish to gain relief from anxiety or other disturbing symptoms. They may know nothing about the trance other than that it is a medical procedure which, according to newspaper reports, was used with great success in the war neuroses. They may be willing to undergo hypnosis in the same way they would expose themselves to a dental extraction for painful teeth. During the trance they will experience an assortment of feelings in the form of varied fears, hopes, expectations and resentments. These are in part dependent upon customary reactions to any close interpersonal relationship. In part, also, they involve the fantasied role of the hypnotist as a powerful authority, as well as the symbolic significance of the hypnotic experience at the particular moment of trance induction.

Because the trance becomes a meaningful emotional experience for the patient (often to his surprise and dismay), he will attempt to deal with it with his customary defenses and reactions. If he has a fear of yielding his control, the trance may have a dangerous or destructive significance, and the patient may fantasy being destroyed or mutilated. If he has a need to be enslaved, the hypnotic experience will be a form of bondage which he will both enjoy and resist. If he has grandiose trends, he may conceive of the trance as a magical means of gratifying his ambitions.

An analysis of fantasies shows that each person possesses a hierarchy of drives and motivations which reinforce or neutralize each other, and which are either gratified or denied by the assumption of the hypnotic state. Desire for hypnosis to ameliorate neurotic suffering may be opposed by a fear of losing control, or of being forced to reveal dreaded secrets, or of being made to perform ridiculous feats compulsively. Should fear of the trance experience become too intense, the patient may awaken. On the other hand an impelling need for gratification of coveted goals may foster further compliance with the commands of the hypnotist and may inspire a deepening of the trance.

As the patient enters a more profound trance, a shift in motivations occurs coincident with removal of repressive cortical controls, which in turn arouses deeper conflicts and needs. The individual may become aware of intense fears, protection from which may be sought through the agency of the hypnotist. He may evidence hostile and destructive tendencies in his speech and actions, or he may wish to be comforted or loved.

As in sleep, hypnosis releases primitive language forms in terms of organ function: oral, anal, and phallic. Sex symbols, even though they probably occur universally, are perhaps not so much the product of a phylogenetic tendency, as they are residues of infantile formulations, when strength and weakness, intactness and dissolution, aggressiveness and passivity, were looked upon in terms of the possession or absence of a male genital organ. Sexual material obtained during hypnosis must always be examined carefully for its symbolic representation of complex forms of human relationship.

Some subjects, even during the first trance induction, have sexual fantasies involving the hypnotist. In such cases, the individual probably regards the hypnosis as he does any other type of interpersonal contact as a sexual experience. He may look upon hypnosis as a physical yielding or sexual seduction. There are other persons in whom symbolization in terms of sex is not apparent. Whether or not this is due to the existence of repression so great as to necessitate the utilization of innocuous symbols shorn of sexual content is difficult to determine. Suffice it to say that in many cases it is impossible to bring to the surface such motivations as a desire for erotic gratification, for omnipotence or for masochistic yielding. These deep motives, while not verbalized, may, of course, exist in the unconscious of the individual, and may possibly be inspired through operation of the transference.

Analysis of fantasies in deep trance states in both normal subjects and neurotic patients frequently shows the hypnotist to be an omnipotent individual vested with protective and punitive powers, whose commands cannot be resisted. Many subjects reveal also that while they feel capable of resisting suggestions, they have no real desire to do so. Conformity creates within them feelings of security and pleasure. Fantasies of being nursed or fed, and of rebirth are also occasionally found. There is evidence that one of the deepest motivations aroused by hypnosis is perpetutation of infantile dependency by leaning on the godlike figure of the hypnotist. The fantasies of feeding and of rebirth are understandable in this light, as are the sexual fantasies which may, in a symbolic manner, represent a close relationship in terms of sexual fusion.

The analysis of some persons who have undergone hypnosis actually reveals the fact that unconsciously they have relished the trance because of gratifications they obtained from rendering themselves dependent after the manner of a small child. However, this motivation appeared only after the induction had started. The original motivation that led them to seek hypnosis was much more superficial. For instance, they might have been induced to yield to hypnosis out of curiosity, scientific interest, exhortations from friends or desire for exhibitionism. They may have sought help for a physical or emotional problem. The wish to make themselves dependent upon a parental representative may, of course, have been present in a latent form, but was not the original motive that caused the person to seek hypnosis and succumb to it. What then, it may be asked, incites and brings to the surface the latent dependency motive during the trance?

Because the process of hypnosis is associated with an inhibition of cortical control, because the subject experiences generalized regression, because boundaries between the ego and the outside world are not clearly demarcated, because the time sense is distorted, it is likely that feelings of helplessness engender the pressing into service of the archaic security mechanism of dependency on the parent in the person of the hypnotist.

During induction the gradual regression of the ego probably produces a regression of defenses and technics of adaptation from those associated with adult self sufficiency to those conditioned by infantile helplessness. The person in his helplessness approaches the period of ego development of the infant in whom dependency on a parental figure is the means of maintaining life. The gradual dissolution of ego boundaries produces an identification with and a yielding to the hypnotist who becomes the agent supplying security and love as well as strength and power. The price for these bounties is compliance, and the need for them apparently is so great that the individual can press into service mechanisms that are beyond voluntary control.

The ability of the individual to invoke vegetative mechanisms is certainly not unique for hypnosis, since, in emotional illness, too, the motivation to escape anxiety causes the elaboration of various symptoms, the development of which is outside the range of normal volition. Under pressure of a sufficiently intense need the person can exert an astonishing control over his psychosomatic resources. One may observe this in the acculturation of the growing child. For instance, the need to win parental approval and love makes it possible for the infant to inhibit the organic reflexes of his rectum and bladder and to regulate the functioning of these organs in conformity with the social pattern.

Suggestion, like hypnosis, is associated with a motivation to gain important objectives through a dependency relationship. The difference between hypnosis and suggestion is that in suggestion the ego operates at a more mature level of integration. We may speculate that the individual who is susceptible to suggestion seeks to attain security and gratification through the agency of a parental figure, or other external authoritative force, consciously, in the same way that the hypnotized subject strives to satisfy these needs in the trance state.

A challenging thought is that all people retain dependency strivings which are residues of the earliest mode of dealing with tension, and that they secretly envisage a Nirvana in which all needs will again be satisfied by some magical agent. It is thus possible that the desire to comply with the hypnotist's suggestions, even at the start, is an expression of hope that dependency needs will be fulfilled. Were we to formulate a theory of hypnosis along these lines, we might regard hypnotizability as a normal trait that has for its ultimate purpose the gratification of security and self esteem by reproducing an earlier developmental stage.

At the start of life each person satisfies his basic needs by dependency on the parent, who appears to have a magical ability of alleviating pain and fulfilling pleasure gratifications. The impulse to be dependent probably never actually dies even though it is supplanted by self sufficiency. Often the dependency striving functions in disguised forms as in religious devotion or in fealty to a superior or ruler. Occasionally it expresses itself openly as a character striving of compulsive dependency. In hypnosis the later adaptational patterns are wiped away by the regressive process associated with inhibition of the higher cortical centers. Dependency becomes the primary security mechanism. The hypnotist then becomes the parental representative.

Rado[61] has pointed out that during the process of hypnosis the hypnotist becomes the intrapsychic representative of the parent or superego. Kubie and Margolin[62] allege that the earlier authorities who constitute the superego are replaced by or merge with that of the hypnotist. The fact that subjects respond compulsively to hypnotic and to posthypnotic suggestions tends to confirm these observations. However, there are among different people varying degrees to which they absorb the hypnotist as a representative of their incorporated parental image or superego. In certain persons, as those with a hysterical makeup, the hypnotist actually seems to displace the habitual superego, and the subject reacts to the hypnotist as if he were actually the parental figure with omnipotent qualities. This may explain why hysterical persons go into the deepest trances, obeying with little resistance the commands of the hypnotist. In other subjects the superego is not so easily displaced and resistance to suggestions is encountered.

It is probable that the subject regards the hypnotist not so much as a real person, but as a symbol of his own superego. The impression that the hypnotist creates in the eyes of the subject is therefore important, for the more closely he symbolizes the powerful or benevolent parent, the more easily will hypnosis be induced and the deeper will be the trance. This explains why some hypnotists will fail and why others will succeed in producing light, medium, and deep trance states in the same subject. It explains, too, how impersonal stimuli which are symbolic of authority may induce hypnosis in the absence of a hypnotist. A written command or sounds of a phonograph record on which sleep suggestions have been dictated will produce the same effects as a flesh-and-blood hypnotist. In some subjects, autosuggestions are responded to in a similar manner. What probably happens here is that the individual reacts as if he were a divided personality with one self as the subject and a more powerful self that phrases commands and becomes representative of the superego.

Thus the hypnotist or symbol of the hypnotist reanimates the power of the subject's own superego. His responses are conditioned by his attitudes toward early authorities. Whether reactions are of defiance, compliance, surrender or contentment depends largely on the character structure the individual has developed out of early relationships with the parents. External authorities merely activate internal superego commands.

In spite of the foregoing facts, the hypnotist is not merely a reanimation of the parental superego. A portion of the subject's ego regards him as a new authority even in deepest hypnosis. In repeated inductions there may be a partial incorporation of the hypnotist's personal attitudes, values, prohibitions and injunctions with subsequent modification of the original superego. The associated reduction in severity of the habitual superego can have a profound therapeutic effect. A relatively long period of psychotherapy is required for this change, during which the patient subjects the standards of the hypnotist to a test, in the end incorporating them as his own values.

Since the hypnotic state is a submission to the hypnotist motivated by the desire to obtain pleasure goals in the form of security and other important gratifications, or to avoid hurt and punishment, any suggestion by the hypnotist that stirs up anxiety does not fall within the framework of this motivation and is apt to remove the need for hypnosis. This explains why, when the subject is enjoined to do anything he believes is against his best interests, he will either refuse to obey or will wake up. In therapeutic hypnosis this factor is important, for the facing of unconscious fears and conflicts entails the generation of a considerable amount of anxiety. The ability to comply with anxiety-provoking commands is in direct proportion to how completely the hypnotist is able to replace the early superego authorities.

In therapeutic hypnosis it is interesting to observe how motivations change. At the start hypnosis may be regarded as a form of magic, and the patient will openly or covertly expect things to be done for him. As therapy proceeds, and he is trained to work out his own problems and goals, he may find in hypnosis a valuable means of facillitating an understanding of himself and his conflicts through hypnotic dreams and other hypnoanalytic technics. The motivation will thus change with therapy and must be reanalyzed constantly.

Remaining for consideration is the relationship of hypnosis to hysteria. There is not a single manifestation of hysteria that cannot be duplicated during hypnosis. For this reason some persons still consider hypnosis a form of hysteria.

Hysterical symptoms appear to serve a twofold function. First, they are defenses elaborated by the ego to protect it from anxiety. Second, they are vicarious forms of impulse fulfillment, symbolically representative of a repressed striving, but sufficiently disguised to evade the repressive forces.

In analyzing the dynamics of symptom formation in hysteria, we are confronted with the interesting finding that both types of symptoms are elaborated to escape the vigilance of the superego. The primary purpose of such repressive defenses as paralysis, anesthesia and amnesia is to keep walled off from the superego memories, conflicts, hostile and erotic strivings that might incur its displeasure. The purpose of the various conversion phenomena, such as tics, spasms and convulsive seizures is to gain coveted gratifications in as innocuous a manner as possible. In each case the desire is to retain the good will of the superego.

The penalty of violating the superego is anxiety, which at its core represents the helplessness of the infant as he experiences tension, pain and hunger for which he senses no relief, because he has been abandoned by the magical giver of things—the mother. The primary motive in hysteria is to avoid this anxiety. The secondary gain is also motivated by a similar purpose. That some symptoms constitute an actual plea for parental help is an attested clinical fact. Hysterical manifestations often seem to serve the purpose of rendering the individual helpless or defenseless to secure absence of censure or direct pleasure grants from other people. Dieterle and Koch[63] have described cases where hysterical symptoms took the form of a regression to infancy with sucking and grasping movements, gurgling, crowing and the assumption of childlike types of ambulation. It is as if the person says, "I have crippled myself, I am helpless; therefore you must love me and support me. I am punishing myself; therefore you must forgive me for all my transgressions." The "belle indifference" of the hysteric may be accounted for by the fact that his symptoms have an ultimate security function.

The question that may be asked is why, if hysterical symptoms serve a protective purpose or are means of propitiating deep needs, can they so readily be made to disappear by hypnosis, whereas other symptoms, such as phobias, do not disappear upon suggestion. For some reason the superego of the hysterical individual is highly plastic and is capable of replacement by authoritative images from the outside world. Freud recognized this fact in calling hysteria a condition in which transference was readily obtained. Hysterical patients who have been invalided for years and who have not responded to orthodox therapies sometimes miraculously recover under suggestive hypnosis. What possibly happens is that the hysterical individual replaces temporarily his own superego with that of the authoritative image of the hypnotist. The commands of the hypnotist become mandatory, and, at least temporarily, the patient seeks to gain security by complying with his new superego. Whereas he has elaborated his symptom to gain help and freedom from punishment from his old superego, the hypnotist, who becomes the new magical helper, implies that he will give him security if he conforms with the command to lose the symptom. Another factor is that in those hysterical symptoms in which the patient punishes himself for a desired transgression, as in arm paralysis associated with masturbatory or hostile impulses, the hypnotist's exhortations to utilize the paralyzed part amounts to parental forgiveness.

Dramatic cures in hysteria may occur under other conditions than hypnosis, for instance through religious conversion or by a visit to a shrine. What is usually overlooked is that the removal of the hysterical symptoms does not occur in a vacuum, but involves a very important interpersonal element. In almost every instance of miracle cure, we can define a figure singularly overvalued by the patient, one who has become the embodiment of all that is powerful and noble in the universe. It is well known that faith in a shrine, priest, doctor or Christian Science practitioner is of paramount importance. What the patient seeks is security and peace through the medium of dependency or an omnipotent figure who can through magic minister to his demands.

Thus, the removal of the hysterical symptom becomes a condition for which the patient feels he will be loved and helped, in the same way that its development originally had served the same purpose, albeit to the functional handicap of the individual. Both the development of the symptom and its disappearance serve the same purpose in the hysteric of gaining love and security from two different objects; the one, the psychic embodiment of the parent or superego, the other, the image of the hypnotist or healer who has become the new superego. Usually there is a psychic tug-of-war between the various superego images. If the healer is looked upon as a stronger power than the superego for whose purpose the symptoms were originally developed, they will be lost. For so long as the person feels that through the disappearance of his illness he can continue to gain security and love, he will drop his symptoms as easily as he has developed them. This usually involves a continued relationship to the source of worship, reverence or faith, and it explains why in the absence of the healer or shrine the symptoms return.

REFERENCES

[1] BRAID, J.: Neurypnology (Braid on Hypnotism. Ed. by A. E. Waite). London, George Ridway, 1899.

[2] BROWN, W.: Psychology and Psychotherapy. Baltimore, Wm. Wood, 1934.

[3] EYSENCK, H. J.: Suggestibility and hypnosis—an experimental analysis. Proc. Roy. Soc. Med. *36:* 349–354, 1943.

[4] HEIDENHAIN, R.: Hypnotism or Animal Magnetism (Translated by L. C. Wooldridge). London, K. Paul, Trench, Trubner, 1906.

[5] WINN, R. B.: Scientific Hypnotism. Boston, Christopher, 1939.

[6] EYSENCK, H. J.: op. cit., reference 3.

[7] McDOUGALL, W.: Brain, *31:* 118, 1908.

[8] PAVLOV, I. P.: The identity of inhibition with sleep and hypnosis. Scient. Monthly *17:* 603, 1923.

[9] RABINOVICH, P. H.: Semana Med. *47:* 1083–1086, 1940.

[10] KUBIE, L. S., AND MARGOLIN, S.: The process of hypnotism and the nature of the hypnotic state. Am. J. Psychiat. *100:* 613–619, 1944.

[11] BASS, M. J.: Differentiation of the hypnotic trance from normal sleep. J. Exper. Psychol. *14:* 382–399, 1931.

[12] WIBLE, C. L., AND JENNESS, A.: Electrocardiograms during sleep and hypnosis. J. Psychol. *1:* 235–245. 1936. JENNESS, A., AND WIBLE, C. L.: Respiration and heart action in sleep and hypnosis. J. Gen. Psychol. *16:* 197–222, 1937.

[13] LOOMIS, A. L., HARVEY, E. N., AND HOBART, G.: Brain potentials during hypnosis. Science *83:* 239–241, 1936.

[14] NYGARD, J. W.: Cerebral circulation prevailing during sleep and hypnosis. Psychol. Bull. *34:* 727, 1937.

[15] Goldwyn, J.: The effect of hypnosis on basal metabolism. Arch. Int. Med. *45:* 109–114, 1930.

[16] BECK, L. F.: Hypnotic identification of an amnesic victim. Brit. J. M. Psychol. *16:* 36–42, 1936.

[17] DORCUS, R. M.: Modification by suggestion of some vestibular and visual responses. Am. J. Psychol. *49:* 82–87, 1937.

[18] PATTIE, F. A.: A report of attempts to produce uniocular blindness by hypnotic suggestion. Brit. J. M. Psychol. *15:* 230–241, 1935.

[19] HULL, C. L.: Hypnosis and suggestibility. New York, Appleton-Century, 1933, p. 209.

[20] JANET, P.: The Major Symptoms of Hysteria, ed. 2. New York, Macmillan, 1920.

[21] PRINCE, M.: Experiments to determine co-conscious (subconscious) ideation. J. Abnorm. & Social Psychol. *3:* 37, 1909.

[22] BURNETT, C. T.: Splitting the mind. Psychol. Monog. *34:* No. 2, 1925.

[23] SIDIS, B.: Psychopathological Researches. New York, G. E. Stechert, 1902.

[24] PATTEN, E. F.: Does post-hypnotic amnesia apply to practice effects? J. Gen. Psychol. *7:* 196–201, 1932.

[25] LIFE, C.: The effects of practice in the trance upon learning in the normal waking state. Thesis, University of Wisconsin, 1929.

[26] SCOTT, H. D.: Hypnosis and the conditioned reflex. J. Gen. Psychol. *4:* 113–130 1930.

[27] MITCHELL, M. B.: Retroactive inhibition and hypnosis. J. Gen. Psychol. *7:* 343–358, 1932.

[28] DORCUS, R. M.: op. cit., reference 17.

[29] PATTIE, F. A.: op. cit., reference 18.

[30] LUNDHOLM, H.: An experimental study of functional anesthesias as induced by suggestion in hypnosis. J. Abnorm. & Social Psychol. *23:* 337–355, 1928.

[31] BARRY, H., MACKINNON, D. W., AND MURRAY, H. A.: Hypnotizability as a personality trait and its typological relations. Human Biol. *3:* 1–36, 1931.

[32] WHITE, R. W., AND SHEVACH, B. J.: Hypnosis and the concept of dissociation. J. Abnorm. & Soc. Psychol. *37:* 309–328, 1942.

[33] FREUD, S.: The Psychopathology of Everyday Life. In The Basic Writings of Sigmund Freud. New York, Modern Library, 1938.

[34] HULL, C. L.: op. cit., reference 19.

[35] WHITE, R. W.: A preface to the theory of hypnotism. J. Abnorm. & Social Psychol. *36:* 477–505, 1941.

[36] CASON, H.: Conditioned pupillary reactions. J. Exper. Psychol. *5:* 108–146, 1922.

[37] HUDGINS, C. V.: Conditioning and the voluntary control of the pupillary light reflex. J. Gen. Psychol. *8:* 3–51, 1933.

[38] MENZIES, R.: Conditioned vasomotor responses in human subjects. J. Psychol. *4:* 75–120, 1937.

[39] JACOBSON, E.: Am. J. Psychol. *44:* 677, 1932.

[40] PAVLOV, I. P.: Conditioned Reflexes. New York, Oxford Univ. Press, 1934, p. 407.

[41] PLATONOW, K. I.: The word as a physiological and therapeutic factor. Psikhoterapiya *11:* 112, 1930.

[42] EYSENCK, H. J.: op. cit., reference 3.

[43] YOUNG, P. C.: Experimental hypnotism: a review. Psychol. Bull. *38:* 100, 1941.

[44] ESTABROOKS, G H.: Hypnotism. New York, Dutton, 1943, p. 130.

[45] HULL, C. L.: op. cit., reference 19.

[46] FERENCZI, S.: Introjektion und übertregung: Jahrt. Psychoanalyse *1:* 422–457, 1909.

[47] FERENCZI, S.: Contributions to Psychoanalysis (Translated by E. Jones). Boston, Badger, 1916.

[48] JONES, E.: Papers on Psychoanalysis. London, Bailliere, Tindall & Cox, 1913, chap. 12.

[49] Freud, S.: Group Psychology and the Analysis of the Ego (Translated by J. Strachey). New York, Boni & Liveright, 1922.

[50] SCHILDER, P. AND KAUDERS, O.: Hypnosis (Translated by S. Rothenberg). New York, Nervous & Mental Disease Publ. Co., 1927.

[51] SPEYER, N., AND STOKVIS, B.: The psycho-analytical factor in hypnosis. Brit. J. M. Psychol. *17:* 217–222, 1938.

[52] LORAND, S.: Hypnotic suggestion: its dynamics, indications, and limitations in the therapy of neurosis. J. Nerv. & Ment. Dis. *94:* 64–75, 1941.

[53] PAVLOV, I. P.: op. cit., reference 40.

[54] KUBIE, L. S., AND MARGOLIN, S.: op. cit., reference 10.

[55] ROSENOW, C.: Meaningful behavior in hypnosis. Am. J. Psychol. *40:* 205–235, 1928.

[56] LUNDHOLM, H.: op. cit., reference 30.

[57] DORCUS, R. M.: op. cit., reference 17.

[58] PATTIE, F. A.: The genuineness of hypnotically produced anesthesia on the skin. Am. J. Psychol. *49:* 435–443, 1937.

[59] WHITE, R. W.: A preface to the theory of hypnotism. J. Abnorm. & Social Psychol. *36:* 477–505, 1941.

[60] McDOUGALL, W.: Outline of Abnormal Psychology. New York, Scribner, 1926.

[61] RADO, S.: Das okonomische Prinzip der Technik. Internat. Ztschr. f. Psychoanal. *12:* 1926.

[62] KUBIE, L. S., AND MARGOLIN, S.: op. cit., reference 10.

[63] DIETERLE, R. R., AND KOCH, E. J.: Experimental induction of infantile behavior in major hysteria. J. Nerv. & Ment. Dis. *86:* 688–710, 1937.

Part Two
THE TECHNIC OF HYPNOSIS

IV
INTRODUCTION TO HYPNOTIC TECHNIC

THIS chapter will concern itself with certain collateral aspects of hypnosis such as susceptibility to hypnosis, suggestibility tests and criteria of trance depth. The remaining chapters in this section will deal with the more practical topic of trance induction.

SUSCEPTIBILITY TO HYPNOSIS

Hypnotizability is a normal trait, and, theoretically at least, every person can be hypnotized. In actual practice, however, only approximately ninety per cent can be inducted into a trance state. What determines the resistance to hypnosis in those persons who are not amenable to induction is not entirely clear. No correlation has been found between hypnosis and body build, extroversion, introversion, race, sex, or social position. On the other hand, age apparently plays some part in susceptibility, children being slightly more amenable and older people slightly less amenable to hypnotic suggestion than young adults.

Many efforts have been made to establish a correlation between mental traits and susceptibility to hypnosis. Findings have been contradictory and hence are not reliable. For instance, Baumgartner[1] found a slightly positive correlation between sympathy, "sweet temper," tactfulness and honesty, and a slightly negative correlation with optimism and suggestibility. R. W. White[2] reported a correlation with extroversion as determined by the Neymann-Kohlstedt test, while no such correlation could be found by Barry, MacKinnon and Murray.[3] Friedlander and Sarbin[4] were unable to find a relationship between hypnotizability and intelligence, extroversion, ascendance, neuroticism or affectivity. R. W. White[5] believed he could detect a positive correlation between hypnotizability and a need for deference, and a negative correlation with a need for dominance. Although suggestibility has been found to correlate highly with hypnotic susceptibility by Estabrooks,[6] Hull,[7] Aveling and Hargreaves,[8] Beck,[9] Saltzman,[10] Dorcus,[11] Jenness and Wible,[12] and R. W. White,[13] such workers as Barry, MacKinnon, and Murray[14] and Williams[15] could find no such correlation.

Brenman and Reichard,[16] utilizing the Rorschach test, report that hypnotizability is positively correlated with "free-floating anxiety," labile affectivity and "extra-tensiveness." Rosenzweig[17] states that hypnotizability is associated with repression as a preferred mechanism of defense and with "impunitiveness," which is rationalization and withdrawal from aggression as a characteristic type of immediate reaction to frustration. Rosenzweig and Sarason[18] add that those persons who are nonhypnotizable do not utilize repression as a mechanism of defense, and are characteristically "extrapunitive" or expressive in their aggression. R. W. White[19] contends that the patient's susceptibility to hypnosis may be predicted by his responses to the Thematic Apperception Test, although he admits of the crudity of the procedure.

These conflicting ideas are, to a large degree, due to defects in our present understanding of what actually constitutes a personality trait. Many so-called character traits are by no means basic to the individual. They may be nothing more than surface compensations for more dynamic underlying strivings. A power drive may thus be a mask for a deep sense of futility and selflessness. Deference and ingratiation may be the conscious counterbalances of inner arrogance and aggression. A compulsive drive for autonomy or independence may be a means of escaping impulses of passivity and dependence. Most personality tests and scales do not consider these unconscious drives which usually become apparent to the analyst only during deep therapy with removal of superficial defenses.

Hypnotizability appears to be a normal characteristic which may be counteracted and successfully neutralized by motives to be unhypnotizable. When an emotionally ill person applies for therapy, he is motivated to receive help from the physician. Should the physician suggest hypnotherapy the patient will usually have a motivation to be hypnotizable, since he has a desire to rid himself of uncomfortable symptoms. However, because the patient has problems in his relations with people, he may fear injury at the hands of the physician during the trance. He may also resist relinquishing his neurotic symptoms due to the spurious values they have for him. The latter factors may provide motivations not to be hypnotizable, and will interfere with the assumption of the trance state. This explains why neurotic persons are, with standard technics, less susceptible to hypnosis than non-neurotic people.

The most important factor in susceptibility to hypnosis is, then, the motivation to be hypnotizable. It is usually impossible to hypnotize a subject if he wills otherwise. He must either want to obey the orders of the hypnotist, or he must feel that regardless of his own will he cannot resist following the hypnotist's commands. An unconscious motivation to be hypnotizable may be stronger than the conscious desire to resist hypnosis. Many persons fight against succumbing to a trance, yet are unable to stay awake once the induction process is started.

On the other hand, the motivations which produce non-hypnotizability may be completely unconscious. Some patients who apply for hypnotherapy are intensely earnest about being hypnotized; but for reasons not known to them, they are unable to enter a trance state.

How a motivation not to be hypnotizable can operate without awareness of the subject is illustrated by the following experiment. Several well-trained somnambules were, during a trance, given the posthypnotic suggestion that they would not be susceptible to hypnotic induction by anyone but myself. Amnesia for this suggestion was then induced. An acquaintance, adept at the art of hypnosis, known also to the subjects since he was a witness to the experiments, informed them, one afternoon, that I was ill and would not be present. He inquired of the subjects whether they would be willing for him to carry on with the work. They were eager to continue. However, his efforts to induce hypnosis were entirely unsuccessful, even though the subjects appeared to cooperate. Each subject remarked later that he could not seem to fixate his attention on what the hypnotist said. One stated: "A million thoughts entered my mind. I couldn't keep my thoughts on what you said. It suddenly occurred to me that I would be unable to fall asleep no matter how hard you tried. I thought this was strange because I really did want to be hypnotized." Another subject was instructed that no one, including myself, would thereafter be able to hypnotize him. He had a similar experience, although his resistance lasted only a few days. Thus, an unconscious motive to be unhypnotizable can be artificially induced in the subject, or may arise spontaneously, blocking all attempts at hypnosis.

The existence of unconscious motives explains why hypnotizability is so difficult to predict. For example, we might expect that dependent, helpless people would be much more susceptible to hypnosis than self-sufficient or power-driven persons. To our surprise we often find the reverse to be the case. The reason for this is that while dependent persons are quite positively motivated to hypnosis, there may exist in them coordinate strivings and fears that neutralize this motivation. A dependent individual may have a tremendous unconscious fear of being engulfed, injured and destroyed in a dependency relationship. His conflict often hinges on those ambivalent feelings. He may be able to satisfy his dependency only so long as he can maintain a certain amount of control or detachment. Hypnosis implies a loss of control, and this realization may motivate him to resist hypnosis. Or the dominant individual may actually be a very submissive dependent person underneath, one who would like to lay down his facade of strength if he could find someone on whom to lean. In hypnosis he may sense a means of gratifying this unconscious need. Thus, the traits that the individual shows on the surface may not be the ones that actually determine his motivation to enter the trance state. The examination of the personality structure usually reveals so many ambivalent character strivings that it is difficult to predict from the strivings which manifest the susceptibility of the individual to hypnosis.

The ability to be hypnotized will depend on a greater balance of forces that produce a motivation to be hypnotizable as compared to forces that oppose the assumption of the trance state. The skillful physician can build up the desire for hypnosis by creating proper incentives in the patient and by undermining the patient's fear of hypnosis.

Suggestibility Tests

A correlation exists between some forms of suggestibility and susceptibility to hypnosis. In therapeutic hypnosis, suggestibility tests may be utilized as a preparatory stage to trance induction. They often get a patient into a suitable frame of mind, developing in him confidence in his ability to respond to suggestions that will lead to a trance. There are many kinds of suggestibility tests, the most common being the postural-sway test, hand levitation, hand clasp and the pendulum test.

The Postural-Sway Test. The patient stands with his feet together, his body held rigid, and his eyes fixed on a spot on the ceiling directly overhead. The hypnotist stands behind the patient and asks him to close his eyes, but to remain rigid. The patient is then instructed as follows: "I want to test your capacity to relax. I am going to place my hands on your shoulder blades." The hands are placed on the medial part of the shoulder blades and the patient is told: "Now as I press my hands against your shoulders, you will feel a force pulling you back toward me. Do not resist. I will catch you when you fall. You are falling, falling, falling. You are being drawn back . . . falling . . . falling." The hands of the operator are then drawn back. Usually the patient will start swaying. If he does not, the hands are placed on the patient's shoulders and he is rocked back and forth with the comment that he is resisting and that he should loosen up. The same suggestions relating to falling back are then repeated, and the pressure of the hands suddenly released.

As soon as the patient starts swaying, suggestions become more forceful. "You are falling back, back, back—all the way—back, back, fall back. I shall catch you when you fall." The physician must, of course, be sure to catch the patient before he falls.

Hand levitation. The patient is asked to sit at a table, his elbow resting on the surface, the palm of the hand down. The operator says, "I am going to put my hand on yours, and I want you to pay attention to the feelings in your hand." The operator then presses the hand of the subject lightly and remarks: "Now you are going to feel your hand growing very light as if it has no weight. It is growing lighter and lighter. It feels very light." This is repeated several times. "Do you feel it growing light?" If the subject replies in the negative, the suggestions are continued. If he has a sensation of lightness, the hand pressure is relaxed lightly, and the subject is told: "Your hand is so light that it has no weight. It gets lighter and lighter. It gradually begins to leave the table, and it comes up right off the table as if it has no weight. It is rising higher and higher."

Hand clasp. The patient sits in a chair and is asked to clasp his hands firmly together. The hypnotist demonstrates this to the patient. Then he says, "I want you to close your eyes for a moment and visualize a vise, a heavy metal vise whose jaws clamp together with a screw. Imagine that your hands are like the jaws of the vise, and as you press them together tighter, they are just like the jaws of the vise tightening. I am going to count from one to five. As I count, your hands will press together tighter, and tighter, and tighter. When I reach the count of five, your hands will be pressed together so firmly that it will be difficult or impossible to separate them. One, tight; two, tighter, and tighter, and tighter; three, very tight, your hands feel glued together; four, your hands are clamped tight, tight; five, so tight that even though you try to separate them, they remain clasped together, until I give you the command to open them—Now open them slowly."

Pendulum test. A ring is attached to a string twelve inches long. The patient seated at a table holds the end of the string with his arm outstretched, the ring dangling above the level of the table. The patient is instructed as follows: "As you support the ring imagine that you are looking at a large circle which is etched into the table top. Let your eyes travel around the circumference of the circle and keep your eyes moving around in a circle. The ring will begin going around in a circle even though you pay no attention to it." When the patient follows these suggestions, he is asked to concentrate on an imaginary line running directly in front of him; then on a line running directly across the table. The pendulum will swing in the direction his eyes travel.

The fact that the patient executes suggestibility tests does not always mean that he will make a good hypnotic subject. However, where he resists these suggestions, he will probably not be susceptible to hypnosis.

THE DEPTH OF TRANCE

A number of attempts have been made to classify the symptoms of hypnosis into stages of varying depth.[20-24] These attempts have not proven themselves to be completely satisfactory because of the extreme variability of the responses among different patients and even in the same patient on different induction days.

There is some objection to classifying hypnotic "stages." All phenomena are due to implied or direct suggestion. Subjects vary in their ideas as to what constitutes the hypnotic state. Some persons are unable to develop posthypnotic amnesia even after attaining a somnambulistic stage. Others may respond to suggestions to dream or to write automatically in merely a light state of hypnosis. There is never in any subject a steady progression of all hypnotic phenomena. As a matter of fact the level of consciousness constantly shifts in the trance state.

With these precautions in mind, the following table (Stages of Hypnosis) will be found useful in estimating the trance depth and anticipating the phenomena that can be expected at different stages of the trance. In therapy, it is useful to know what therapeutic technics may be utilized at the depth of hypnosis a patient is able to attain. For example, it is useless to attempt regression and reorientation to an earlier phase of development in the event the subject is only able to enter a light or medium trance. Similarly, one cannot expect a patient to do play therapy or dramatics unless hypnosis is sufficiently deep. Attempts to produce phenomena beyond those that can be expected at a certain hypnotic level may damage the confidence of the patient in hypnotic therapy.

Stages of Hypnosis
(With a standard trance induction using a fixation object)

Smarting of eyes Watering of eyes Heaviness of eyes Fluttering of lids	WAKING STATE
Heavy sensation in extremities Drowsiness *Psychobiologic therapy (Reassurance, persuasion,* *re-education, confession and ventilation)* *Hypnoanalysis (Free association, Fantasy induction)*	PREHYPNOTIC STAGE (HYPNOIDAL STATE)
Closing of eyes Physical relaxation Catalepsy of eyelids Catalepsy of the limbs Rigid limb catalepsies Inhibition of voluntary movements Automatic movements *Psychobiologic therapy (Guidance)*	LIGHT TRANCE
Disturbances in cutaneous sensibilities *Ability to learn technic of autohypnosis* Partial analgesia (glove anesthesia) Automatic obedience *Hypnoanalysis (Dream induction)* Partial posthypnotic anesthesia Induced personality changes	MEDIUM TRANCE
Hypnoanalysis (Automatic writing) Simple posthypnotic suggestions Extensive anesthesias Emotional changes Hallucinations Regression *Symptom removal by prestige suggestion* *Psychobiologic therapy (some desensitization technics)*	DEEP TRANCE

Complete posthypnotic amnesia
Ability to open eyes without affecting trance
Psychobiologic therapy (Reconditioning)
Hypnoanalysis (Crystal and mirror gazing,
  dramatics, play therapy, induction of   SOMNAMBULISTIC
  experimental conflicts, regression and   TRANCE
  revivification)
Bizarre posthypnotic suggestions
Posthypnotic positive hallucinations
Posthypnotic negative hallucinations

Again it must be emphasized that the table, like any other scale, must not be accepted literally. Various subjects may show different phenomena at certain stages. Some patients may dream vividly on command and may follow posthypnotic suggestions even though they have never progressed beyond light stages of hypnosis. Other patients in somnambulistic states may not dream or follow posthypnotic suggestions. Emotional changes may be evoked in certain patients in medium stages of hypnosis, and in other subjects may not develop even in somnambulism. These exceptions occur frequently enough to prevent dogmatic statements regarding successive phenomena at different trance depths.

Relatively few people are able to achieve the deeper stages of hypnosis. Hull[25] has summarized the work of a number of observers covering over ten thousand subjects, and has found the mean percentage to be 10.48 per cent uninfluenced, 32.68 per cent capable of developing a light trance, 34.58 per cent a deep trance and 22.26 per cent a somnambulistic trance.

These figures indicate that only a small percentage of subjects are able to achieve a somnambulistic depth in hypnosis. An aptitude for somnambulism seems to be a factor which is apparently quite distinct from the factor of susceptibility. The exact nature of the aptitude for deep hypnosis is not entirely clear, but some persons believe it to be constitutional. There is some association between the capacity to achieve somnambulism and the development of hysterical symptoms in the face of conflict. This is by no means a universal rule, and it does not necessarily follow that all somnambules are hysterical. Persons who are sleep walkers, automatic writers, crystal gazers, or who are very adept at using the "ouija board" are frequently somnambules.

That the capacity for somnambulism is not exclusively dependent upon constitution is borne out by the fact that many subjects who otherwise are capable of entering only light trance states, can, under certain conditions, with the proper hypnotist, achieve somnambulism. Neurotic patients whose customary defenses no longer protect them, or who have been exposed to overwhelmingly traumatic environmental conditions, as in the war neuroses, may so intensely desire dependency on a protective parental figure that they will comply punctiliously with hypnotic commands to the point of developing somnambulism. When ego stability is achieved, or when the environment becomes more secure so that helplessness vanishes, the patient seems to lose the motivation to enter the somnambulistic state.

There is evidence that fully fifty per cent of hypnotizable subjects can, with the proper technic, be trained to achieve the somnambulistic state. There are, however, relatively few hypnotists who have the patience or the skill required to train the average individual to the level of somnambulism.

For practical purposes, therefore, we must assume that the physician will be able to develop one somnambule out of every ten patients that he sees. This fact might appear discouraging from a therapeutic viewpoint. Fortunately, however, a deep trance is not essential for most forms of therapeutic hypnosis. Indeed, in many cases, a very light trance is all that is required, the power of suggestion being effective even though the patient retains a complete memory of events that have occurred during hypnosis. In most of the psychobiologic therapies, such as guidance, reassurance, persuasion, re-education, and confession and ventilation, a light trance or a hypnoidal state is sufficient. It is possible also to work hypnoanalytically with technics of free association and fantasy induction under a hypnoidal condition. Indeed experience soon proves to the physician that depth of trance is not at all related to therapeutic effectiveness.

Nevertheless, there are advantages to a deep trance state in some conditions, as in symptom removal by authoritative suggestion. Since the image the physician wishes to create in the mind of the patient in this therapy is one of a powerful, omniscient personage, a deep trance can have a more profound effect on the patient than a light trance. In some psychobiologic technics, as desensitization and reconditioning, and in the hypnoanalytic technics of crystal and mirror gazing, dramatics, play therapy, induction of experimental conflicts, and regression and revivification, a somnambulistic trance will be required. It behooves the physician, consequently, to achieve as high a skill as possible in the technic of trance induction. For this reason detailed induction technics will be presented in the following chapters.

REFERENCES

[1] BAUMGARTNER, M.: The correlation of direct suggestibility with certain character traits. J. Applied Psychol. *15:* 1–15, 1931.

[2] WHITE, R. W.: Prediction of hypnotic susceptibility from a knowledge of subjects' attitudes. J. Psychol. *3:* 265–277, 1937.

[3] BARRY, H. JR., MACKINNON, D. W., AND MURRAY, H. A. JR.: Studies in personality: A. Hypnotizability as a personality trait and its topological relations. Human Biology *3:* 1–36, 1931.

[4] FRIEDLANDER, J. W., AND SARBIN, T. H.: The depth of hypnosis. J. Abnorm. & Social Psychol. *33:* 453–475, 1938.

[5] WHITE, R. W.: An analysis of motivation in hypnosis. J Gen. Psychol. *24:* 145–162, 1941.

[6] ESTABROOKS, G. H.: Experimental Studies in Suggestion. London, Hippolyte Bailliere, 1929.

[7] HULL, C. L.: Hypnosis and Suggestibility. New York, Appleton-Century, 1933.

[8] AVELING, E., AND HARGREAVES, H. L.: Suggestibility with and without prestige in children. Brit. J. Psychol. *12:* 53–75, 1921–1922.

[9] BECK, L. F.: Relationships between waking suggestibility and hypnotic susceptibility. Psychol. Bull. *33:* 747, 1936.

[10] SALTZMAN, B. N.: The reliabilities of tests of waking and hypnotic suggestibility. Psychol. Bull. *33:* 622–623, 1936.

[11] DORCUS, R. M.: Modification by suggestion of some vestibular and visual responses. Am. J. Psychol. *49:* 82–87, 1937.

[12] JENNESS, A., AND WIBLE, C. L.: Respiration and heart action in sleep and hypnosis. J. Gen. Psychol. *16:* 197–222, 1937.

[13] WHITE, R. W.: op. cit., reference 2.

[14] BARRY, H. JR., MACKINNON, D. W., AND MURRAY, H. A. JR.: op. cit., reference 3.

[15] WILLIAMS, G. W.: Suggestibility in the normal and hypnotic states. Arch. Psychol., vol. 19, no. 122, 1930.

[16] BRENMAN, M., AND REICHARD, S.: Use of the Rorschach test in the prediction of hypnotizability. Bull. Menninger Clin. *7:* 183–187, 1943.

[17] ROSENZWEIG, S.: The experimental study of repression. In MURRAY, H.: Explorations in Personality. New York, Oxford University Press, 1938, pp. 472–491.

[18] ROSENZWEIG, S. AND SARASON, S.: An experimental study of the triadic hypothesis: reaction to frustration, ego defense, and hypnotizability. I. Correlational approach. Char. & Pers. *11:* 1–19, 1942–1943.

[19] WHITE, R. W.: Hypnosis Test. In Murray's Explorations in Personality. New York, Oxford University Press, 1938, pp. 453–461.

[20] BRAID, J.: Neurypnology (Braid on hypnotism), edited by A. E. Waite. London, George Ridway, 1899.

[21] BERNHEIM, H.: Suggestive Therapeutics: a treatise on the nature and uses of hypnotism (Translated by C. A. Herter). New York, Putnams, 1900.

[22] WINGFIELD, H. E.: An Introduction to the Study of Hypnotism, ed. 2. London, Bailliere, Tindall & Cox, 1920.

[23] DAVIS, L. W., AND HUSBAND, R. W.: A study of hypnotic susceptibility in relation to personality traits. J. Abnorm. & Social Psychol. *26:* 175–182, 1931.

[24] LeCRON, L. M., AND BORDEAUX, J.: Hypnotism Today. New York, Grune & Stratton, 1947, pp. 64–67.

[25] HULL, C. L.: op. cit., reference 7.

V

THE FIRST HYPNOTIC SESSION

A T THE first hypnotic session the aim is to give the patient confidence in his ability to enter the trance state. To achieve this aim the physician may execute the following steps in order: (1) encourage motivations that will lead to hypnosis; (2) remove as fully as possible misconceptions, fears, and resistances that oppose hypnosis; (3) give the patient a suggestibility test to demonstrate that he can follow suggestions; (4) encourage relaxation by a suggestive preparatory talk; (5) induce a trance; (6) deepen the trance; (7) awaken the patient; (8) discuss with him his reaction to hypnosis.

MOTIVATING THE PATIENT TOWARD HYPNOSIS

The ability to be hypnotized depends on a preponderance of motivations to be hypnotizable as compared with motivations not to be hypnotizable. Before hypnosis is attempted the physician must build up motivations for hypnosis.

One way of doing this is to encourage the patient to talk about how inconvenient his symptoms are to him, and to get him to verbalize a desire to get well at all costs. He is asked whether he is sure he really wants to get over his difficulties, because in some cases a person's neurosis yields important dividends for him. Yet with the discomfiture he experiences, and the suffering he undergoes, it is understandable that he will want to conquer his symptoms even if they do give him some secondary gains. If he is really serious about getting well, he will want to cooperate in the relaxing hypnotic exercises which will help him to overcome his problems.

The patient is informed that hypnosis is an experience

that can have important values for him besides shortening the treatment period. It enables many people to relax and to gain poise and self mastery.

Removing Misconceptions, Fears and Resistances

It is extremely important to remove misconceptions about hypnosis at the first session. The patient may be asked what he knows about hypnosis and what his feelings are about being hypnotized.

If the patient has observed a trance, it is essential to get him to describe what he has seen and to correct any false ideas he may have gained. Many patients have observed stage hypnotists in action and may expect to be put into a somnambulistic state at the first trance induction. The frontal assault on the subject conducted by stage hypnotists is contraindicated in therapeutic hypnosis. Stage hypnotists operate under dramatic circumstances, and susceptible subjects, who are carefully chosen by rapid tests for suggestibility, such as the postural sway test, usually enter a somnambulistic state. The physician deals with an entirely different situation in his office and furthermore cannot select his patients. Consequently he will rarely achieve somnambulism at the first session even in patients who are potential somnambules. The patient, if he has been intrigued by the antics of the stage hypnotist, may get the false idea that all people can go into a somnambulistic state with complete amnesia for trance events. Unless this idea is corrected, he may lose confidence in the physician and in himself.

The following is from a soundscriber record:

Dr. Have you ever seen anyone hypnotized?

Pt. Yes, I saw a hypnotist put a person to sleep on the stage, and then he made him do everything he told him to. He stuck needles in him and the man couldn't feel pain. He made him go swimming in an imaginary lake.

Dr. The kind of hypnosis that is performed on the stage is different from therapeutic hypnosis. If we were to do the same kind of hypnosis here, it would not help your nervous condition and even might have a harmful effect. You will not be knocked out or forced to do distasteful things. Unlike stage hypnosis you will cooperate with me in bringing about certain effects. And you will remember almost everything that has happened. The technic is different; we want you to get well, not to do fancy tricks.

The following questions and answers are from transcribed records:

Don't you have to have a weak mind or a weak will to be hypnotized? "Not at all, as a matter of fact hypnosis is a perfectly normal phenomenon, and more than ninety per cent of all people can be hypnotized. The only people who cannot be hypnotized are those who have a mistaken notion that it will hurt them, or who, for one reason or another, have a resistance against it."

Isn't it dangerous to be hypnotized—can't it hurt a person? "Hypnosis has been associated with crystal balls and magic for so long that it is natural for you to ask this question. Hypnosis is a perfectly scientific phenomenon which can help a person overcome many problems. Hypnosis is not possible unless a person participates in it. He will, therefore, not do anything that is harmful to himself. Suggestions can always be vetoed which are distasteful. Stories about a person's being robbed of his will power and becoming a slave to the hypnotist are fantastic. Such things do not happen. Instead, hypnosis can have a very beneficial effect in strengthening a person's will."

I am afraid I can't be hypnotized. "In spite of the fact that you have such a fear, you are probably hypnotizable. All people can be hypnotized, if they relax and do not resist. Just make your mind passive and do not try too hard to follow suggestions. All we are after the first time is a drowsy relaxed feeling, and you do not have to try too hard to get this."

If I am hypnotized and fall asleep maybe I won't awaken. "Most people confuse sleep and hypnosis. They are two different things. A person may be hypnotized and be just as wide awake as you are. Hypnosis is merely an increased capacity to follow suggestions made by the physician. If suggestions are given to a person in hypnosis that he will fall asleep, he may become sleepy and act sleepy. If other suggestions are given that he be wide awake, he may be able to open his eyes and still be hypnotized. If a person happens to fall asleep as the result of suggestion, it is very easy to wake him up by suggestions."

Suggestibility Tests

One or more suggestibility tests are given the patient to convince him that he has the capacity to follow suggestions. He is told:

"Hypnosis is a form of relaxation during which it is possible to follow therapeutic suggestions more easily. There is nothing mysterious about it. It is a scientific phenomenon and perfectly normal. I am going to give you an idea of what suggestion is like. This is not hypnosis, but it will acquaint you with how easy it is for the mind to follow suggestions."

The patient is then given the hand clasp test, the technic of which will be found in the previous chapter. The postural sway test may be given instead or in addition, or any of the other tests may be used. Suggestibility tests help pave the way for hypnosis and are often instrumental in removing some resistances to the trance. Should the patient succeed in opening his hands in the hand clasp test, the physician must not act dismayed, but should quickly add: "You notice some stiffness and slight resistance to opening them. This is normal. Later on you will develop the capacity to keep them closed longer." Similar comments may be made pertinent to the other tests, should they be used without full success.

PREPARATORY TALK

A short preparatory talk is given the patient along the following lines:

"I now would like to give you a general idea of what happens in hypnosis. You will notice that you will relax and probably will begin to feel just a little drowsy. It will not be necessary for you to try too hard. Just make your mind passive and relax. Then you will become aware of certain things that are happening as you relax, and I want you to concentrate on them. As a matter of fact, I will bring them to your attention. You will, perhaps, not experience all the phenomena I may bring to your attention. That is perfectly normal. Hypnosis is a normal experience and every person seems to go through a state that resembles it—a hypnoidal state—each night before dozing off. I do not want you to go to sleep, because I want you to be aware of what I say and aware of your thoughts. However, if you do happen to start dozing off and are comfortable, let yourself go. I will awaken you. I want this experience to be relaxing and pleasant for you, and no questions will be asked that will embarrass you. Make your mind passive, and do not analyze your thoughts and sensations. Do you understand?"

TRANCE INDUCTION

Hypnosis is easily induced in most patients, and the physician must start out confident that he will be successful. This feeling of confidence cannot help but reflect itself in the physician's voice and will be rewarded by a maximum of successes. Where the physician's tone is hesitant and faltering, or where he anticipates failure, he will probably be unable to induce a trance. He should be reassuring and persuasive. Suggestions must be repeated rhythmically and monotonously in a steady tone of voice.

The personality of the hypnotist and his ability to inspire faith and confidence is thus a determining factor. There are certain qualities such as appearance, eloquence and a kindly firmness which build up a desire in the patient to be hypnotizable, or which motivate him toward an inability to resist the hypnotist's commands. The reputation of the hypnotist, his reported successes in being able to hypnotize other people, also has a profound effect on the subject. One of the most potent influences is for the subject to see the operator hypnotize other people in a group. The old-time hypnotists had, at all times, one or more patients in a sleep-like trance in their waiting rooms for the subject to observe.

Before inducing the trance the patient should be made as comfortable as possible. He should be seated in an armchair, his head supported by a pillow, both feet resting on the floor. The room should be free of glaring lights or drafts. The patient may be asked if he is completely comfortable and relaxed. If he complains of any discomfiture which is remediable, like being too warm or too cold or needing to go to the bathroom, it should be corrected before induction begins.

There are various methods of trance induction. Practically all of them aim for a gradual restriction of consciousness by limiting sensory impressions. This is accomplished by fixation of attention either on a material object or on a limited group of ideas. Sensory restriction is reinforced by a rhythmic monotonous repetition of commands and suggestions. Four alternative methods will be presented here. Each has certain advantages and disadvantages.

1. *Hypnosis by Means of Hand Levitation.* I believe this is the best of all induction procedures. It permits of a participation in the induction process by the patient and lends itself to nondirective and analytic technics. It is, however, the most difficult of methods and calls for greater endurance on the part of the hypnotist.

A transcribed soundscriber record of an actual induction follows to illustrate the method. In this patient, who was suffering from an anxiety neurosis, misconceptions regarding hypnosis were corrected, the hand clasp test executed and prehypnotic suggestions made. These were followed by this explanation:

"I want you to sit comfortably in your chair and relax. As you sit there, bring both hands palms down on your thighs—just like that. Keep watching your hands, and you will notice that you are able to observe them closely.

"What you will do is sit in the chair and relax. Then you will notice that certain things happen in the course of relaxing. They always have happened while relaxing, but you have not noticed them so closely before. I am going to point them out to you. I'd like to have you concentrate on all sensations and feelings in your hands no matter what they may be. Perhaps you may feel the heaviness of your hand as it lies on your thigh, or you may feel pressure. Perhaps you will feel the texture of your trousers as they press against the palm of your hand; or the warmth of your hand on your thigh. Perhaps you may feel tingling. No matter what sensations there are, I want you to observe them. Keep watching your hand, and you will notice how quiet it is, how it remains in one position. There is motion there, but it is not yet noticeable. I want you to keep watching your hand. Your attention may wander from the hand, but it will always return back to the hand, and you keep watching the hand and wondering when the motion that is there will show itself."

(At this point the patient's attention is fixed on his hand. He is curious about what will happen, and sensations such as any person might experience are suggested to him as possibilities. No attempt is being made to force any suggestions on him, and if he observes any sensations or feelings, he incorporates them as a product of his own experience. The object eventually is to get him to respond to the sug-

gestions of the hypnotist as if these too are parts of his own experiences. A subtle attempt is being made to get him to associate his sensations with the words spoken to him so that words or commands uttered by the hypnotist will evoke sensory or motor responses later on. Unless the patient is consciously resisting, a slight motion or jerking will develop in one of the fingers or in the hand. As soon as this happens, the hypnotist mentions it and remarks that the motion will probably increase. The hypnotist must also comment on any other objective reaction of the patient, such as motion of the legs or deep breathing. The result of this linking of the patient's reactions with comments of the hypnotist is an association of the two in the patient's mind.)

"It will be interesting to see which one of the fingers will move first. It may be the middle finger, or the forefinger, or the ring finger, or the little finger, or the thumb. One of the fingers is going to jerk or move. You don't know exactly when or in which hand. Keep watching and you will begin to notice a slight movement, possibly in the right hand. There, the thumb jerks and moves, just like that.

"As the movement begins you will notice an interesting thing. Very slowly the spaces between the fingers will widen, the fingers will slowly move apart, and you'll notice that the spaces will get wider and wider and wider. They'll move apart slowly; the fingers will seem to be spreading apart, wider and wider and wider. The fingers are spreading, wider and wider and wider apart, just like that."

(This is the first real suggestion to which the patient is expected to respond. If the fingers start spreading apart, they do so because the patient is reacting to suggestion. The hypnotist continues to talk as if the response is one that would have come about by itself in the natural course of events.)

"As the fingers spread apart, you will notice that the fingers will soon want to arch up from the thigh, as if they want to lift, higher and higher. *(The patient's index finger starts moving upward slightly.)* Notice how the index finger lifts. As it does the other fingers want to follow—up, up, slowly rising. (*The other fingers start lifting.*)

"As the fingers lift you'll become aware of lightness in the hand, a feeling of lightness, so much so that the fingers will arch up, and the whole hand will slowly lift and rise as if it feels like a feather, as if a balloon is lifting it up in the air, lifting, lifting,—up—up—up, pulling up higher and higher and higher, the hand becoming very light. (*The hand starts rising.*) As you watch your hand rise, you'll notice that the arm comes up, up, up in the air, a little higher—and higher —and higher—and higher, up—up—up. (*The arm has lifted about five inches above the thigh and the patient is gazing at it fixedly.*)

"Keep watching the hand and arm as it rises straight up, and as it does you will soon become aware of how drowsy and tired your eyes become. As your arm continues to rise, you will get tired and relaxed and sleepy, very sleepy. Your eyes will get heavy and your lids may want to close. And as your arm rises higher and higher, you will want to feel more relaxed and sleepy, and you will want to enjoy the peaceful, relaxed feeling of letting your eyes close and of being sleepy."

> (*It will be noticed that as the patient executes one suggestion, his positive response is used to reinforce the next suggestion. For instance, as his arm rises, it is suggested in essence that he will get drowsy because his arm is rising.*)

"Your arm lifts—up—up—and you are getting very drowsy; your lids get very heavy, your breathing gets slow and regular. Breathe deeply—in and out. (*The patient holds his arm stretched out directly in front of him, his eyes are blinking and his breathing is deep and regular.*) As you keep watching your hand and arm and feeling more and more drowsy and relaxed, you will notice that the direction of the hand will change. The arm will bend, and the hand will move closer and closer to your face—up—up—up—and as it rises you will slowly but steadily go into a deep, deep, sleep in which you relax deeply and to your satisfaction. The arm will continue to rise up—up—lifting, lifting—up in the air until it touches your face, and you will get sleepier and sleepier, but you must not go to sleep until your hand touches your face. When your hand touches your face, you will be asleep, deeply asleep."

> (*The patient here is requested to choose his own pace in falling asleep, so that when his hand touches his face, he feels himself to be asleep to his own satisfaction. Hand levitation and sleepiness continue to reinforce each other. When the patient finally does close his eyes, he will have entered a trance with his own participation. He will later be less inclined to deny that he has been in a trance.*)

"Your hand is now changing its direction. It moves up—up—up toward your face. Your eyelids are getting heavy. You are getting sleepier, and sleepier, and sleepier. (*The patient's hand is approaching his face, his eyelids are blinking more rapidly.*) Your eyes get heavy, very heavy, and the hand moves straight up towards your face. You get very tired and drowsy. Your eyes are closing, are closing. When your hand touches your face you'll be asleep, deeply asleep. You'll feel very drowsy. You feel drowsier and drowsier and drowsier, very sleepy, very tired. Your eyes are like lead, and your hand moves up, up, up, right towards your face, and when it reaches your face, you will be asleep. (*Patient's hand touches his face and his eyes close.*) Go to sleep, go to sleep, just asleep. And as you sleep you feel very tired and relaxed. I want you to concentrate on relaxation, a state of tensionless relaxation. Think of nothing else, but sleep, deep sleep."

This technic will prove satisfactory for most patients. Slight variations may be introduced for special effects as will be noticed in the transcribed case histories in Volume Two.

2. *Hypnosis through Use of a Fixation Object.* A much

simpler alternative method of trance induction, useful in most conditions, but in my opinion not as good as hand levitation, is by a fixation object. The method is somewhat more directive than hand levitation and somewhat more rapid. Most operators use this method, which consists of holding an object sufficiently close to the eyes of the subject to produce convergence. The nature of the object is immaterial and may consist of a key, a coin or a pencil. A large ball bearing mounted on a rod or a Christmas tree ball ornament on a string make excellent fixation objects, concentrating light sources in the room on the surface. Where a metallic object is used, a light behind the patient may be reflected into his eyes. The fixation object is held about ten to twelve inches from the eyes and a little above them. A card with a black spot painted on it, propped up against a book on the physician's desk, or a spot on the ceiling may serve as substitute fixation points even though the distance is greater.

The following suggestions are from a record of an induction.

"I am holding an object above your eyes, look at it steadily. You may pick out a spot of light on it, if you desire, and focus on that intently. At the same time relax and do not resist suggestions. Keep concentrating on the idea of sleep and do not permit any other thoughts to enter your mind. Just focus your eyes on the object. You may possibly notice that your eyes may want to travel in one direction or in another direction, but they will always return to a spot on the object. Keep your eyes fixated on this object, keep looking at it as long as you want; and as you keep looking at it, I want you to relax yourself and make your mind passive. Stop resisting; relax.

"As you relax you will begin to notice that your arms get heavy, your legs get heavy, your eyes get tired, you get heavier all over. A sense of drowsiness is creeping over your entire body. Keep looking at the object and blink as much as you like. Let your eyes get as tired and drowsy as possible.

"You are getting drowsy now. Soon your eyes will tire and water. Wink if you wish. Your lids will get so heavy they will start shutting. Relax and get sleepier. Your eyes are watering. Your lids keep closing. Your eyes get tired, watery and they burn. They become fatigued. Your eyelids are heavy, and get heavier and heavier. Your eyes are very tired. Soon they will close.

"Keep thinking about sleep, how it would feel to be asleep. You notice that you are getting sleepier and sleepier. Keep staring at the object as hard as you can and as long as you can, and you notice that your eyelids are getting heavier and heavier. Your eyes burn, feel tired and a sense of sleepiness creeps over you. You are getting sleepier and sleepier and sleepier. You are getting very, very sleepy, and your eyelids get heavier and heavier, and they will close and you will go into a quiet restful sleep.

"Now your arms and legs are heavy like lead. A warm feeling spreads over your body, a drowsy feeling as if you are floating on a cloud. Let yourself relax and sleep, go to sleep. It is pleasant to relax. Let yourself get sleepy. Sink into a deep, deep sleep. You are relaxed and comfortable. Breathe deeply, very deeply and slowly, just like that. With each breath your sleep gets deeper and deeper. Your eyes have practically closed. You are almost asleep, deeply asleep. Go to sleep, relax and sleep, just sleep, sleep, sleep."

In most cases a repetition of suggestions such as the above for several minutes will result in the closing of the patient's eyes. The physician may press his fingers on the patient's closed eyes to emphasize their closure. In the event the eyes do not close spontaneously a counting technic is sometimes successful. The patient is told:

"You notice that your eyelids become heavy, and I am going to count from one to ten. As I do, your eyelids will get heavier and heavier, and when I reach the count of ten your eyelids will close, and you will keep them closed until I tell you to open them up. One—they are getting very heavy. They are getting heavier and heavier and heavier. Two—your eyelids are getting very heavy. You feel sleepy all over. You get sleepier and sleepier. You feel sleepy all over. You get sleepier and sleepier. Your eyes are getting very, very tired. They burn, they smart and they water, and as I approach the count of ten, your lids get so heavy that you cannot keep them open. Three—they are getting heavier and heavier. Four—you go into a deeper and deeper and more quiet state of relaxation. You become sleepier and sleepier all over. Five—you're getting sleepier and sleepier and sleepier. Six—you notice that your eyelids have become very heavy. It is very, very difficult to keep them open. They are beginning to close. They are closing, closing, closing. Seven—they are getting very, very heavy. Eight— they are getting so heavy that when I reach the count of ten they will close, and you will go into a very restful sleep. Nine—they are getting very heavy. They begin to close. They are getting heavier and heavier. Ten—they close, and you keep them closed until I tell you to open them up."

If the eyes still remain open, the physician may bring his hand to within several inches of the patient's eyes, then, moving his hand up and down, he remarks, "Follow my hand up and down, up and down, and as you do you will get sleepier and sleepier—up and down." This is repeated for about two minutes. If the eyes do not close the patient is told, "Now you can close them." At the same time the fingers of the operator press the eyelids down lightly. Another technic is to instruct the patient to look at the index and third fingers which are brought close to the eyes and separated to correspond with the space between the eyes. He is told: "Your eyes are getting very heavy and sleepy . . . .

Continue to look at my fingers, I am going to bring them closer and closer to your eyes, and as I do they will shut." The patient will, of course, be unable to resist closing his eyes as the fingers approach them. The operator may then press the eyelids together remarking that they are stuck together and that they will remain shut until he is instructed to open them again.

3. *Hypnosis with Sleep Suggestions.* In a third alternative method, which is useful in many of the psychobiologic technics, the patient is requested to lie down on a couch and to close his eyes. He is instructed as in the following transcription:

"I should like to have you lie down on the couch and relax yourself all over. I should like to have you become aware of any tensions that exist in your muscles. First concentrate on your forehead, loosen up your forehead. Loosen up the muscles in your face, straighten out your neck, loosen that up too. Now the shoulders. Loosen up your body; stretch out your arms and legs. Let yourself get lazy all over, from your head right down to your feet. Now fold your hands on your chest, and as I talk to you try to visualize things exactly as I talk about them. First become aware of the pressure of the pillow against your head. Concentrate on the back of the head and become aware of how the pillow presses against it. Now the pressure of the pillow against your shoulders, the pressure of the couch against your back. Now shift your attention to your thighs and think of how the couch supports your whole body. It is as if your body sinks into the couch and is supported by it completely. Now I want you to visualize yourself in a comfortable place, the most comfortable place you know, a place where you would like to stretch out, forget your worries and your cares, so you can sleep. Perhaps it will be at the seashore or in the mountains or some other place if you prefer. (*The patient here prefers to think of the mountains.*)

"As you lie there I want you to start breathing deeply and slowly. As you do, relax yourself even more. Make your body limp so that when I raise your arm it will come down limp of its own accord. (*The arm is raised, and it falls down unsupported when released.*) I want you to relax the rest of your body the same way, from your forehead to your toes. Stretch out and breathe deeply. Good, like that.

"Now as you lie there, relaxed, breathing deeply, imagine you are on a mountain top on a sunny day. Everything is peaceful and serene. You are lying in the shade in tall soft grass. You watch the deep blue sky overhead. Perhaps you see one or two billowy clouds floating lazily by. Everything is peaceful and serene like your mind must be now. All around you are tall fir, spruce and pine trees. The scent of pine penetrates your nostrils and makes you feel fresh and relaxed. And in the distance there are lakes, the surface as smooth as glass. Watch the lakes and your mind will become peaceful and quiet like the surface of the water. Your body is relaxed. Your mind is relaxed. Relax and sleep, deeper and deeper. Sleep more deeply, go to sleep.

"As you start getting sleepy, your arm, your right arm will get light, like a feather. It will get lighter and lighter, and then it will lift—up—up—up. The sleepier you get, the lighter your arm will feel, and the higher it will lift until it touches your face. As you relax, your hand and arm lift and rise higher and higher, and when your hand touches your face, you will be asleep, deeply asleep. Your arm is rising slowly now, just like a feather—up—up—up—higher and higher and higher. It is getting close to your face, you will be asleep, deeply asleep. Now your hand has touched your face and you are asleep."

4. *Hypnosis through Eye Gaze.* This method which is used by stage hypnotists is completely directive and authoritarian and hence should rarely be used, except where it is essential for therapeutic reasons to establish a strong authoritarian

relationship with the patient, as in symptom removal and some forms of alcoholism, drug addiction and psychopathic personality.

The hypnotist must practice to develop a steady eye gaze. This can be done by staring fixedly at a small object placed about one foot from the eyes for several minutes each day. If eye strain occurs during the practice session, the eyes should be closed and moved from side to side. Eventually the hypnotist will be able to stare at a close object without blinking.

In hypnotizing a patient with the eye gaze method, the operator stands facing the patient with his eyes approximately twelve inches away. He must stand above the patient, and if the latter is the taller of the two, the patient may be seated while the operator stands. The operator grasps the shoulders of the patient and rocks him slowly back and forth while staring at the bridge of the patient's nose. The operator then repeats:

"Look steadily into my eyes. As you do your eyes will get heavy. Your arms are getting heavy, very heavy. Your legs are getting heavy, heavy, heavy. Your body is getting heavy. You are getting heavy all over. You are getting sleeply, sleepy, sleepy. Your eyes are heavy and tired. Don't close them until you can't keep them open any longer. Your eyelids are heavy like lead. You are going into a deep, deep sleep."

The operator may pause for a moment, and when the patient's eyes begin to blink his tone becomes even more commanding. "Now your eyes are blinking. You are going to sleep. Nothing can stop you. Sleep, sleep, sleep." As soon as the eyes have closed the operator may press the eyelids with his fingers, saying: "The lids are glued together, they cannot open until I tell you to open them. Sleep until I give you the command to wake up." After the patient has closed his eyes, he should be helped into a chair.

In the event the operator finds his own eyes tiring in the course of induction, he may place his fingers on the patient's eyelids closing them, repeating at the same time, "Sleep, sleep, sleep; go to sleep." This will give him a chance to rest his own eyes for a moment.

DEEPENING THE TRANCE

As soon as the patient has closed his eyes, or has indicated that he is in a trance by successful hand levitation to a point of contact with his face, further suggestions are given him to deepen the trance state. In patients who are obviously in a medium or deep trance some of these suggestions may be omitted. Suggestions are given for rigid limb catalepsy, lid catalepsy, skin hyperesthesia, skin anesthesia, free association under hypnosis, fantasy and dream induction and, in some cases, for minor posthypnotic suggestions.

1. *Limb Catalepsy*. While the left arm rests on the thigh, the patient is given the following suggestions:

"I am going to stroke the left arm. As I stroke it, you will experience a feeling of weight in this arm, so that it begins to feel heavy like lead. The heaviness in this arm will get so that it will resist movement. It won't budge as you sit there. Your arm will feel heavier and heavier and heavier. I'm going to count from one to five, and at the count of five the arm will have gotten so heavy that it will be as if a hundred pound weight is pressing down on it. It will press against your thigh and get heavy and heavier and heavier. One, heavy; two, heavier and heavier; three, as heavy as lead; four, heavy, heavy; five, when you try to budge it, it will resist movement. It feels so heavy that when I bring it up in the air, it falls down because it feels so heavy you cannot keep it up. It is getting heavier, heavier and heavier."

The arm is then raised in the air and permitted to drop. If the patient is able to support his arm, suggestions are repeated. It is rare that this test fails. Should the patient be able to move his arm, he is not hypnotized, and he may be told that some people find it a little difficult at first to experience anything other than a slight heaviness. He will undoubtedly succeed the next time. He is then asked to open his eyes.

Should the test be successful, which it will be in most instances, rigid catalepsy is next attempted. The patient's left arm is extended by the operator horizontally, and pulled out while stroked downward.

"You notice that your arm has become as heavy as lead, and now it will become rigid and stiff, too, just like a board. It will get heavy like lead and stiff like a board. As I stroke it, it gets stiffer, stiffer, more rigid. The muscles contract and it stiffens up. (*The stroking of the arm continues until the muscles are felt to stiffen.*) Now, your arm is so stiff, it will remain as it is. You cannot raise it. Try as hard as you like, you are unable to raise your arm. It is as heavy as lead and stiff as a board. It is stiff, stiff, stiff. It is so stiff, it cannot bend, and it gets stiffer and stiffer and stiffer. You notice how stiff it is? You cannot bend it, it is so stiff. The harder you try to bend it, the stiffer it gets."

If rigid catalepsy is successful, the patient is told: "Now relax yourself completely. Relax your eyes. Relax your arm. Relax all parts of your body, and you will go into a deeper and deeper sleep, deeper and deeper. The next time I talk to you, you will be more deeply asleep." The patient is then allowed to sleep for two minutes. If the patient succeeds in raising his arm, he is awakened with the same explanation as in failure to experience heaviness of the arm.

2. *Lid Catalepsy.* Further suggestions are continued as follows: "As you lie here thinking about sleep, you begin to relax your muscles. The muscles in your entire body relax. The muscles of your head, neck, shoulders, back, arms, thighs, legs, and even fingers and toes relax. You get drowsier and drowsier. Your breathing is getting deep, slow and regular, in

and out. Inhale deeply and then exhale. You feel very warm, comfortable and relaxed. You feel very sleepy, very, very sleepy. You begin to notice that you pay no attention to anything but the sound of my voice. You notice that your eyelids, too, have become so heavy that they feel as if they are made of lead. They feel glued together so that even though you try hard to open them, they stay shut. They remain closed until I give you the command to open them. Now your eyelids are shut tight, tight, tight. They are clamped together. So tight that you cannot open them even if you try. The harder you try to open them, the heavier they feel. Try and you will see that you cannot. They are very, very tight."

In most cases the patient will be unable to open his eyes even though he may struggle very hard to do so. If he manages to open his eyes, it is best to remark immediately: "Now you can open them. You notice there was some resistance. This is perfectly normal and indicates that sleep suggestions are working. Continue to concentrate on sleep, and try not to keep your eyes open nor to close them voluntarily." The fingers are then pressed down on the patient's eyelids, closing them, and the patient is told that the next session will enable him to go into a deeper relaxed state that will resemble sleep. Sleep suggestions then are repeated and suggestions for inhibition of voluntary movements made. There are some persons who go into a fairly deep trance state, yet resist lid catalepsy.

3. *Inhibition of Voluntary Movements.* As the state of hypnosis gets deeper, the subject becomes more and more amenable to suggestions to lose control of groups of muscles, ranging from isolated small groups to muscles involving the entire body. The hand clasp test may now be repeated.

"Now you put your fingers together, and interlock them. You keep them tightly locked together, tighter and tighter and tighter. When I count to five, you will find that you are unable to separate your fingers. One—they are getting tighter and tighter. Two—they are getting very tight. Three—tight, tight. Four—very tight. Five—they are locked together now, and you cannot separate them. Try as hard as you like, you will find that you are unable to separate your fingers."

Another suggestion may be given the patient that as he grasps the physician's hand, he will be unable to let go. "You will notice that as you hold my hand, your hand is getting fast to mine. The harder you try to remove your hand from mine, the firmer you will grasp it." After the patient does this he is told, "Now you can let go." A book may then be given the patient with the following suggestions: "Clasp the book between your thumb and first finger. Clasp it hard, tight, tight, tight, harder, harder. You will notice that as you clasp the book tight, you are unable to open your hand and drop the book. The book remains in your hand, and you are unable to drop it until I tell you to let go.—Now let go."

If these tests are successful, the following suggestion is made: "Now you will find that you are unable to pronounce your name. You are unable to say your name no matter how hard you try. Even though you try to say your name you are unable to do so."

Suggestions involving larger groups of muscles may then be made as follows: "Relax completely now; relax completely. Your body muscles remain relaxed. Your body seems to be floating in space, and you will be unable to move your muscles. You are getting more and more relaxed. You are unable to get out of your chair, (or couch) and you remain relaxed, very comfortable. Try as hard as you can, you are unable to get up. You remain quiet and relaxed."

4. *Automatic Movements.* Automatic movements indicate a somewhat deeper state of hypnosis. The patient's two hands are revolved one around the other with the suggestion that he is unable to stop them. "I take your two hands, and

I revolve them around each other. They go around faster, faster, and faster. They keep going faster and faster. Keep them going. They cannot stop even though you try to stop them. They keep going around and around. Faster and faster. You cannot stop them. Try. Try as hard as you can, they will not stop. Now your hands stop, and come back to where they were. You go into a deeper and deeper and more relaxing sleep."

5. *Disturbances in cutaneous sensibility*. Hyperesthesia may be produced by giving the patient suggestions as in the following transcribed record:

"Imagine that you are walking down a corridor and you notice in the far end corner of the corridor, a pail of hot water. You realize it is hot because the steam issues from the surface of the water. As you visualize that in your mind, you will indicate to me that you see it by lifting up your left hand about six inches. As you visualize the pail of hot water, your hand will rise up about six inches. Now, it comes up. Bring it down. Good. Now you become curious about how hot the water is, so you walk over to the pail of water, take your right hand and you plunge it into the water. As you plunge it into the water, see if you can make this vivid in your mind so you feel the heat, the smarting and pain in your hand. Let yourself go. Your hand will tingle or feel warm or tender. As soon as you feel a sensation, your left hand will rise about six inches to indicate this to me. It rises and now it comes down. Good. As you sit there, I am going to touch the right hand with a pin. You will notice that the hand has become so tender that when I touch it with a pin, it will be as though I am poking a nail through it. I will show you. It is very tender and sensitive. I am going to touch it with a pin now. It will feel as though I am poking a nail through it. Just like that. You notice how tender that feels? (*Patient nods*) You will notice the difference when I touch this tender hand here, and when I touch the other hand with the pin. I will touch the other hand first, and now I am going to touch the tender hand here, this way. Do you notice the difference when I poke it?" (*Patient nods.*)

Good hypnotic subjects will actually flinch with pain when the hand is touched with a pin. It is important to get some acknowledgment of difference in sensitivity in the two hands. If the patient feels no difference, he is told that it requires some practice to feel a difference and that he undoubtedly will feel the difference at the next session. The trance is then terminated.

Following successful hyperesthesia, anesthesia may next be attempted. Very rarely is complete anesthesia obtained at the first session, so that the physician must be content to get from the patient an acknowledgment of relative insensitivity. The patient may be given the following suggestions:

"You notice that whereas your right hand is sensitive, the left hand becomes less and less sensitive. Now imagine that you go to a doctor's office because a finger on the left hand, the forefinger, has a boil and needs treatment. The doctor injects novocaine around the wrist to create a wrist block and to remove the pain, like this. (*The physician circles the wrist with slight pin pricks.*)

"Slowly you notice that the hand becomes numb, and that soon it will be come so numb that when I poke it with a pin there will be no real pain as compared with the right hand. The feeling will leave the hand and it will get numb. As you think about your hand, imagine that you are wearing a thick heavy leather glove on your left hand. Picture it in your mind and get a feeling that the glove is on the hand. As soon as you visualize yourself wearing the glove and feel as if you have the glove on your hand, indicate that to me by your hand rising up about six inches. Your hand will feel as if you are wearing a thick heavy leather glove so that when I poke it with a pin it will feel as if I am poking leather. No pain, just a dull feeling. As soon as you experience the sensation of wearing a thick heavy glove on your hand, indicate it by your hand rising. (*These suggestions are repeated until the hand rises.*)

"Now I am going to show you the difference by poking first the right hand, the sensitive one, and then the left. Do you notice the difference? (*With this acknowledgment further suggestions are made.*) Now there is more and more difficulty in feeling pain. The hand is getting more and more numb. The pain is fading away. (*The hand is again pricked.*) "The dullness extends over your entire hand, includes the back of your hand, the fingers, the thumb, and the front of your hand. The feeling gets duller and duller. It feels almost as if it were made out of wood. I am able to pinch it, to stick it with a pin, and you will feel no real pain. Now it is becoming so numb that you feel no real pain. (*At this point the hand is either pinched or pricked with a pin and the subject is questioned again.*) Do you notice the numbness? (*If the patient remarks that he feels pain, he is reassured.*) You feel slight pain, but it is less than in the other hand, isn't it? (*He will usually remark that there is a difference.*) Good, that shows that the suggestions are beginning to work. Now relax yourself more and go into a deeper sleep. (*Further suggestions for deeper sleep are then given.*)

"Now you are sinking into a deeper and deeper and more profound sleep. You will stay asleep until I give you the command to wake up. Even though you are asleep you are able to hear my voice, to follow commands, and you will stay asleep until I direct you to wake up. When you awaken you may remember everything that has happened or you may forget some things. You will decide that for yourself. The next time we try hypnosis you will fall asleep faster and more easily. Do you understand?" (*The patient is permitted to sleep for a few minutes and then awakened, unless it is desired to proceed further in the trance, whereupon suggestions for deepening the trance, which are included in the next chapter, are continued.)*

In some patients the response to this procedure is so good that the depth of trance can proceed to somnambulism. However this is rare, and several trance sessions will be required before the patient is capable of reaching his limit of trance depth.

In some patients, particularly compulsion neurotics, it may be advisable to try to induct the patient deeply during the first session, allowing sufficient time, one and one-half or two hours, for this purpose. At the first session, compulsive patients are often very much impressed with the changes occurring in themselves, and, not knowing what to expect next, they cannot marshal their defenses. It may be possible to get a person to enter a deep trance the first time, but thereafter, since he knows what to expect, he can mobilize his defenses and resist. Once he is in a deep trance, posthypnotic suggestions may be made that he will, at a given signal, enter again into a deep trance thereafter.

Awakening the Patient

To arouse the patient a technic aiming at slow awakening is best. The following suggestions may be given:

"Relax yourself completely. I am going to start waking you up. I will count slowly from one to five, and as I do you will gradually become more and more awake. At the count of five your eyes will open. You will have no headache, no dizziness, no confusion or any other uncomfortable symptoms. One, you are getting more and more awake now; two, slowly awaken; three, you begin to feel more awake; four, you are getting wider and wider awake; five, your eyes begin to open gradually; wake up completely."

Some patients, upon awakening, show untoward psychosomatic effects in the form of shivering, confusion, nausea, and headache. In very rare cases overactivity and excitement may occur. Where these sequelae are present, it is best to rehypnotize the person, and to suggest that his symptoms will not be present when he awakens. These effects are most often present when the patient has been given a posthypnotic suggestion that he attempts to resist, either because it is opposed to his standards, or because he desires to maintain control of his actions without yielding to the commands of the physician. In such cases, rehypnosis and suggestion that symptoms will disappear are usually without avail. During rehypnosis the physician had best inform the patient that he will not have to follow the suggestions given to him. In some cases even this release will not neutralize the former suggestion, and psychosomatic symptoms will not disappear until the subject carries out the posthypnotic suggestion that has been made. At any rate all unusual symptoms following hypnosis disappear spontaneously in the course of several hours after the termination of the trance.

In isolated cases the patient will refuse to awaken from hypnosis following suggestions that the trance be terminated. Sometimes the reason for this lies in an expressed or unexpressed posthypnotic suggestion that the patient refuses to fulfill. Escape from conflict is sought in sleep. Sometimes the patient feels such great pleasure in the trance that he wants the state to continue. Where the patient persists in sleeping, he may be asked why he refuses to awaken and what the physician may do to wake him up. The physician must be firm, but never threatening. If exhortations fail to arouse the patient, there is no need for alarm, since the person will always awaken spontaneously following a nap. Sleep in resistive patients does not extend beyond several hours. During this period of sleep, it is best to have another person present with the patient to protect him if somnambulistic activity occurs. However, refusal to awaken is so rare that the physician will probably never encounter a case of this kind.

DISCUSSION OF TRANCE EXPERIENCES

The reaction of the patient to his trance experiences will range from intense amazement and satisfaction to profound disappointment and depression.

The following questions are commonly asked and answers for them may be along indicated lines:

I do not believe I was hypnotized because I could hear everything you said. "Hypnosis is no bludgeon that knocks a person out. It would be totally without value if the subject couldn't hear what was said. It is true that in the deepest states of hypnosis some things are not remembered, but deep states of hypnosis, while useful for stage tricks and the like, are not necessary in most forms of therapeutic hypnosis. As a matter of fact in your particular case a light form of hypnosis may be advantageous. If a deeper form is necessary, we will achieve it by training you to enter the deeper states in later sessions. It takes time for a person to learn how to enter into a deep trance, and we will go as deep as necessary with your cooperation."

I am afraid hypnosis will not help me because I wasn't able to do everything you suggested. "In the next few sessions I am going to suggest that you observe a number of different kinds of phenomena. You will be able to observe some, but not all of them. It is not necessary for you to be able to observe everything that I bring to your attention. All hypnotized people are capable of doing certain things in the trance and not others. What you have experienced is perfectly normal."

I do not believe I was hypnotized because I was in full control at all times and could have resisted suggestions. "Hypnosis is a cooperative enterprise and we have no desire for you to lose control of yourself. Indeed, we are aiming to give you better control of yourself and your functions, so you will get stronger. If you have a desire to resist suggestions, there are reasons for this resistance, and I shall try to help you to understand them. In the next few sessions you will develop greater confidence in your ability to enjoy the experience of hypnosis which will be of value to you in overcoming your problems."

When you tell me to do things should I do them voluntarily? "It is not necessary for you to do things deliberately. If you make your mind passive, things will happen in the natural course of events. Just relax and enjoy the experience of watching how things come about as the result of suggestion. You don't have to try too hard."

The patient should, following clarification of his doubts, be questioned as to how he felt emotionally, and he may be asked what went through his mind both as he started entering the trance state and while he was in the trance. Notes may be made of the patient's experiences which can be mentioned in the course of subsequent inductions. Each patient reacts to hypnosis in his own unique way, and when he is presented with a picture of his experiences in his own terms, this facilitates the induction process. The physician may mention casually that at the next session the patient will experience other phenomena and that he will be able to enter the trance more easily.

VI

THE SECOND HYPNOTIC SESSION

THE MANAGEMENT of the second hypnotic session will depend on the depth of the first trance, and the patient's emotional response to it. The induction of hypnosis cannot help but mobilize feelings which in part are a reflection of the individual's basic problems in interpersonal relationships. The activity of the physician inherent in hypnosis, and the feelings of closeness that develop in the patient toward the physician during the trance, bring out in sharp focus the patient's fears, demands, expectations and conflicts. Success in hypnotherapy will depend upon the correct evaluation and proper handling of these reactions.

For example, a patient may have a deep fear of close relationships with people which cause him to control himself rigidly in various areas of his functioning. His inability to establish close contacts with others produces a desperate loneliness for which he seeks therapy. At the first trance session his desire for help may have been intense enough to produce a motivation to be hypnotizable, thus enabling him to achieve a medium trance. However, the very assumption of the trance state opposes his character defense of absolute self control. Following the first session, therefore, his response may be hostility toward the physician or anxiety at having exposed himself to possible hurt. These emotions may be completely repressed. The only response the patient may show is an intensified desire for detachment which will reflect itself in resistance against further hypnosis.

The patient should therefore be questioned about his reaction to the last session and particularly about subsequent dreams. His dreams, interpreted correctly, frequently reveal not only his immediate emotional attitude toward the physician, but also may contain the essence of his neurotic problem. It may be necessary to postpone further hypnotic sessions until his fears have been clarified, or suggestions can be made in the second trance which take into account his reactions.

If the patient resisted entering the first trance, his subsequent waking productions and his dreams will often yield clues to his resistance. Such clues utilized adroitly may make the second induction attempt a success.

TRANCE MANAGEMENT IN RESISTIVE PATIENTS

Should the patient have failed to enter a trance state in the previous session, a modification of technic will be necessary in order to overcome his resistance. Among the more common resistances are defiance of the authority of the hypnotist, a fear of yielding one's will or independence, a need to prove oneself superior, or a fear of failure.

Where the nature of the resistance is known it may in some cases be circumvented. For example, where the patient spontaneously admits that he fears giving up his independence, the physician may assure him that no suggestion will be made without first gaining his consent. It may be stressed that it is impossible to obtain any effect that he, himself, is unwilling to produce. During hypnosis the patient is repeatedly assured on this score, and, as he consents to deeper and deeper states, he may finally become a very apt hypnotic subject.

Where the patient defies the authority of the physician, he may sometimes admit that hostile, challenging and depreciatory impulses, or strivings to be negativistic, invade his mind during the attempted induction process. The ventilation of these feelings may possibly make him more susceptible.

One of the most difficult resistances to handle is that of a fear of failure. Here the individual looks upon hypnosis as a test of his ability to perform. Because of a deep sense of self devaluation, or because success in achievement creates anxiety, he may find it impossible to reach any significant trance depth. This resistance is usually associated with a profound character disorganization, and prolonged therapy may be necessary before self esteem is strengthened. A kindly attitude of reassurance helps certain patients circumvent this problem. When they feel that they need not be terrified if they do not succeed at once, they may become more self tolerant and relax better during the trance. A modified form of this resistance is seen in the patient who has tried many other forms of therapy without success. He is so desperate for hypnosis to succeed that he may want to reach somnambulism at once. Inability to do so fills him with hopelessness and causes him to fight off suggestions. A careful explanation that somnambulism is neither necessary nor desirable may permit the patient to relax enough to undergo induction.

In certain persons, trance induction and satisfactory depth may be achieved only when their aptitudes are challenged. Such patients want to be told that a person's ability to be hypnotized depends upon a considerable amount of intelligence and concentrative capacity. Because there is present a compulsive need to function perfectively, or a competitive desire to excel, the patient may succumb to such appeals when every other approach has failed. The entire hypnotic procedure must be couched in language to challenge the subject's ability to perform well. For instance, instead of the command that his arm is going to become rigid and stiff, the following suggestion may be made: "See if you can make your arm stiff and rigid, and, as I count from one to ten, see if you have the ability to make your arm so stiff that you will be unable to bend it." Or, if there is a desire to produce paralysis, the patient may be told: "See if you can hold your arm so that it becomes paralyzed. It takes a great deal of effort and concentration to do this. Concentrate steadily on holding your arm so that it is unable to move." All suggestions are phrased so that the subject feels that his capacity to perform is questioned. After the first few trance inductions, he may be challenged to follow the physician's suggestions directly. The orthodox procedure may then be instituted.

One of the most frequent causes of resistance to hypnosis is a fluctuating attention. Distractibility prevents the patient from concentrating on the physician's suggestions. A counting technic may be helpful here. The patient is instructed as follows: "I want you to start counting. When you say, 'one,' close your eyes. When you say, 'two,' open your eyes. At 'three' close your eyes, at 'four' open them, and so on." As the patient counts while opening and shutting his eyes, the physician should make comments on how sleepy he will get, how tired his eyes will be, how heavy his eyelids are, and how he will go into a deep, restful sleep.

In emergencies, as, for example, psychopathic personalities who are destroying themselves with drink and who are negativistic to all forms of psychotherapy or appeals to reason, it may sometimes be possible to use their defiance or resistance to reinforce sleep suggestions. Using the eye gaze method the patient is told:

"As you sit here looking into my eyes, you begin to resist falling asleep. You say to yourself, 'It isn't possible to fall asleep. I can't fall asleep.' But you will find that the more you resist, the more difficult it is to keep from falling asleep. The harder you fight, the sleepier you get. Try it, and you will see that the more you resist falling asleep, the sleepier you are. Fight hard against falling asleep. Try not to fall asleep, and the harder you try, the sleepier you get. The more you fight, the sleepier you get. Fight hard to keep awake. Try to defy me, try to keep awake; but the more you defy me, the sleepier you get. Your eyelids are getting heavier and heavier until they close."

Such methods of browbeating the patient into a hypnotic state are, of course, contraindicated except in emergency conditions.

It is sometimes possble to circumvent resistance by giving

the patient relaxing or sleep suggestions without any indication that he is being hypnotized. Hypnosis has so many unfortunate associations that some patients are terror stricken
even when explanations attempt to correct their misconceptions. Instead of telling the patient an attempt will be
made to hypnotize him a second time, he is told that he will
get instead an exercise in relaxation. No mention should be
made of the words "hypnosis" or "trance." The physician
should merely remark that he wishes to see how well the patient can relax. A blood pressure apparatus may be applied
to the arm, or the pulse may be tested regularly, with the explanation that the degree of relaxation will be registered in
blood pressure or pulse rate. The technic for hypnosis by
sleep suggestions may then be given the patient, explaining
to him that his pulse rate will come down and his blood pressure will fall if he can relax as in sleep.

Mechanical devices. Hypnosis may be resisted on the basis
of a conscious or unconscious fear of the physician. This occurs mostly in detached people who have built a shell around
themselves, and who attempt to ward off contacts of an interpersonal nature. When the physician approaches the patient,
terror may become so extreme that hypnosis is impossible.
To obviate this a mechanical contrivance may be utilized.
Mechanical devices are also helpful in impressionable people
who expect the mysterious in hypnosis. They are furthermore
successful in distractible persons who are unable to concentrate their attention on words.

Listening to a monotonous auditory stimulation may be
successful where other methods fail. The beat of a metronome
or a clock may be utilized as a fixation stimulus, the suggestion being given the patient that he will get sleepier and
sleepier as he listens to the rhythmic beat. If he is unable to
concentrate on the idea of sleep, it may be possible for him
to visualize in his mind a very peaceful scene, or a monoto-

nous drowsy mental picture. If musical, he may mentally reproduce a musical composition.

The effectiveness of the metronome may be increased
by gluing a one inch cardboard circle on top of the lever and
covering it with tin foil or silvered paper. An electronic
metronome with a small light on the front panel that flashes
on and off with each beat can be purchased and is excellent
for the same purpose. The metronomes should be regulated
to a slow frequency.

Another device I have found extremely effective is a
slowly revolving disk on which is painted a spiral. An electri-
cian or radio man can reduce the speed of revolution of an
electric fan by inserting a resistance in series. A heavy cardboard or plywood disk of about eight inches may be mounted
in place of the blade with a white and a black spiral painted
on it. The spiral must correspond in direction with the direction of fan rotation to produce the proper effect. The patient
is instructed to watch the revolving wheel with the following
instructions which are repeated until the eyes close:

"Keep your eyes fastened on the wheel. As you watch it,
you will notice that it vibrates. The white circles become
more prominent, then the black. Then it seems to recede in
the distance and you feel as if you are drawn into it. Your
breathing becomes deep and regular. You get drowsy, very
drowsy. Soon you will be asleep."

Hypnotic Drugs (Narcosynthesis). In some instances, a resistant subject may be hypnotized successfully after taking a
hypnotic drug. The patient may be given six to nine grains
of sodium amytal one-half hour prior to hypnosis, or he may
get one to two drams of paraldehyde five to ten minutes
before hypnosis is attempted. Where the patient has tremors,
spasms, hiccups, or other symptoms which make it impossible
for him to relax sufficiently to concentrate his attention, a
hypnotic is indispensable.

When other methods fail, the intravenous injection of a solution of hypnotic drug may be used. This method,[1-3] which has been called narcosynthesis or narcoanalysis, produces in itself a hypnotic-like state which resembles, but is not similar to hypnosis.

Hypnosis involves the assumption of a trance state on the basis of a particular type of relationship to the hypnotist. Because the person is motivated to go into a trance state, he submits himself to sleep suggestions, in the course of which there is a temporary deadening of higher cortical centers and an entering into unconscious layers of mental activity. In narcosynthesis, the relationship situation is not so apparent at the start. The drug, however, acts as a cortical depressant and produces the same phenomena as a hypnotically produced deadening of the cortical centers. The psychologic regression in narcosynthesis, as well as cognizance on the part of the patient of his helplessness, incites archaic dependency feelings toward the operator. Transference phenomena become apparent as emotionally charged repressed experiences come to the surface.

Repressed conflicts and traumatic memories are released, often with a cathartic effect. For this reason narcosynthesis is particularly applicable to acute traumatic neuroses, war neuroses and certain hysterical conditions. The material released must be accepted and integrated by the waking ego to insure permanent results.

In the chronic neuroses, narcosynthesis is not so effective as in the acute neuroses since the neurotic condition is too deeply imbedded and too structuralized. In addition to the toxic effects of the hypnotic drug, there are other distinct disadvantages to narcosynthesis as compared with hypnosis in the treatment of chronic neuroses. The relationship in narcosynthesis is too directive and it is often difficult to get the patient to participate in and to take responsibility for his own development.

While it has important values as a temporary procedure, narcosynthesis must always be combined with psychotherapy on a waking level. During narcosynthesis, it may be possible to give the patient suggestions to the effect that he will be susceptible to hypnosis. Suggestions must be detailed and specific, covering every aspect of the induction process. For example, the patient may be told that when he is shown a fixation object, he will gaze at it, and as he does he will notice that his eyes will water, his lids will get heavy, his breathing will deepen, and he will fall asleep. He will sleep deeper and deeper until he is as deeply asleep as at present. These suggestions should be repeated and the patient may be asked if he understands thoroughly what he is to do. If he seems confused, the suggestions should be repeated when the drug effect is not so pronounced. As soon as the patient understands what is expected of him, he is asked to repeat what will happen at the next session. After the narcosynthesis session, and before the patient is fully awake, he may be shown the fixation object and sleep suggestions are given to him with the added suggestion, after he closes his eyes, that the next time he is shown the object he will go to sleep faster and more deeply. Again before leaving the room this procedure is repeated. The technic works best when positive transference phenomena are operative in the narcotic state. It may not succeed in the event the patient does not understand what he is to do, or if he is in a state of hostile resistance.

Sodium amytal, in my experience, has advantages over other drugs. There are various technics of administration. One method is to dissolve one gram of sodium amytal in thirty or forty cc. of sterilized distilled water. A small gage intravenous needle attached to a large syringe is used for the administration which is made slowly at the rate of about one to two cc. per minute. Caffeine with sodium benzoate should be kept at hand and used in the event of respiratory embarrassment At the termination of the interview, seven and one-half grains of caffeine may be injected subcutaneously to facillitate awaking. Sodium pentothal may be used also, dissolving seven and one-half grains in twenty cc. of sterilized distilled water. In the course of administration a conversation is carried on with the patient and drug injections should be halted temporarily in the event the patient is too incoherent. Should the patient become too alert, more drug is introduced. It goes without saying that adequate preparations must be made for the patient so that he can sleep off the effects of the drug.

I have utilized prolonged nitrous oxide and oxygen inhalations with a special respirator, but see no advantages over sodium amytal for the purposes outlined above. There are certain emotional conditions which seem to be responsive to nitrous oxide from a therapeutic standpoint, but a description of these and an account of the technic is outside the purpose of this volume.

INCREASING TRANCE DEPTH

Once the patient is brought to a point in the trance where he experiences a disturbance in cutaneous sensibility, he may proceed to the next phase in the training process. In nonresistive patients, the second trance session may proceed from this point on. Where the patient prefers it, he may lie on a couch rather than sit up in a chair. Many patients prefer the couch position because it allows them to relax better.

The patient first is inducted into a trance and rapidly carried through limb and lid catalepsy, inhibition of voluntary movements, automatic movements and disturbances in cutaneous sensibility. Then he is given the following suggestions, successful execution of which indicate greater trance depth.

Ability to Talk in the Trance without Awakening. It is desirable to get the patient to a point in hypnosis where he is able to carry on a conversation without arousing from the trance. In a number of cases this ability can be developed in the subject through training even though he may not have the aptitude of developing analgesia. Suggestions such as these may be used: "Even though you are asleep, you will be able to hear my voice very distinctly and to talk to me without awakening. You will talk back just like a person in his sleep. You will be able to answer my questions without awakening and without difficulty."

At this point, simple questions can be asked which do not arouse conflicts or fears, such as whether he feels comfortable, where he lives, how old he is, and so forth. "Now you see you are able to talk to me even though you are drowsy. Your eyes still are shut fast, you cannot move your limbs, and you remain asleep even though you talk to me. As you talk, you may want to open your eyes or move your limbs, but you will feel you do not desire to do this until I tell you to open your eyes or to move your limbs." Later on, as the patient becomes better trained in hypnosis, he will be able to answer questions even though they invoke considerable anxiety.

The patient may also be trained in free association.[4] He is informed that he is to express every thought or feeling, no matter how insignificant or ridiculous these may seem, and to talk about anything that comes to his mind. To do this he must allow his mind to wander and he must keep nothing back. The patient may then be asked, "Supposing you make your mind a blank for a moment, then tell me the first thing that pops up in your mind." The patient may not succeed very well at first, but with training he may become facile in talking about his associations.

Hallucinatory Suggestions. To produce hallucinations by suggestion the patient may be trained as follows: "As you sit there I'm going to suggest to you that you imagine yourself and myself walking out of the door together. We approach a church yard. We walk into the church yard and as we look directly overhead, we notice the church steeple. I want you to picture this in your mind and as soon as you see the church, indicate it to me by your left hand rising about six inches off your thigh."

When the hand rises, suggestions continue: "Now look at the church building and steeple and notice a bell, a large bell. As soon as you see the bell, indicate it to me by your hand rising again." When the patient responds, he is told, "Watch the bell, and you will notice that it begins to move. Watch it move, and as it moves you get a sensation as if the bell is ringing. As soon as you hear the bell ringing or get a sensation as if the bell is ringing, indicate it to me by your hand rising again."

If the patient is responding readily, and if he seems to be in a good trance, the following suggestions may be given to him: "Now listen very intently. You will be able to hear the sound of the church bell tolling. It rings loud and clear. Listen carefully, and you will hear it. As soon as you do raise your hand."

Should the patient fail in the last test, he is told: "You are responding well to suggestions, the next time you will be able to hear the bell more distinctly."

Following this the patient is told: "I'm going to pick up a small bottle. Visualize me doing that. You are curious as to what is in the bottle. You look at the label and notice a flower on the label. You realize perfume is in the bottle. Visualize a flower, and, as you do you will smell the perfume. I am going to place the bottle under your nose and you will smell perfume." The physician may then remove the cork from a small empty bottle for the sound effect. Then he places the bottle under the patient's nose, remarking, "As soon as you smell the perfume, indicate it to me by your left hand rising about six inches."

Fantasy and Dream Induction. These are extremely valuable technics which permit the physician to work much more dynamically with the patient's problems. Instructions such as follow are given the patient: "Now as you sit there, I'm going to ask you to visualize yourself inside a theater. You are sitting in a seat in the second or third row. You are observing the stage. You notice that the curtains are drawn together. Raise your hand about six inches when you visualize this." When the patient raises his hand, suggestions continue. "You are curious as to what is going on behind the curtain. Then you notice a man (*or woman if the patient is a woman*) standing on the stage at the far end of the curtain. He has an expression of extreme fear and horror on his face as if he is observing behind the curtain the most frightening and horrible thing imaginable. You wonder what this may be, and you seem to absorb this man's (*or woman's*) fear. In a moment the curtain will open suddenly and you will see what frightens the person. As soon as you do tell me about it without waking up. As soon as you see action on the stage, tell me exactly what you see."

After the patient describes what he sees, he is told: "You continue to sit in the theater observing the stage. The curtain again is closed. You see the same man, but this time, instead of having a fearful expression on his face, he has a happy expression. It is as if he is filled with unbounded happiness and joy, and as you watch him, you begin to participate in his happy feelings. You wonder what causes him to be so happy. In a moment the curtain will open suddenly, and you will see what makes him feel so happy. You will see the happiest and most delightful thing that can happen to a person. As soon as you see action on the stage, tell me exactly what you see."

Upon describing his fantasy, the patient is told: "What you have observed are fantasies. Fantasies are thought processes in a state of reverie. They are related to dreams. As a matter of fact dreams are nothing more than fantasies in a state of sleep. Whenever in the future I ask you to dream while you are in a trance, it will be possible for you to let your mind wander and to have a series of thought processes similar to those I have just described. Or you may have an actual dream. When I give you the suggestion to dream, just let yourself sleep deeply enough so that a series of images comes to your mind. If you find it difficult to dream, imagine yourself in a theater, sitting in the second or third row, looking at the stage. As you watch the drawn curtain, it will suddenly open, and you will see action. For example, as you sit there now, I want you to go into a deep sleep and to have a dream, anything that happens to come to your mind. As soon as you have had this dream, tell me about it without waking up."

The fantasies that the patient has produced in reference to situations of fear and happiness can yield important clues as to his own conflicts. Later on, with this technic perfected, it is possible to get the patient to dream or to produce fantasies relating to any special topics, such as existing anxieties, resistance manifestations, and transference feelings toward the physician.

Psychotherapeutic Suggestions. Before the second trance session, the physician will probably have made an appraisal of the patient's problem, and in consideration of such factors as the time available for therapy, the depth of personality modifications desired, the motivations of the patient, and his ego strength, an estimate will have been made of the therapeutic goal. Depending upon the goal, suggestions may be made during the second trance session toward symptom removal, guidance, reassurance, persuasion, desensitization, re-education, reconditioning, or towards an analytic understanding of the dynamic sources of the patient's difficulty.

Once the therapeutic objective has been determined, the physician must work in the trance toward establishing the type of relationship which will permit the achievement of this objective. For instance, if symptom removal through prestige suggestion is the goal, and no structural changes in the personality are planned, strong directiveness and authoritarianism will have to be maintained in the trance. If, on the other hand, deep changes are desired in the personality structure, a cooperative, nondirective type of relationship will probably be necessary, and the conduct of the trance session must be of a type where the patient participates actively.

Posthypnotic Suggestions. Where the patient has been told, prior to the induction of hypnosis, that he will remember all events that have occurred, specific directions to forget the events during hypnosis should not be given him. Despite the statement that he remember, if he has developed a somnambulistic trance, a partial or complete amnesia will probably exist. A very simple way of determining the presence of amnesia is to have the patient repeat a six digit series without instructing him to remember this. In recounting his trance experiences the patient, in failing to recall the numbers, may give indication as to the presence of amnesia.

There are two posthypnotic suggestions which are more or less easily produced. The first involves posthypnotic dreaming, the second, posthypnotic blinking.

Posthypnotic suggestions to dream may be phrased as follows: "After you go to bed tonight, you will have a dream which you will probably remember. You will also probably dream on other evenings after tonight. I want you to remember the dreams, if possible, and bring them to me when you come here next time. Do you understand?"

In giving the patient suggestions for posthypnotic blinking, he is told: "I am going to awaken you soon by counting slowly from one to five. At the count of five, open your eyes and look at me. You will notice that your eyes will begin blinking spasmodically, and that no matter how hard you try to control blinking, it will be impossible to prevent your eyes from blinking as you look at me. I will then ask you to close your eyes, and I will count from one to three. At the count of three I want you to open your eyes, and this time it will be possible for you to look at me steadily without blinking. Now start waking up slowly. One, two, three, four, five."

Awakening the Patient

The regular counting suggestions for awakening the patient are then given to him, and, if the suggestion for post-hypnotic blinking has been made, this suggestion is repeated immediately prior to the completion of the count. After the patient awakens, he may be asked what he remembers of the trance, and his reaction to it. In many instances the patient will express a fear that he is not responding to suggestions, or that he has not been asleep. He should be quickly reassured, and told that he is responding quite satisfactorily, and that he will become more and more convinced of this as time goes on.

REFERENCES

[1]Horsley, J. S.: Narco-analysis.   London, Oxford University Press, 1943.
[2]Kubie, L. S., and Margolin, S.: The therapeutic role of drugs in the process of repression, dissociation and synthesis.
[3]Brenman, M., and Gill, M. M.: Hypnotherapy.   Publication of the Josiah Macy, Jr. Foundation, vol. II, no. 3, 1944, pp. 21-25.
[4]Wolberg, L. R.: Hypnoanalysis.   New York, Grune & Stratton, 1945, pp. 175-182.

VII

SUBSEQUENT HYPNOTIC SESSIONS

Subsequent hypnotic sessions are concerned with the following: (1) Continued training in trance depth to the limit of the patient's capacities; (2) Teaching the patient to enter a trance state rapidly at a given signal; (3) Administration of therapeutic suggestions, (4) Training in hypnoanalytic procedures in cases where a modified analytic approach is indicated.

Continued Training in Trance Depth

While the great majority of patients will not require more than a light or medium trance for hypnotherapy, a somnambulistic state is necessary in some forms of symptom removal, in reconditioning, in the induction of experimental conflicts, and in such hypnoanalytic technics as regression and revivification, play therapy, dramatics, automatic drawing and mirror gazing.

Approximately one out of ten patients will, with very little training, be capable of entering a somnambulistic trance with posthypnotic amnesia. As many as five out of ten patients can, with proper training, be taught to enter a deep trance with varying degrees of posthypnotic amnesia. Success will depend upon the personality and persistence of the physician, as well as upon his skill in detecting and overcoming specific resistances of the patient. People differ in their capacity to comply with hypnotic suggestions. There are some persons who develop deep anesthesias and hallucinations on command within a few minutes after the first induction. Other persons may need an hour of preparatory suggestions before they succumb to a trance. They may require another half-hour before they enter a deep trance, and even more time to achieve the deepest somnambulistic state. Most people are, with the usual technics, unable to achieve somnambulism until the third or fourth trance.

Training a person to reach a somnambulistic state may require a tremendous amount of patience. Most failures in achieving depth are due to the fact that the physician is too hurried in his approach. Where the therapeutic method requires a very deep trance, a sufficiently long time must be set aside for the patient so that he can enter gradually into a state where he responds automatically to suggestions without injecting into the situation his usual waking reactions. At the beginning, one and a half or two hours or even more time may be needed. With proper training this may be brought down to one hour, and finally, after the patient is so trained that spontaneous activity is inhibited without resistance, it may be possible to obtain a stuporous trance and somnambulism in a relatively few minutes.

Where definite resistances to trance depth crop up which cannot be overcome by ordinary training procedures, the technics applying to resistive subjects, outlined previously, may be tried. In some cases the required depth of trance may not be obtained except with supplementary hypnotic drugs.

As a general rule, successive trance states make for a deepening of hypnosis. There are, however, important exceptions to this rule. Compulsive personalities with an ambivalent attitude toward authority, as well as magical expectations of what the trance will do for them, often display hostility that manifests itself in a successful defiance of hypnotic suggestions. Patients with a markedly devaluated self esteem, in whom there is a compulsion to fail, may transfer the need to fail to the achievement of a deep trance.

At successive inductions the deepening of the trance may be enhanced by introducing periodically, during the trance, sleep intervals ranging from five to fifteen minutes. The production of more and more vivid hallucinations and of cataleptic phenomena help impress on the patient the fact that he is capable of achieving a deep trance. Where there is hesitation in obeying any command, this command should be worked at, and no suggestions should be given corresponding to a deeper state of hypnosis until the command is executed freely. There are times when this rule has to be disregarded, since some subjects seem to be unable to develop certain types of phenomena. For instance, a patient may be able to go into deep hypnosis even though he is unable to develop analgesia. In one somnambule, resistance to development of hallucinations was found to be due to a belief that anyone who heard voices or saw visions was incurably insane. Only after this misconception was removed were hallucinations possible.

Patients vary in their susceptibility to hypnosis from day to day. A refractory patient may suddenly go into a deep hypnotic state for no apparent reason. How long to continue attempts at hypnosis in order to induce somnambulism is difficult to say. For practical purposes where there is no response to several successive inductions, attempts may be halted with the statement that the patient is in a sufficiently deep trance for effective therapeutic suggestions.

The ultimate aim of training in depth is to get the patient to a point where he is able to open his eyes in a trance without awakening, to develop amnesia, and finally to respond to complicated posthypnotic suggestions.

Opening the Eyes without Awakening. In teaching the patient to open his eyes without awakening, he may be given the following suggestion: "As you sit there, imagine that I am holding a bottle of water close to your eyes. You notice that it is colorless; but as you watch it, it slowly changes to a pink color, and finally to a reddish color. As soon as you see the color change, as soon as you visualize the color changing to red, indicate that to me by your left hand rising about six inches."

When the patient responds, he is told: "Even though you

are asleep, deeply asleep, it will be possible for you to open your eyes slowly without awakening. At first things will be hazy, then they will become more clear; but you will still be asleep, deeply asleep, even though you have your eyes wide open. You will continue to stay asleep with your eyes wide open until I give you the command to awaken. It will be possible for you to stand up and walk around the room just like a person walks in his sleep. It will be possible for you to observe things that I point out to you. When you open your eyes, you will notice that I hold a bottle of clear fluid in front of your eyes. As you watch the bottle, it will slowly change to a pinkish color and finally to a reddish color, similar to the experience you just had with your eyes shut. As soon as you see the color change, indicate that to me by your left hand rising about six inches. Now slowly open your eyes; very slowly open your eyes. Things will be blurred at first, but as you look at the bottle, they will clear up, and you will notice that the color will change to a pinkish, then to a reddish color. Slowly open your eyes, open them wider and wider." A bottle containing water may then be brought close to the patient's eyes, and he may be asked to gaze at the bottle until he notices that the color changes to pink or red.

As soon as the patient acknowledges the fact that he sees the color change, he may be given another hallucinatory suggestion. "Look at the table in front of you and you will notice that there is a candlestick there with a burning candle. Go over and blow it out." This direction should be repeated several times.

Developing Amnesia. If a patient has reached the somnambulistic state, he will probably awaken from the trance with a spontaneous amnesia. In some cases the patient may need special training in forgetting certain aspects of the trance or the entire trance experience. The first step is ascertaining how much of the trance has been forgotten.

Should the patient recall everything, he may be told immediately preceding termination of the next trance session that he will imagine he is at home asleep, that he will have a short dream following which his eyes will open, and he will awaken with a start. As soon as he awakens, he will get the impression that he has just aroused himself from a sound sleep. He will remember the dream vividly, but immediately after recounting it, he will have a hazy recollection of the other events in the trance. He may even forget some of them when questioned.

If the patient develops a partial amnesia as a result of these suggestions, he may be told during the next trance: "Forgetting is a perfectly normal experience and is a means of preventing an overburdening of the mind. It is easy to forget by shifting attention from some things. For instance, last time you forgot certain experiences that happened in the trance. (*The specific experiences should be mentioned.*) This is perfectly normal. Today you will probably forget many, most or even all of the experiences you are having now. You will, before you awaken, have a dream. As soon as you dream, awaken with a start, as if you are at home in bed, and have just awakened from a sound sleep. You will remember the dream, but you will forget all or most of the other events that have happened."

There are some patients who seem unable to develop the capacity to develop amnesia. For one reason or another they have a need to retain sufficient control of their faculties to remember what has occurred in the trance state. Injunctions that they forget are met with an embarrassed or defiant remembering. For this reason a suggestion that the patient remember some minor aspect of the trance may be included in the suggestions for amnesia.

Posthypnotic Suggestions. It is best to proceed slowly with posthypnotic suggestions. If the patient responds positively to suggestions for posthypnotic eye-blinking and dreaming, he may be given a suggestion that he will exhibit, at a given signal, phenomena which were produced in the trance. For instance, hyperesthesia of the right hand and anesthesia of the left hand may be induced during the trance, and the patient may be told: "After you awaken and have been awake a while, I will tap three times on the desk. At the third tap you will notice that your right hand will tingle and be sensitive, while the left hand will be numb. This will last until I tap once more on the desk, when the hands will return to a normal sensation." The hyperesthesia and anesthesia are then removed and the suggestion repeated immediately prior to awakening the patient.

Another posthypnotic suggestion that is often effective is requesting the patient to dream in the trance, to awaken upon completing the dream, but to forget the dream on awakening, as if he has just come out of a very deep sleep. He will be unable to remember the dream until the physician taps on the desk three times, whereupon the dream will suddenly pop into his mind and he will repeat it.

The patient accordingly is given the following suggestion: "I want you now to have a dream. As soon as you have the dream, your right hand will rise straight up in the air until it touches your face. As soon as it touches your face your eyes will open, and you will awaken with a start. But you will have forgotten the dream completely. Every time you think of it your mind will go blank. However, I will rap on my desk three times, and when you hear the third rap, the dream will suddenly pop into your mind and you will tell me about it."

In giving the patient posthypnotic suggestions, these should be as specific as possible, and must be repeated several times. It is often desirable to ask the patient whether he understands what he is to do upon awakening. His ability to recount what is expected of him will usually insure success. Where a specific action is suggested, it is usually helpful to give the patient a cue, such as the tapping above, following which he is to perform the posthypnotic act. Where therapeutic posthypnotic suggestions are given, it is not necessary to inject a cue. It is best to forumulate posthypnotic suggestions in such a manner that they will not conflict too drastically with the patient's personality or customary activities. Under no circumstances is the patient to be made to perform a ridiculous act, since resistance may be provoked that will interfere with a proper relationship. It is also desirable, especially with a patient who is a somnambule, to give him posthypnotic suggestions to the effect that he will not be hypnotizable by any person except the physician.

Conditioning the Trance to a Given Signal

As a general rule successive inductions are associated with an ability on the part of the patient to sink into a trance more and more easily. It is usually best at the second or third session to condition the patient to enter a trance upon a given signal. The nature of this signal can vary. It may be a certain word or sentence, or an auditory stimulus such as a bell or buzzing sound, or a visual stimulus like a blinking electric light. The patient is given a suggestion, such as follows, while he is in a trance:

"You are deeply asleep at the present time. Now listen to me carefully. From now on it will not be necessary to go through the process of hypnotizing you each time you come here. When I give you a certain signal like tapping on the desk (*any other signal may be introduced here if desired*), you will very easily and immediately enter into a state of sleep as deep as the one you are in now."

This suggestion is repeated and then the patient is told: "I am now going to awaken you. As soon as I awaken you, I am going to give you the signal. The moment you hear the signal, you will again fall asleep as deeply as you are now. Do you understand?" After this the patient is awakened and immediately thereupon the signal is given him, to demonstrate to him that he will be responsive to it. As soon as he falls asleep again, the suggestions are repeated, and the patient is then requested to acknowledge the fact that he understands that he is to fall asleep at any time when the signal is presented to him.

At the next trance session the patient is told that he will be given a signal whereupon he will automatically start falling asleep. The signal is then presented, and after the patient has entered a·trance state, the suggestion is reinforced.

When the patient is later trained in self hypnosis, he may be taught to give himself a verbal signal in order to achieve a trance state.

Administration of Therapeutic Suggestions

The point in the induction process where therapeutic suggestions are introduced will vary with the patient's problems, his aptitude for hypnosis and his personality makeup. In some cases of symptom removal it may be expedient to confine therapy to a prolonged single session, slowly and progressively inducting the patient into a very deep trance prior to the termination of which therapeutic suggestions are introduced. In other cases a half dozen sessions may pass before therapy is started. As a general rule therapeutic suggestions should be made when the patient has achieved his maximum in trance depth.

Because of the heightened suggestibility in the trance, psychotherapeutic efforts are usually responded to more readily than in the waking state. The close relationship to the physician which is a product of hypnosis carries over into waking life, and the patient will continue to respond better to therapy even when hypnosis is discontinued.

There are some patients who regard hypnosis as a miraculous cure-all, and who are inclined toward hostility and depression when their problems do not dissolve in thin air after a series of trance sessions. Persons suffering from severe character disturbances with markedly devaluated self esteem particularly expect that the physician will produce in them, through the medium of hypnosis, vigor and self confidence without any effort of their own.

In such patients it is best to halt hypnosis at a point where the patient has reached his deepest level of trance depth with an explanation such as the following:

"As you sit (or lie) there relaxed and drowsy, I am going to talk to you to explain the technics that will be necessary to help your condition. You have certain problems and symptoms that are the product of fears and conflicts that probably go far back in your life. We are anxious that you achieve permanent, not temporary, relief. Therefore, it will be necessary to learn everything we can about your symptoms, what they mean, how they started, and under what conditions they appear today. Because most conflicts are unconscious, it is difficult to get at them. In a drowsy, relaxed state such as you are in now, it will be possible to make suggestions to you so that you will, after you awaken, from now on, for as long as it will be necessary, be able to help me to help you understand what is behind your symptoms. No matter what resistances or doubts you may have, you will find yourself doing what is necessary to get well. We have now achieved the important thing in hypnosis of enlisting the aid of your unconscious. For the time being hypnosis will not be necessary, and we will continue with psychotherapy on a waking level. You will be responsive to this therapy, even though we never again use hypnosis. Doubts, anxieties and resistances may crop up in the course of treatment. In spite of these, you will be able to make progress. Do you understand and are you willing to cooperate in our treatment plan?"

Even though hypnosis is discontinued, the few trance sessions the patient has had may effect so positive a relationship with the physician that therapy in the waking state will proceed with fewer resistances and with greater rapidity. Sufficient emphasis cannot be placed on the fact that many of the beneficial effects of hypnosis accrue from the emotional feelings toward the physician which are expedited by the trance.

A question that is often asked refers to the effect on the patient's capacity to follow therapeutic suggestions after he has been unable or has refused to experience certain suggested phenomena in the trance. Should the patient resist successfully some of the physician's suggestions, might this not lower the latter's prestige and cause the patient to refuse to follow therapeutic suggestions? When the physician sets himself up as an omniscient personage whose mandates the patient dare not resist, there is definite danger of this. The patient who is antagonistic to such a relationship will pit his resistive powers against the strength of the physician's commands. In such a struggle the patient will usually emerge victorious to the detriment of the therapeutic plan.

In some programs of psychotherapy, an authoritarian directive relationship may be deemed necessary. In order not to jeopardize this relationship, the physician should always instruct the patient that there are some kinds of phenomena he may be unable to experience in the trance, there are others he will experience partially, and still others quite vividly. This is to be expected since the nervous make-up of different people varies, and they show varying apti-tudes in achieving certain feelings and sensations. The important thing is not how many of the suggested kinds of phenomena he experiences, but rather that he is in a relaxed, drowsy state and experiences some of the things brought to his attention. It is this state that will make him amenable to those suggestions that will be valuable to him in over-coming his disturbing symptoms. Because he realizes their importance, he will be unable to resist these therapeutic suggestions. The stronger his desire to get well, the greater will be his determination to follow these therapeutic suggestions that will make him well.

Where the therapeutic goal demands a nondirective or analytic approach, the matter of the patient's failing to experience suggested phenomena need not affect the therapeutic relationship. The conduct of the trance session here encourages the patient's active participation. It is suggested to the patient that he will be increasingly curious as to the different kinds of phenomena he can observe in himself. It does not matter whether such phenomena occur or not. The important thing is that the patient enjoy the experience of going into a trance and of experiencing things that will prove to be of value in making him an emotionally healthy person. Should the patient fail to experience any phenomenon in the trance, he will believe this to be his prerogative, and he will not be so apt to feel frustrated.

Patients who are able to achieve only light trance depths are particularly susceptible to a fear that their therapy will prove to be a failure. Where it is obvious that no more than a light trance is possible, the patient's fear must be anticipated. He may be given an explanation such as follows:

"You are drowsy and relaxed as you sit (*or lie*) there, and are fully aware of what I am saying to you. It will not be necessary for you to be more deeply asleep, and it may be inadvantageous. In the state you are in now, of being relaxed and slightly drowsy, therapeutic suggestions are particularly effective in penetrating into the subconscious mind. The conscious mind often has resistances to curative suggestions. In a state such as you are in at present, we can approach your unconscious mind, which governs your fears and your symptoms. You will respond to the therapeutic suggestions I give you, even though you may doubt your capacity to be responsive. No matter how much you fear that suggestions will be ineffective, you will find that they will work nevertheless.''

It may also be wise to repeat the fact that while sleep sug-

gestions are being given, he will not really be asleep, since he
will be conscious of everything that occurs. Although it may
seem to him as if he is wide awake, nevertheless, he will actually be in a relaxed drowsy trance state which renders his
unconscious mind remarkably susceptible to suggestion.
He may be told that unconscious mental activities influence
the development of symptoms, and that hypnotic therapy
gets deep into the unconscious strata of mind.   In this way
it can have a definite therapeutic effect even in cases where
the person does not believe it can help him. It is necessary
not to promise a cure, but to state that improvement will
depend largely on the patient's cooperation and desire to
be helped.

Where symptom removal, reassurance, guidance, persuasion, and re-education are to be used, such an explanation is
often effective. The patient may be told in the waking state,
should he continue to evidence doubts, that there are certain
advantages to a light trance, since it combines a control of
functions with a conscious willingness to cooperate. The
person is able to remember, to criticize and to maintain
freedom and activity in his thought processes. This makes
him an ally and does not force him into actions which might
create antagonism. Under deep hypnosis, he may automatically obey, but his compliance will not change his inner strivings, motivations and convictions. What is essential is that
he, himself, see the necessity for doing those things that will
lead to his cure.

Where an analytic approach is indicated, and the patient
is unable to achieve somnambulism, he may be taught the
technic of free association and fantasy and dream induction
under light hypnosis. In the trance the patient is encouraged
to participate actively in getting to the bottom of his fears
and conflicts. He is told that his symptoms have a cause and
a meaning. He will have a desire to inquire into his relationships with people, to see under what circumstances his symp-

toms appear or become exaggerated. He will begin to understand how his difficulty originated and the conditions that brought it about. While free association and dreams under hypnosis will help him achieve these aims, he will also find himself more capable of establishing a continuity between his symptoms and his deeper personality problems in waking life. This insight will enable him to adjust to his inner needs and to external demands without the fears and misunderstandings that have plagued him up to the present. His relationships with people will then become more productive and congenial.

HYPNOANALYTIC PROCEDURES

Where the patient's problem is such that it requires analytic probing, and where his motivations and ego strength will allow of such an approach, he may be trained in the various hypnoanalytic procedures.

The technics of free association, of fantasy and dream induction, will require no more than a light or medium trance. The specific directions for these technics have already been discussed, and more complete details on the latter procedures, as well as on the other hypnoanalytic methods to be outlined, may be obtained elsewhere.[1]

The technics of automatic writing, hypnotic drawing, play therapy during hypnosis, dramatics under hypnosis, regression and revivification, crystal and mirror gazing, and the induction of experimental conflicts will require a deep if not somnambulistic trance.

The patient may be trained in automatic writing by being told during a trance that it will be possible for him to write without being completely aware of what his hand is doing. A suggestion such as the following may be made:

"I'm going to stroke your hand, and you will begin to experience the feeling as if it is detached from your body. I will place a pencil in your hand and then put the pencil on a pad of paper. Your hand will begin moving along, writing on the paper, as if an outside force were pushing it along. Your hand will continue to move even though you concentrate your attention on something entirely apart from the writing."

Because the productions in automatic writing are fragmentary and cryptic, it will be essential to train the patient to translate what he has written. This can be done by giving him a suggestion that he will be able to open his eyes without awakening, and that he will be able to translate the meaning of what his hand has written. Posthypnotic suggestions may be given the patient that it will be possible for him to write automatically in the waking state, that he may do this while engaged in another activity, such as reading a book. What he has written during the waking state, may, of course, require translation under hypnosis.

Training the individual to draw hypnotically requires some patience. The patient is told in a trance that it will be possible for him to open his eyes and to sketch freely anything that he wants to draw. He may also be requested to draw pictures of various people or of certain emotional situations. It may be possible to get him to illustrate a dream or an experience. The drawing technic may be utilized with suggestions for age regression in an attempt to arrive at an understanding of the genetic determinants of the patient's problems. Under hypnosis the patient can be asked to translate the meaning of his drawings or to associate freely to them. A story telling technic may be combined with hypnotic drawing.

Play therapy under hypnosis is often highly effective inasmuch as the individual is much more facile in expressing his emotions in the trance state. With his eyes open while in the trance, the patient is given a variety of play materials and encouraged to build or to play in any manner that he desires. Story telling can be combined with play therapy. The patient also may be enjoined to identify with one of the dolls and to construct situations out of his life experiences. Regression may be utilized with technics for play therapy.

Dramatics under hypnosis are frequently an effective means of getting the patient to "act out" his difficulties with a cathartic effect. In the last war hypnosis was frequently utilized for this purpose, the patient being urged in the trance to relive the traumatic battle scene. The patient is given suggestions during the trance that he will be able to imagine himself re-experiencing the traumatic event. In the course of this he may open his eyes and misidentify the physician as an important personage who played a prominent role in his past. Immediate life situations and problems in present relationships may also be dramatized.

There are several methods of producing regression, one way being as follows: "As you lie there, listen carefully to what I say to you. Time is a relative thing. The individual always incorporates within himself every action, every event of his past. No memory is ever forgotten. It resides within, and can be brought up again by going back to the time of the memory. As you lie there imagine that we are turning back time like the pages of a book. You will feel yourself beginning to go back in time, and you may actually experience the sensation of your body beginning to get smaller, smaller and smaller. Your head will feel small, your arms and legs will feel small. You will feel small all over, and when I talk to you next, you will be exactly six years of age. (*Any other age may be introduced here.*) As you lie there, you will begin to feel yourself growing smaller and smaller, and as soon as you feel yourself to have grown small, as soon as you get the sensation that you are six years of age, your left hand will rise from your thigh about six inches." Should the patient have a specific symptom or fear, the origin of which he cannot remember, he may be given suggestions to regress to the time of the first development of the symptom, and to recount all the details.

Where the technic of crystal or mirror gazing is required, the patient is requested to open his eyes without awakening. He is presented with a crystal, with a glass of water, or with a mirror which reflects the blank ceiling. He is then given the following suggestions: "As you look into the mirror (*or crystal, or glass of water*) you will begin to see things vividly in it. You will see action as if you are watching a play. Describe to me exactly what you see." Specific situations, forgotten memories, or significant relationships with past authorities may be visualized dramatically through this technic.

In inducing an experimental conflict, the patient is given this suggestion: "As you sleep deeply, I am going to bring back to your mind an event that occurred to you some time ago, but which you have forgotten. There are reasons why you forgot this event, but as I recall the event to you, you will remember the circumstance in great detail. You will recall fully the event just as it happened, and you will re-experience the feelings relating to the event exactly as when it occurred the first time."

A fictitious situation that is built up around the patient's difficulty is then introduced as an event that had once occurred. He is told: "After you have awakened, the situation as I have described it will be on your mind. You will not be aware consciously of the situation, but it will govern your actions and your speaking. I have told you about an experience which happened to you. You recalled this in great detail; and after you awaken, the entire situation will be on your mind, but you will not be conscious of what it is. Nevertheless you will react to it. Do you understand?"

The reactions of the patient to such a fictitious situation may provide valuable clues to the nature of his real conflict, and guide the course of subsequent therapy.

REFERENCE

[1]WOLBERG, L. R.: Hypnoanalysis.   New York, Grune & Stratton, 1945.

VIII

SELF HYPNOSIS AND GROUP HYPNOSIS

An EFFECTIVE psychotherapeutic plan may consider the following four stages in succession: (1) inducting the patient into as deep a trance as possible; (2) utilizing the trance to expedite the type of psychotherapy most suitable for the patient; (3) teaching the patient, once the cure, improvement, or symptom relief is obtained, that he can bring about the same effects through his own efforts; (4) demonstrating to him, as soon as the latter is achieved, that therapeutic results can be maintained without need for further recourse to hypnosis.

One means by which the patient is taught that he can duplicate therapeutic effects through his own efforts is by the technic of self hypnosis. Self hypnosis, as the term is employed here, means an actual trance induced by the patient as a result of posthypnotic suggestions given him by the physician.

The aim of self hypnosis is to convince the patient that there is nothing magical about hypnosis, and that he can obtain benefits of suggestion through his own efforts. In this way he conceives of himself as capable of functioning without the need for a dependent relationship on the physician. Self hypnosis is a means of reinforcing indefinitely hypnotic suggestions. Eventually it is a way of proving to the patient that the trance is no longer necessary for permanent improvement.

The capacity to induce a trance through self suggestions and to experience certain phenomena in the trance, has, in itself, little effect on the patient's neurosis, on his self esteem, or the strengthening of the ego. However, where the individual is capable of mastering his symptoms through psycho-

therapy aided by hypnosis, the conviction that he can produce the same effects without the agency of another person
can contribute to his self confidence. The influence it exerts
on the ego is wholly dependent on the effect it has on the
patient's sense of self mastery.

Various technics may be used to produce self hypnosis.
While in a trance the patient is given the suggestion that he
will, by repeating a signal, be able to go into a deep hypnotic
sleep, during which he is conscious of everything. He may
then give himself whatever therapeutic suggestions are prescribed, and thereafter awaken himself by another signal.

The following is a transcription of two successive sessions
in which a patient was taught the technic of self hypnosis.

First Session

Dr. Now as you rest, I am going to train you how to utilize
the effects of hypnosis to improve your self confidence. I am
going to teach you how to produce the same effects that
have been produced by my suggestions through suggestions
that you give yourself.

When I give you a signal, you will awaken. I will then ask
you to bring your right hand down to your thigh. When you
have brought your hand down to your thigh, I should like
to have you give yourself the suggestion that you will gaze
at your hand intently. Then you will notice feeling various
sensations in your hand. You will become observant of what
those sensations are, no matter what they are. You tell yourself, as you watch your hand, that you are going to notice
that it will get lighter, that the fingers will move, and that
the hand will rise and lift up, up, up, straight up towards
your face. When your hand touches your face you'll be asleep,
deeply asleep, the same as you are now. I'm going to count
from one to five; at the count of five open your eyes and
awaken. Bring your hand down to your thigh, and then give
yourself the suggestions that I mentioned to you to put
yourself to sleep. One, two, three, four, five.

(Patient opens his eyes, brings his hand down to his thigh, observes it closely as it wiggles, rises and moves up towards his face, following which his eyes close.)

Now you notice that as you brought your hand down to your thigh, the fingers moved, that they spread apart, that the hand lifted, that the arm rose, that your eyes got heavy, your eyelids closed, and that you fell asleep again. In the state of drowsiness that you are in now, I'm going to stroke your left arm, and as I stroke the arm, it will suddenly become heavy and stiff and rigid to a point where it will not bend. I'm going to stroke your arm now this way, and I'm going to hold it out in front of you, this way. I'm going to stroke it and count from one to five. When I reach the count of five, your arm will have gotten so stiff that it will be impossible to move it or bend it. One, two, three, four, five. Stiff and rigid and firm, just like a board, so that even though you try to bend it with all your might, the harder you try, the heavier and stiffer and more rigid it is, until I give you the suggestion, by counting from one to five, that it will loosen up. At the count of five, the rigidity will leave it, and you will be able to bring your arm down to your thigh. One, two, three, four, five. The rigidity disappears; it comes down to your thigh in exactly that way.

This time, I shall give you the suggestion to open your eyes and awaken again at a certain signal. Then I want you to put yourself to sleep in the same way that you did before. Upon putting yourself to sleep, I want you then to give yourself suggestions that your left arm will become heavy and stiff and rigid, that it will stick right out in front of you. You will try to bend it, and you will notice that it will be impossible to bend it until you count from one to five. And when you count from one to five, the rigidity will leave the arm; it will come down to your thigh in exactly the same position that it is now. You still will be deeply asleep. I am going to count from one to five, and when I reach the count of five, open your eyes and bring your hand down on your thigh. Put yourself to sleep and give yourself the suggestion to produce rigidity in your arm. Then by counting to five, remove the rigidity. One, two, three, four, five.

(*Patient follows these suggestions and after producing arm rigidity, he counts.*)

Pt. One, two, three, four, five. (*The arm rigidity disappears.*)

Dr. Now you notice that you have put yourself to sleep again and that you induced arm rigidity. You tried to bend the arm. It would not bend, so that you gave yourself a suggestion that the arm would loosen up by counting from one to five. The arm lost its rigidity, came down, and now you are deeply asleep. As you sit there, I'm going to give you a suggestion that you be able to sit in your chair with your chin down, fully asleep and to bring your right hand down to your thigh while you sleep. Now imagine yourself walking along a corridor. You see a pail of hot water in the corner. You look at the pail of hot water. You wonder exactly how hot that water is, and as you wonder how hot the water is, you decide that you're going to take your hand, your right hand, and plunge it in the water to determine how hot it is. You do, and the hand is burned. It will feel a little tender and achy. When you visualize yourself doing that, indicate it to me by your left hand rising about six inches. Visualize yourself walking along, taking your hand, plunging it into the water, so that it feels as if it's burned and achy. Indicate to me that you have done this by your left hand rising up about six inches. (*Long pause.*)

Your hand rises and now it comes down. I'm going to pinch it, and you'll notice that when I pinch it, there will be a difference in the sensitivity of your right hand as compared with your left hand. I'll show you. You've just plunged it into this pail of hot water and it is raw and red and tender. As I pinch it, you notice the sensitivity as compared with

the normal hand on the other side. You notice the difference when I pinch it?

Pt. Yes.

Dr. You notice that? Good. Now imagine that you've gone
into a doctor's office for an infection involving one of the
fingers of the left hand. The doctor injects novocaine all the
way around the wrist producing a wrist block. You begin to
develop the sensation of your hand becoming numb, almost
as if you're wearing a thick heavy leather glove. As soon as
you get the sensation that you're wearing a thick, heavy
leather glove, as soon as you visualize yourself wearing a thick
heavy leather glove, indicate it to me by your left hand rising
up about six inches. Just imagine that you're wearing a thick
heavy leather glove, and then the hand will start feeling
numb. When the hand becomes numb, it will rise about six
inches. (*Pause*)

Your hand rises, and it comes down. I'm going to pinch
the two hands now. This right one will continue to remain
quite sensitive, and this left one will remain numb, the pain
will have disappeared. When I pinch it, there won't be any
real pain. Do you notice that? But when I pinch the right
one the pain will be almost excruciating. You notice that, the
difference in the two? Now, I'm going to ask you to pinch
your own hands alternately as you sit there. Pinch them and
see the difference. (*Patient pinches his hands alternately.*) You
notice the difference?

Pt. Yes.

Dr. Good. As you sit there, I'm going to give you the suggestion that you open your eyes. When I give you the signal,
proceed to put yourself to sleep. As soon as you are asleep,
give yourself the suggestion that your left arm will become
rigid and extend in front of you, so that it will be impossible
to bend it. As soon as you have achieved that, you will count
from one to five. On counting from one to five, the arm will
then loosen up, and you will be able to bring it down to your

thigh. Thereupon you will take your right hand and bring it down to your thigh. You will still remain deeply asleep. And then you will give yourself a suggestion that you're walking along a corridor. You see a pail of hot water. You take your right hand and plunge it in the water. It begins to feel achy and tender and painful. As soon as you get that sensation, then this left hand here will rise a little to indicate that you get that sensation. Immediately you'll get a feeling of wearing a thick heavy leather glove on the left, following which the hand will become numb. You will test both hands by pinching yourself to prove that the difference is there.

Right now I'm going to remove the numbness in the left by stroking your hand, and remove the sensitivity on the right too. When I pinch both hands they feel exactly the same, when I pinch here and when I pinch here. You notice that now?

Pt. Yes.

Dr. Good. They're restored to normal sensation. I'm going to ask you, when I reach the count of five, to open your eyes, put yourself to sleep, produce arm rigidity, produce hypersensitivity of the right hand, and produce numbness of the left hand, through your own efforts. Then by pinching them you will find that they are materially different. One, two, three, four, five.

(*Patient follows these suggestions and is able to notice a difference in the feelings of his hands.*)

You notice the difference, good. You have been able, by self suggestions, to put yourself to sleep, to produce arm rigidity, to produce hypersensitivity of the right hand, and to produce anesthesia of the left hand. You are going to notice an extremely interesting thing when you wake up. The hypersensitivity and the anesthesia, the numbness, will remain. The moment you wake up, test your hands and you will notice that they are materially different in feeling. However soon afterward they will return to normal.

As you sit there I'm going to give you a suggestion that you imagine yourself walking along a street approaching a churchyard. You walk into the churchyard and you notice the church, its steeple and bell. You see the bell. The bell begins to move, and as the bell moves, you get a distinct sensation of ringing, clanging. As soon as you get the impression of the clanging of the bell, indicate it to me by your hand, your left hand, rising up about six inches. (*Patient's hand rises.*) Your hand rises and it comes down.

Now I'm going to give you a suggestion that you imagine me approaching you with a bottle in my hand. I remove the cork from the bottle. You notice that the bottle has a flower on the label, and you wonder if the bottle contains perfume. I put the bottle under your nose, and you actually smell the fragrance of perfume as you watch the flower on the label. As soon as you smell the fragrance of perfume, indicate it to me by your hand, your left hand rising about six inches. (*After a pause, patient's hand rises.*)

I'm going finally to ask you to awaken when I reach the count of five. When you awaken, rapidly put yourself to sleep, produce arm rigidity, hypersensitivity of your right hand, anesthesia of your left hand, imagine yourself going into the churchyard and hearing the bell ring distinctly, and finally smell the odor of perfume. As soon as you do these things, wake yourself up by counting from one to five. After awakening you will notice that when you pinch your hands, they will still be hypersensitive on the right side and dull on the left side. Upon testing this to your satisfaction, give yourself a suggestion that they return to normal. I'm going to count from one to five, when I reach the count of five, you will be able to put yourself to sleep rapidly, to produce arm rigidity, to produce hypersensitivity of the right hand, anesthesia of the left hand, to be able to hear the bell ring, to smell perfume, and then finally to awaken.

From now on, you will be able to give yourself suggestions at any time and place, such as you've given yourself here.

You will be able to reproduce the effects such as you've produced here. You will be able to achieve those effects through your own efforts. And the effects will persist with you as long as you want. Each time you practice doing this it will reinforce your ability to do it better the next time. You will also be able to give yourself therapeutic suggestions that I have given you, that I will repeat next time. One, two, three, four, five.

(*Patient follows all of these suggestions, tests his hands and remarks that they are different in sensation.*)

Dr. You still feel the numbness and the sensitivity? When do you wish them to return to normal?

Pt. Now.

Dr. Try the sensations now. (*Patient retests hands.*) How are they?

Pt. They feel exactly the same now.

Dr. Good.

SECOND SESSION

Dr. Today I'd like to have you do this. Start in by giving yourself suggestions to put yourself to sleep. And as soon as you are asleep, I'll talk to you. (*Patient observes his arm rise and then his eyes close.*) Now I'm going to extend your left arm out in front of you, and as I stroke it, it will get stiff and rigid, heavy and firm, just like a board. At the count of five, it will be just as heavy and rigid as a board. One, two, three, four, five. Heavy and firm and rigid just like a board, and it will get heavier and heavier as you sit there. Even though you attempt to move it with all your might, the harder you try, the more rigid and firm it will become. Finally, you, yourself, upon my suggestion, will be able to remove the arm rigidity. I'm going to ask you to count from one to five, and when you reach the count of five, you will be able to move your arm back to your thigh.

Pt. One, two, three, four, five.

Dr. Your arm comes down. Now listen carefully to me. I'm going to give you a suggestion now that you go into a sufficiently deep sleep so that you have a fantasy or a dream. If dreams do not come spontaneously, you will then be able to visualize yourself sitting in the second or third row in a theater. You will notice the closed curtain on the stage. Then suddenly the curtain will open and you will see action on the stage, no matter what that may be. As soon as you see action, I want you to tell me about it without waking up. On the other hand it may be possible, as you sit there, for your sleep to get sufficiently deep so that you actually dream. In either case, tell me about it without waking up, no matter how long it takes. (*Pause*)

Pt. On a stage, the head of a newspaper office. Many people sitting at their desks using typewriters. Many other people using telephones, and one character, one voice louder than the others, that of the City Editor, who is taking a story on a particular telephone.

> (*The character of this patient's fantasies and dreams have changed remarkably during his treatment. A persuasive method seems to have brought about a different attitude toward himself. Whereas previously he has been withdrawn and timid, he has become expressive and outspoken. The editor in his fantasy undoubtedly refers to himself.*)

Dr. I see. Now listen carefully to me. I'm going to outline for you a proposed plan from this point on. It is extremely necessary for you eventually not only to have the benefits that accrue from feeling you can function well in one respect or in another, but this feeling must extend to your whole activity as a person. You will want to experience a feeling that you are able to be more outspoken, more aggressive, more active than you have ever been before. You will want to liberate yourself from the restraints and the shackles that have, up to this time, forced you to assume a submissive role, to abdicate your rights to self expression and to creative self fulfilment. You will want to develop a stature that will be very gratifying to you. You will be less concerned with a fear that you are not going to perform well, and more concerned with a desire to find pleasure in close human relationships. You will want to feel that ability growing in you. You will want to do what is necessary for you to be more extroverted and outspoken in your attitudes towards people.

I am teaching you the technic of self hypnosis, which will enable you to get to the point where you can do what is essential to develop the stature we're after. More and more you will develop a feeling that you can and will be able to succeed in having a good normal life, in being a demonstrative and successful person in your activities with other people.

Listen carefully, the suggestions I have given you, you must give yourself after you put yourself to sleep and immediately before you awaken. Do you understand?

Pt. Yes.

Dr. We have a session scheduled here for tomorrow. I'm going to give you a suggestion that instead of your coming here, you spend the session alone in your office or at home. Perhaps you will have a better opportunity of being alone at home, where you can induce self hypnosis and give yourself the therapeutic suggestions I have given you.

I will go through the whole technic with you, so that you can practice this by yourself tomorrow. Imagine that the session that you spend with yourself is equivalent to the session you were supposed to spend with me. I want you to practice this so that you can carry it out on your own, afterward. You will be able to put yourself to sleep by following the suggestions that I have given you. You will sit in a chair, and then, making sure you are going to be comfortable, you give yourself the suggestions that your hand will start moving, that it will get light, that it will lift and rise until it touches your face. Then you will go to sleep. Upon falling asleep you will give yourself the suggestion that your left arm will extend in front of you, straight out in front of you, and become rigid and firm like a board. As soon as it becomes firm and rigid, you'll notice that even though you try to move it, that will be impossible. Then you'll count from one to five, and at the count of five, the arm rigidity will disappear. The left hand will come down to your thigh. Then you will bring your right hand down from your head to your thigh.

Following this you give yourself the suggestion you imagine yourself walking along a corridor, that you see a pail of hot water in the corner, that you notice the steam issuing from the surface of the water, that you take your hand and plunge it into the water. As soon as you plunge it into the water, you feel it become sensitive, hypersensitive. The next suggestion you will give yourself will be to produce hand anesthesia. You will imagine yourself going into a doctor's office. He gives you an injection of novocaine around the left wrist. Then you get the sensation of wearing a thick heavy leather glove. You notice the difference in feeling in the two hands by pinching them alternately.

Following this I want you to give yourself those suggestions referring to your desire to overcome your panicky feelings, timidity and stage fright, which I have given you, and which you have found so useful. The suggestions you give yourself will enable you to continue wanting to correct those things in your relations with people that have caused you difficulty. They will enable you to get more self confidence and assuredness. As soon as you give yourself those suggestions, you will then sleep for about two or three minutes and then spontaneously awaken.

In the event anybody walks into the room, you will then be able to wake up by giving yourself the suggestion that you want to wake up immediately. You might mention the fact that you happened to doze off, that you felt a little sleepy. Or, if anything occurs that needs your waking attention, you will be able to awaken immediately. After this when the opportunity presents itself you can put yourself to sleep again and continue with the suggestions.

Now I'm going to count from one to five. At the count of five your eyes will open. Then I want you to put yourself to sleep, to produce hand rigidity, to remove the rigidity, to produce hand anesthesia on the left and hyperesthesia on the right, then notice the difference between the anesthetic hand on the left and the hyperesthetic hand on the right by pinching both. Then begin giving yourself therapeutic suggestions that will enable you to feel better and stronger. Following that I want you to wake yourself up. One, two, three, four, five.

> (*Patient carries out these suggestions. At the next session he is taught to put himself into a trance deeply merely by saying, "Sleep deeply now," and counting from one to five, and to give himself therapeutic suggestions without the need to produce arm rigidity or differences in cutaneous sensibility.*)

Following this he was taught to give himself the same suggestions in the waking state without hypnosis and to notice that the effect continued. Finally he was shown that his attitude toward people and toward himself had changed so materially that his gain could continue without further suggestions by virtue of the fact that he was leading a different kind of life.

GROUP HYPNOSIS

Group hypnosis is utilized for two purposes: first, to increase susceptibility to hypnosis in prospective patients; second, as a form of psychotherapy.

Although the physician will rarely have the opportunity to prepare prospective patients for hypnosis by introducing them to a group, the technic is a useful one to know. In employing group hypnosis as a means of demonstrating the phenomena of the trance, it is always helpful to include in the group one or two good hypnotic subjects.

One of the most effective means of producing group hypnosis is to tell the group that a number of nervous symptoms are caused by an inability to relax. It is possible by simple suggestions to learn how to relax and even to enter a hypnotic-like sleep. A suggestion such as the following may be used:

"I should like to demonstrate to you how easy it is to relax. I should like to have you bring down your arms and your hands, resting them on your thighs. Place your feet firmly on the floor. Settle back in your chair, start loosening the muscles in your body, close your eyes; breathe in deeply and regularly and relax.

"Relax your body and your mind. Relax yourself all over. Begin by relaxing the muscles of your forehead. Loosen up the muscles of your forehead. Then take the wrinkles out of your face. Shrug your shoulders. Notice how tense your back is. Shrug your shoulders and loosen your back. Let your arms feel as if they weigh a ton. Let them fall and rest on your thighs so that you have no inclination to move them. Then shift your attention to your legs. Let your legs feel heavy.

"As you sit there breathing deeply, you will feel your arms growing heavy and your legs growing heavy. Your eyes will feel tired, and your eyelids will be as heavy as lead. Your body is getting heavier and heavier. Your eyes are getting tired, very tired. They are closed and you have no desire to open them. You are going to fall asleep, deeply asleep. As you relax, it is impossible for you to help sleeping. It is impossible for you to open your eyes. They are glued together firmly. They are heavier and heavier, and they continue to stay stuck together as you feel yourself sinking into a deeper and deeper sleep. Keep breathing in deeply and go to sleep, deeply asleep. You will find now that your eyes are so firmly glued together that it is impossible to open them. The harder you try to open them, the heavier they feel. Try and you'll see that the harder you try to open them, the heavier they feel."

These suggestions should be made in a firm, confident tone of voice. As a general rule a good number of the members of the group when challenged to open their eyes, will not be able to do so. The physician may then walk over to those who have their eyes closed and place two fingers on the eyelids, pressing them together firmly with the comment: "Continue to sleep."

After this the following statement is made: "From now on whenever I give you the suggestion to sleep, your eyes will become heavy, they will close and you will sink into a state of sleep quickly and easily. You will relax all over, and your sleep will get deeper and deeper. As you sit there with your eyes closed, I am going to give you a suggestion now that you slowly awaken. Slowly your eyes will open, and you will be awake. However, whenever I suggest that you sleep, your eyes will close rapidly, and you will go into a deep restful sleep."

Following this, the patients who have responded positively are brought to the front of the room, or seated in chairs facing the remaining members of the group. Should the physician have present one or two trained hypnotic subjects, he may proceed to induct them into a deep trance, demonstrating each step carefully. Then, the members of the group who have been selected are given the suggestion that they will relax, that their eyes will close and that they will go into a deep sleep. These suggestions are repeated until a trance has been produced. Thereafter several members may be inducted further into a trance state as deeply as they will go.

The remaining members of the group, among whom there may be patients the physician wishes especially to hypnotize, are then told that they too can easily learn to relax and sleep in the same way, and that the next time the procedure is tried, they will find it easier to sink into a state of sleep. At this point they may be enjoined to close their eyes, to relax and to go to sleep deeply. Almost invariably a certain number of the members of the group who had previously resisted falling asleep will enter a trance state. This demonstration will have a positive effect on the patient's trance susceptibility when later inducted into a trance through individual effort.

The second use of group hypnosis, involves its employment for psychotherapeutic purposes. In attempting to use group hypnosis for psychotherapy, the physician must realize its limitations. It must not be confused with real group psychotherapy which is nondirective and which permits the patient to interact freely with other members of the group and with the group leader. In this interaction he expresses his customary character trends and personality patterns and gains insight into his problems and difficulties in interpersonal relationships.

The psychotherapies employed with group hypnosis are those of a directive nature, involving principles of guidance, reassurance, desensitization and persuasion. Once the trance has been produced in susceptible patients by the technics outlined above, other members of the group are urged to relax themselves, to close their eyes, and to absorb the suggestions that will be given to them. Following this suggestions are given to the group. The following persuasive suggestions from a record are exemplary:

"You have acquired faulty emotional habits that need correction. Such habits are the result of the wrong kind of thinking. You can be happy, free from worry and tension, by establishing the right habits of thinking and acting. You must tell yourself, 'I will correct those difficulties that can be remedied. I will face those that cannot be remedied. I may be unable to change the world, but I can change myself so that I will not get emotional about things. I will abolish worrying and thinking too much about myself. If anything comes up that needs solution, I will immediately review all possible courses of action and choose the one that seems to be best. Once I have made up my mind, I shall follow the plan I have evolved. I shall stop thinking and talking too much about my troubles. I shall be pleasant in my relationships with people, and shall not permit myself to be upset. I shall direct my thoughts to pleasant things, and keep in mind the kind of person I would like to be. I must think I am well, and then I will get better. If worrisome ideas keep coming up in my mind, I shall control my thoughts by picturing in my mind a time in my life when I was really happy.' "

Group hypnosis with directive psychotherapy has definite limitations, being oriented as it is around a leader who establishes himself as an omniscient personage, whose pronouncements he expects the patient to follow. What is perpetuated here is essentially the authoritative magical figure of a parental substitute. Symptom relief is brought about as a result of a repression of conflict, and a desire on the part of the patient to comply with suggestions as a means of gaining status in the eyes of the leader. The group exists to a large extent as an appendage of the leader, and beneficial results are maintained so long as the patient is capable of maintaining an image of the former as completely powerful and protective.

Psychotherapy with group hypnosis is often effective in dependent persons whose chief motivation for therapy is to find an invincible authority on whom they can pin their faith. So long as they feel that the personage whom they endow with power will protect them, they may be capable of functioning without symptoms.

In justification of this kind of therapy, there are some individuals whose inner will to live and to develop is so diminutive that the most one can expect from them is a relief of symptoms without any real reorganization of their personality. Such persons flourish under an approach in which they are able to establish a submissive relationship to a leader. The mastery of symptoms, the institution of self discipline, the tolerance of anxiety and tension, the repression of inexpressible impulses and drives, may often result from a relationship of this type.

However, it is necessary not to over-rate the permanency of this type of therapy, inasmuch as success depends upon the ability of the patient to maintain a notion of the leader as noble, good and protective. Furthermore a clinging relationship to the leader may encourage the patient's dependency and may make it difficult for him to take up life on his own.

For these reasons attempts must always be made to encourage free interaction in the group, to get all patients who show a semblance of ego strength to enter into individual psychotherapy, or into a more dynamic form of group psychotherapy which is aimed at rehabilitating the individual in his attitudes toward life, toward people and toward himself. The emphasis should be on improving the stature of the person to a point where he is capable of dealing with his inner needs and conflicts without having to depend upon the beneficences of a protective, authoritarian figure.

Part Three
APPLICATIONS OF
HYPNOTHERAPY

IX

THE PRINCIPLES OF PSYCHOTHERAPY

THE ADEQUATE treatment of an emotional problem by any method including hypnosis presupposes an understanding of dynamic psychotherapeutic principles. Hypnosis is no magical entity that can in itself invoke drastic emotional change. It must always be utilized in conjunction with some form of psychotherapy which is best adapted for the patient.

In applying psychotherapy to the problems of the patient, it is essential to remember that manifest symptoms are not the best criteria on which to base the treatment plan. Emphasis on symptoms in therapy was in the past largely the product of traditional methods of classification which designated the various syndromes chiefly by their component symptoms. This practice has proved itself to be quite arbitrary and inadequate.

Emotional problems usually spread themselves over a wide pathologic area and only in the rarest instances do they confine themselves to one syndrome. For instance, a man may apply for psychiatric help with the complaint of numbness, paresthesia and spasticity of an arm, for which there is no organic cause. On the basis of his symptoms, we may justifiably suspect that he has a hysterical condition, and we may be tempted to classify his disorder as conversion hysteria. However, in talking to the patient at length, we are apt to discover that he suffers, in addition to symptoms relating to his arm, well defined phobias of the dark and of closed spaces, symptoms which would fall into the classification of anxiety hysteria. Additionally, there may be complaints of tension, fatigue, headaches, and dyspeptic attacks, which manifestations we would consider as psychosomatic in nature. Upon further investigation we may also find that he is withdrawn and shy, and that he has definite problems in his relations with people. We would then be inclined to feel that he also has a character disorder. How to classify him accurately would thus constitute a problem. It is extremely difficult to classify the majority of patients in one or another disease category exclusively.

More significant than this is the fact that symptoms, though upsetting to the patient, are initiated by difficulties and conflicts of which the patient is largely unaware. Indeed the symptoms may not reflect in the least the inner conflicts and dynamic disturbances in adaption from which they issue. These disturbances are perhaps less dramatic than the complaints for which treatment is sought, but from the standpoint of therapy they must be considered primary.

Among the disturbances in psychobiologic adaptation which are probably universal to all psychoneuroses are disorders in security, self esteem, relationships with people and expression of inner impulses and demands. An understanding of how and why such disturbances operate in the patient is basic to successful treatment.

Feelings of insecurity are always present in greater or lesser degree in neurotic persons. The individual feels menaced by some intangible danger which threatens him at all times. He is hemmed in by forces with which he feels powerless to cope. He may consequently adopt a number of defense mechanisms which are calculated to bolster up his morale or which remove him temporarily from what he considers are the sources of his difficulty.

Common to all neuroses is also a disturbance in self evaluation. The neurotic individual is apt to consider himself different or inferior to other people. He has contemptuous attitudes towards himself that make him feel unloved and unlovable. Self devaluation reflects itself in a lack of assertiveness and self confidence. It engenders deep dependency strivings, hostile attitudes, perfectionistic and grandiose tendencies. In some instances it leads to desperate attempts at self sufficiency, to compulsive independence, and to a peculiar detached attitude towards other people as if to avoid a realization of one's own lack of worth.

Present in all neurotic syndromes are difficulties in the individual's relationships to other people. There are many kinds of relationship problems. The person may become excessively dependent upon others and seek a clinging alliance by attaching himself to a stronger person. He may attempt to domineer other people, attempting to wrest from them love and support by sheer force. He may feel that people are not to be trusted, and he may then try to detach himself from others and function within an isolated shell, thus veering away from any form of intimate relationship. He may develop tendencies towards perfectionism or ambitiousness or masochistic suffering.

As a general rule, relationship difficulties involve all persons with whom the neurotic individual is associated. They are reflected particularly towards authority. The neurotic patient's feelings about authority are largely the product of incorporated attitudes in relationships to the earliest authorities. The consequence of these attitudes may be a peculiar overevaluation of all authoritative people and a minimization of his own capacities and abilities. The patient may become obsequious or ingratiating in an attempt to win favors from those he believes are stronger than himself. On the other hand, he may adopt an extremely hostile, destructive attitude towards authoritative persons, in a violent attempt to liberate himself from the tyranny of their influence. Because he both overvalues authority and feels subjugated by it, he suffers intensely in his adjustment.

Another disturbance common to the neuroses is an incapacity on the part of the individual to express his inner basic demands and needs. Very frequently he will repress normal strivings, as for affection, love, recognition, or sexual satisfaction, on the basis that these gratifications are either denied him or involve such great dangers to himself that he is willing to forego them. An analysis of impulses discloses that sexual and hostile feelings undergo the most rigorous taboo. The inability to express inner strivings is usually associated with an overevaluation and fear of authority, and with feelings of self devaluation and helplessness.

When we analyze the genetic origin of neurotic disturbances of security, self devaluation, interpersonal relationships, and ability to express inner impulses and demands, we find these rooted, as a general rule, in experiences and conditionings in childhood. While it is true that hereditary influences play a signal role in personality development, it is also true that the individual with the most intact heredity will react catastrophically to inimical influences in his early childhood, particularly to improper handling and to disappointments engendered in his relationships with his parents.

Where experiences with the parent and with the early environment are harmonious, the child is able to evolve a system of security which regards the world as a bountiful place, and to develop a self esteem which encourages assertiveness and self confidence. He will be convinced of his capacities to love and to be loved. He will most probably possess character strivings that permit him to relate himself constructively to other persons, and to express, through culturally condoned outlets, social and biologic needs. On the other hand, where the child has been rejected, overprotected or unduly intimidated, the world will constitute for him a place of menace. He will be devastated by fears and tensions. His self esteem will be warped to a point where he is overwhelmed by feelings of helplessness, by lack of assertiveness and loss of self confidence. His relationships with people will be disturbed and he may harbor markedly destructive attitudes toward authority. Finally, inner strivings and demands will suffer repression in greater or lesser degree.

The failing psychobiologic adjustment of the neurotic individual is registered by generation of tension and anxiety that reflect themselves on various levels of nerve integration. On the psychic level, the individual will be overwhelmed by catastrophic helplessness, by fear and depression. On subcortical levels, there may result a profound autonomic disturbance in the form of psychosomatic symptoms. Where feelings of helplessness or expectations of injury are profound, anxiety may be especially prominent. Anxiety is a universal symptom in neuroses and constitutes a danger signal of imminent collapse. Anxiety is the motor that brings into play all the instrumentalities the ego has at its disposal to adjust the individual to psychic equilibrium. Anxiety and its attendant physiologic reactions are so destructive to the person that attempts to cope with it are always made.

Many symptoms the person displays in response to anxiety serve to defend him against the effects of this emotion. They constitute also a type of defense against the initiating conflicts themselves. What determines the kind of symptom, and consequently the syndrome from which the person suffers, is not entirely known. Why individuals should react differently and adopt varying defenses to the same dynamic conflicts is a challenging question. For instance, one person who is struggling with strong dependency strivings and associated hostile feelings may develop depressive manifestations; a second with the same kind of conflict may show psychosomatic symptoms of a gastrointestinal nature; while a third may display alcoholic addiction. Indeed, when we come to analyze various neurotic problems, we find the difficulties that generate them to be strikingly similar. However, the reaction of individuals to these difficulties, the types of defenses adopted, the method utilized to cope with inner conflicts and fears, vary. The problem of symptom determination is an interesting one and calls for further investigation and clarification.

From a therapeutic standpoint, however, as has been indicated, the kind of symptom the individual elaborates to cope with anxiety is not nearly so important as the difficulties which create anxiety. It is essential to understand thoroughly the sources of anxiety, since an understanding of why the individual is failing in his psychobiologic adjustment will make it possible to outline for him an adequate therapeutic plan.

For instance we may take the case of a patient who seeks help for symptoms of a peptic ulcer. A psychiatric examination reveals the presence of a pervasive depression and sense of hopelessness which the patient attributes to the unremitting pain and discomfort of his gastric disturbance. The history shows that his symptoms became exacerbated when his fiancée terminated their love affair. From his associations and dreams it is apparent that he is an extremely dependent person who always has sought a relationship with a maternal person. The extent of his dependency is not known to him. In his own estimation, he is a totally effective, self confident, well functioning individual. But underneath these feelings there is obviously a profound sense of helplessness. So long as he can cling to a maternal person, so long as he feels loved by this person, he is able to function well and efficiently. However, in instances when he is rejected, or whenever he imagines that he is rejected, he collapses. And because he feels so trapped by his dependency, he has hostile impulses which threaten his security.

When this man applies to a physician for treatment, he

may be so concerned with his gastric complaints that he will minimize or even be unaware of his disturbed life adjustment. Nevertheless, in a short while the physician will be able to diagnose his psychosomatic problem as incident to a disturbance in his adaptational pattern. The physician may discover, for instance, when he begins to analyze his character strivings, that the patient actually feels as helpless as an infant who has been abandoned by his mother, and that his symptoms are the consequence of the departure of his fiancée who is the psychic equivalent of his mother.

The knowledge of what is behind the patient's symptoms will best enable the physician to outline an appropriate treatment plan which can deal with the causes as well as with the effects.

DYNAMICS OF PSYCHOTHERAPEUTIC CHANGE

The knowledge that symptoms arise out of failure of the individual in his dealings with life displaces the emphasis in therapy from the treatment of symptoms to the rehabilitation of the patient in his functional relationships with life and with people. The ultimate objective in all rational psychotherapy is to build security in the individual so that he no longer feels menaced by fears of the world. In addition self esteem must be enhanced to the point of self confidence, assertiveness and creative self fulfillment. The person must gain respect for himself without strivings for perfectionism or superiority. His relationships with people must become harmonious and shorn of such impulses as dependency, detachment, and aggression. Finally, he must become capable of satisfying his inner needs and demands without anxiety and in conformity with the standards of the group.

Such goals, unfortunately, are not always obtained easily because of absence of adequate motivations in the patient, and because of resistances that inevitably arise when neurotic personality drives are challenged. The skill of the therapist is determined by his ability to create the proper incentives for deep character change and to solve resistances that block progress.

The first step in the treatment process where the therapeutic goal is rehabilitation of the personality, is a demonstration to the patient that his symptoms do not occur at random, but are exacerbated by definite life situations which involve his attitudes toward people and his estimate of himself. It is necessary that he realize that his symptoms are surface warnings of inner problems of which he is only partially aware.

Some patients have managed, through their own efforts, to come to this conclusion even before they seek therapy. However, the majority of neurotic persons are confounded by their symptoms which they regard as extraneous and unjustified. Patients with psychosomatic problems are particularly unable to see a connection between their physical complaints and their deeper conflicts.

Considerable time may therefore have to be spent in getting the patient to establish a continuity between his symptoms and his conflicts. Once the patient accepts the physician's explanation that his symptoms have a specific meaning, and once he is willing to abandon his hopes for immediate symptom removal by some spectacular performance on the part of the physician, the discomfort of his symptoms will provide the incentive for a deeper inquiry into himself. The four most common methods of making this inquiry are through free association, the interpretation of dreams, the observation of happenings in one's daily life which either exaggerate or relieve symptoms, and the transference situation that develops with the physician.

As soon as the patient realizes that his symptoms are stirred up as the result of certain occurrences in his life situation and in his contacts with people, emphasis will be shifted from his symptoms to his conflicts and difficulties in inter-

personal relationships. When he observes that he suffers
because he detaches himself, or makes himself excessively
dependent, or ingratiates himself in a submissive way, or
lashes out defensively at people, we have taken the first
step in therapy.

It may require a tremendous amount of work on the part
of the physician to bring the patient to a realization that he
does have problems in his attitudes toward others and toward himself. His character traits are so integral a part of
himself that he can scarcely conceive of the possibility that
his attitudes and feelings are disturbed. To him they constitute life and he may be surprised to discover that most
people do not have the same values and reactions as himself.

Virtually he reacts like the man in the story who visited a
psychiatrist and was asked by the latter to recount his
troubles. "But I have no troubles," exclaimed the man.
"Then why are you here?" replied the psychiatrist. "Because
my wife insisted I see you." "But do you have any unusual
psychologic or physical symptoms?" queried the doctor.
"None whatsoever," expostulated the patient. "I lead a
normal and complete life as is evidenced by my daily routine." "Tell me about your routine," invited the psychiatrist.
"Well," remarked the man, "I awake in the morning, dress,
shave, go downstairs for a satisfying, hearty breakfast, go
back upstairs, brush my teeth, vomit up my breakfast, comb
my hair, put on my coat. . . ." "Wait a minute," exclaimed
the doctor, "what did you say about vomiting up your
breakfast?" "Sure I do," replied the patient. "Doesn't
everybody?"

There is scarcely a neurotic person who does not believe
sincerely that his fears of the world, his strivings and traits,
no matter how unusual they may be, are not most natural,
if not universal. If he recognizes that he is unique in the way
he feels, then he is certain that he is especially constituted and
that life can offer him no other course than the one he is
pursuing.

This conviction is one of the strongest resistances to change that the patient displays in the course of treatment. Usually he doubts that he projects his fears and his attitudes indiscriminately no matter what the circumstances may be.

A potent means of displaying to the patient how he endows life with his own prejudices and fears is through the medium of the transference. In the immediate relationship with the physician it may be possible to demonstrate conclusively to the patient that he injects into it his basic attitudes and conflicts. For instance, he may become fearful of the physician, or dependent, or hostile. He may have impulses toward destructiveness or masochistic suffering, or he may seek to detach himself by running away from therapy. The physician, by confronting the patient with the facades he utilizes, can demonstrate to him that the reality situation is different from the one he imagines to exist.

This demonstration will occasion much surprise, and the patient will usually respond with further resistance. For his basic character trends are now being challenged, and the patient will resent giving up his way of life, which, though unsatisfying and though productive of anxiety, is still the only way of life he knows. Furthermore, his neurosis has many spurious values for him which he is chary of abandoning. For instance, a compulsive tendency to flay and to deride oneself may be a chief means of gaining sympathy from others. The person may believe that assertiveness or any other course of action will bring rejection or counterhostility.

Insight into the fact that his responses are not justified by present-day reality, that they are residual in misconceptions, is an important step in the process of getting well. It creates the desire to explore more thoroughly the meaning and the origin of impulses and patterns of behavior. The relationship with the physician is the experimental laboratory in which recreated attitudes are nurtured, for the patient constantly tests the physician with his old strivings and demands.

With the help of the physician, the patient will become aware of, as a result of his insight into his distorted attitudes and patterns, the genetic origin of these tendencies. Through the medium of fantasies, dreams and the various hypno-analytic procedures, in the event hypnosis is used, he will be able to remember or to reconstruct the experiences and conditionings in his early childhood which exaggerated his insecurities, generated conflicts and necessitated his various character deviations. The most important catalyst in the process of remembering and reconstructing the past is the transference with the physician.

In the course of his therapeutic work, the patient will often repeat his most traumatic early experiences, usually those with his parents and siblings, which he failed to master as a child, and which were responsible for his deepest anxieties and deviations in his character formation. The unique situation of protectiveness in his relationship with the physician will enable him to recapitulate those fearsome situations which had once overwhelmed his adaptive capacities and blocked his personality growth. Previously, anxiety had prevented any attempt to remember, let alone to repeat his experience. Now he feels he has a better chance to master his fears, and he will strive to recreate the early situation in some symbolic form in an effort to face it realistically.

The consequence of a successful effort, even though minor, is a dawning realization of how his early misconceptions and conflicts have crippled his functioning and have necessitated disturbed attitudes toward people and toward himself. This insight creates the incentive for experimenting with life on new terms, and helps him to master the anxieties that have conditioned his habitual reactions. Life no longer is regarded as a mere arena of past happenings. Situations and relationships are re-evaluated in the light of existing reality.

As the patient liberates himself from the ghosts of his past, the world no longer becomes a place of menace; his sense of security becomes enhanced. Interpersonal relationships become less strained, less blighted by dependency, aggression and detachment, and more cooperative and harmonious. The anxieties surrounding basic needs and demands no longer have the same force in preventing or inhibiting their expression.

With the patient's expanding insight, the physician becomes more and more nondirective in his technic. The patient in turn begins to become more self confident, assertive and expressive. He finds that he has the right to make choices and decisions, to establish his own values and goals. As the ego of the patient expands, the super-ego loses its force and tyranny. The patient becomes stronger and for the first time he appreciates real joy in living and in the experiencing of normal productivity and assertiveness. Finally, he no longer requires help from the physician, and life itself becomes a place where he can gratify his social and biologic needs, which, prior to therapy, he felt were utterly beyond his reach.

PARTIAL THERAPEUTIC GOALS

Unfortunately not all people are capable of achieving this ideal objective of complete personality rehabilitation. There are a number of reasons why this is so, but the two most important reasons involve inadequate motivations and diminutive ego strength.

In appraising the motivations of the patient, one must operate on the basis of the old saw that it is possible to lead a horse to water, but one cannot make him drink. Unless the patient has a desire to change his way of life, to reintegrate himself in his relations with people, it will be difficult, if not impossible, to influence him toward that type of character change that we seek as an ultimate goal in therapy.

There are many patients who are so inconvenienced by their symptoms that they want relief; yet they desire to cling to the dynamic source of their symptoms even at the cost of suffering.

For instance, in the case of the man previously described, who had developed a gastric complaint following a broken love affair, he may desire treatment for this symptom, but he may at first see no connection between his symptom and his dependency, and hence no need for dealing with the latter striving. It is quite obvious that his character disturbance of compulsive dependency is the source of not only his gastric symptoms, but of a diffuse anxiety, depression and a generally disturbed attitude toward life. It is apparent also that no permanent relief can be achieved in his general maladjustment until self growth proceeds to the point of greater assuredness and self sufficiency. Yet the patient may resist desperately any attempt to treat him when he senses that his way of life, his tendency to cling to others for love and support, is challenged.

During therapy, a connection between his symptom and his dependency will be established, but he may still refuse to accept this insight, or he may intellectually accept it and emotionally hang on to his dependency striving as the only possible means of adaptation. Here, while he has the motivation to give up his symptoms, he is not adequately motivated to give up what constitutes for him his sole means of adjustment, his dependency, which underlies his symptoms. In view of this he may resent working with a nondirective or analytic method that throws the burden of responsibility for the therapeutic work on his shoulders. We may actually discover that what he really desires from therapy is some form of dependency on the physician in the hope that this will restore the shattered security he suffered when he was abandoned by his fiancée.

Under these circumstances, symptom relief, on the basis of authoritative suggestion, may be the only therapy that makes sense to the patient. An abandonment of symptoms may result from restoration of the patient's security through his becoming dependent on the physician, who sets himself up as an omniscient parent. The motivations of the patient for support and direction would also make reassurance, guidance, persuasion, desensitization and re-educational approaches possible in the same authoritarian framework. The patient would be enjoined to find a new outlet for his affection or to make an effort toward a reconciliation between himself and his sweetheart. Should persuasion be decided upon, the patient would be encouraged to evolve a plan of action, expanding his assets and relating himself more intimately with people while he stopped thinking painful and destructive thoughts. In desensitization he would be inspired to talk about his unfortunate love affair until it no longer caused him emotional pain. Re-education would strive to get him to relate himself in a less dependent manner to people, and to seek outlets for his hostility in competitive sports or muscular activities.

Thus the motivation of the patient, inadequate as it is, would circumscribe the therapeutic goal. What the patient desires is supportive help for his problem. The kind of relationship he wants with the physician is of an authoritarian nature, in which he is the child-pupil and the physician the master-teacher. So long as this motivation exists, he will shy away from a more mature participating kind of relationship which is the only medium in which real ego change is forged. Yet, because it may be impossible to alter the patient's motivation to accept a deeper type of therapy, a directive therapeutic approach may be the only kind to which he will respond.

As soon as a patient becomes cognizant of the fact that his symptoms are derived from fundamental personality problems, his motivations may change from a mere desire for symptom removal to a desire for an integrated type of relationship to life and to people. This will allow of a more extensive therapeutic goal. However, the mere verbalization of a desire for better relationships is not to be confused with a real motivation for character change, since what the patient may mean by an improved relationship is a fulfillment of those neurotic needs and strivings which have been unfulfilled up to this time.

The patient may be peculiarly resistant toward developing the proper motivation for extensive personality change. One reason for this is that he may believe that the therapeutic goal conflicts with his ability to make a good adjustment. Such ideas are usually unjustified, but occasionally there is a realistic basis for this fear. Where, for instance, his economic security is dependent upon fierce competitiveness, a resolution of his hostility and its channelization into impersonal activities may make him incapable of standing up against his competitors. Although hostile impulses toward people may initiate his anxiety, an attitude of brotherly love may threaten the very foundations of his economic security. Consequently, the patient will shy away from an approach which might make him subject to economic disaster.

More nebulous than motivation, but as important a factor in limiting the therapeutic goal, is the ego strength of the patient. Ego strength is an integrating factor operative in the individual which permits of a mobilization of adaptive physical and psychologic resources. The ability to face inner conflicts and repressed memories requires a certain amount of fortitude which many persons do not possess. The capacity to tolerate the intense emotions liberated in the transference and to recognize the irrationality of these emotions and their genetic origin requires even greater ego strength. Finally, the ability to abandon the spurious values and secondary gains of a neurosis, and to establish patterns of behavior in line with mature goals, calls for a relatively strong ego structure.

Immature ego organizations and those that cling to reality

solely by elaborating neurotic facades are apt to crumble under the impact of the emotions set loose during an analytic form of therapy. Extremely dependent people, or schizoid, prepsychotic or psychotic individuals, are especially vulnerable and are unable to relinquish defenses which bolster up their weakened egos. They are apt to become paranoid, suicidal, or psychotically excited, or to develop alarming psychosomatic symptoms in the turmoil of a transference reaction. In such cases the therapeutic goal of extensive alteration in personality must be abandoned in favor of partial goals, the achievement of which does not encourage the development of a deep and disturbing relationship to the therapist.

It is thus necessary, for various reasons, to abandon, for the time being at least, goals that aim for extensive alteration of the character structure, and, taking into consideration how far the patient is willing and able to go in working through his problems, content oneself with removal of his symptoms, relief of anxiety, or adjustment to existing work and life situations. Even though the patient remains neurotic and the gains are purely palliative, his ability to cope with life can have a stabilizing influence on his ego.

The physician who is sensitive to the inner dynamics of the patient's neurosis may then be able to influence the patient toward developing the proper motivation, and to stabilize the ego so that it can accept the type of nonsupportive and analytic relationship which will allow of a more complete therapeutic objective.

Evaluating the Patient's Problem

An evaluation of the patient's problem at the start of therapy is invaluable in determining the extent of the therapeutic goal that may reasonably be achieved with the patient's existing personality equipment. A correct evaluation may, for instance, help decide whether to aim merely for an adjustment of the individual to his present life situation through such approaches as symptom removal, guidance, environmental manipulation, reassurance, persuasion or desensitization; or to reorganize partially the patient's personality patterns by means of re-education; or to rehabilitate the patient's character structure through reconditioning or by utilization of a psychoanalytically oriented psychotherapy.

In the evaluation process, the severity of the patient's problem is determined by inquiring into the chief complaint, the history and development of the complaint, and the co-existing psychic, emotional, somatic and behavioral symptoms. An exploration is also made of hereditary and constitutional factors and of the developmental history, noting particularly neurotic components and defects in health, habit training, physique, emotional expression, intellect, social and sexual impulses.

The specific areas of the patient's psychobiologic failings are investigated along the following lines:

1. The home situation with an estimate of destructive factors, both remediable and irremediable.

2. Existing somatic malfunctions, especially in relation to appetite, digestion, sleep and sexual enjoyment.

3. Intellectual defects in terms of judgment and reasoning powers.

4. The work, economic and marital adjustment.

5. The extent and nature of the patient's hobbies, recreations, social and religious interests.

6. Ambitions and goals in life.

7. The severity of insecurity feelings.

8. The character structure with emphasis on (a) disturbances in relations with people and authority, (b) disturbances in attitudes toward the self, (c) disturbances of conscience, (d) disturbances in the ability to express inner needs and demands, (e) disturbances in methods of handling conflict.

The dynamics of the patient's illness are estimated further by an inquiry into the nature of his conditionings with important early authorities, particularly the mother and father, and into the adjustment with his siblings. The patient's past and present dreams and his current attitudes toward the physician are explored. Physical and neurologic examinations are performed, while psychiatric examinations contribute important clues as to the severity of the patient's difficulty and the areas of his functioning that are disturbed and require correction.

There are three important items of information which are helpful in planning a therapeutic program. The first has to do with the existing motivations, what the patient actually seeks out of treatment. The second involves ego strength or weakness, the equipment with which the patient can function in treatment. The third is the kind of technic he will be able to utilize most effectively within set limits of time and finances.

The motivations of the patient will soon become apparent to the physician from his verbalized productions, dreams and response to therapy.

The ego strength is more difficult to estimate since adequate criteria have not yet been established. To some extent we may estimate limitations in ego strength from developmental failures of the individual, the incompetence of past and present psychobiologic adaptations, absence of a real precipitating factor, the difficulties in his relations with people, the intensity of dependency, the diminutiveness of self esteem and the inadequacy of his prevailing defenses against anxiety.

Projective tests like the Rorschach, Thematic Apperception Test, Goodenough, and Expressive Handwriting are able to supply some data, particularly when they are interpreted by skilled workers. However, the application of projective materials to therapy has not yet been worked out to a point of reliability, even though progress has been made in this direction at certain research clinics.

With training the physician may be able to administer the Rorschach test himself, and, where necessary, may then have it scored and interpreted by a psychologist expert in the Rorschach method. An amazing amount of information may be obtained from the raw Rorschach responses, and the physician may, at the time of administration, be capable of estimating the integrative capacities of the patient, his sensitivity, originality, intelligence, suggestibility, intensity of anxiety as well as methods of coping with anxiety, reactions to emotional stimuli, schizoid tendencies, and even dynamic problems in interpersonal relationships.

The Rorschach test may, in addition to yielding information on ego strength, be useful in planning a proper therapeutic approach. For instance, where a person's responses break down on the color cards, as when he gives pure color responses and his forms disintegrate, one may rightfully suspect that he cannot stand a great deal of emotional pressure. The therapeutic approach, at least at the start, would best be supportive, avoiding the deeper unconscious content. If the patient's responses concentrate on edge detail and on minutiae, one may be led to assume that the person is extremely rigid and that the chances of getting beneath the surface are not very good. The most that may be done for him is to work within the framework of his particular intellectual way of functioning, until he no longer needs to utilize intellectuality as a compulsive defense against feeling.

THE CONDUCT OF THE THERAPEUTIC SESSION

The treatment of emotional problems takes place in a setting of a most unique interpersonal relationship between physician and patient. In this setting the patient is influenced to change his attitudes toward life and to gain emotional security and self esteem. The patient, however, has a great deal to say about the extent to which the physician is going to influence him. He comes to therapy with certain hopes and expectations. He has a problem that annoys him greatly, symptoms which create unhappiness and interfere with his functioning. He wants the physician to remove his difficulties rapidly and with as little annoyance to himself as possible. He does not usually realize that his symptoms are the product of deep conflicts and disturbances in his relationships with people. And because his particular kind of relation to people, neurotic and destructive as this may be, constitutes for him the only way of living he knows, he may resist desperately any effort at change.

Experience has shown that his resistances can be altered with the right kind of psychotherapy, that it is possible to influence him so that he loses his symptoms and leads a more productive life. The medium through which this transformation occurs is the relationship with the physician which assumes a quality such as he never before has known.

Psychotherapy is, in essence, an interpersonal relationship, and whatever changes occur these develop as a result of the interpersonal experience. The relationship takes many forms and directions, and the patient will always try to manipulate it so that it will suit his own particular needs and purposes. Very often these purposes are completely opposed to the therapeutic objective; as a matter of fact they may destroy that objective if not interfered with. On the other hand the patient has no other way of relating himself to people than with his usual characterologic machinery. We must expect that he will display toward the physician the same inordinate demands, dependency, hostility, detachment and destructive attitudes that he has displayed toward people in general. We must anticipate that he will wedge his relationship with the physician into the framework of his neurosis.

Success in therapy depends on the physician's ability to forestall the patient's intentions, to break up neurotic patterns before they go too far, or to bring the patient to a realization of how he is functioning in the relationship with the physician and the neurotic consequences of his behavior.

The manipulation of the therapeutic relationship will depend on the role the physician desires to play in the patient's life. If the therapeutic approach is to be one of symptom removal by authoritative suggestion, guidance, reassurance, persuasion, desensitization, reconditioning and directive re-education, the physician will have to establish and to maintain himself as a wise, strong, or benevolent authority. It will be essential to diagnose and to remove hostilities which crop up and threaten this relationship. Should the therapeutic approach be nondirective or analytic, a more cooperative relationship will be required, the physician disposing of the inordinate dependency demands made of him, resolving the patient's inner paralysis, dissipating resistances to change, and helping the patient to understand his inner conflicts and fears.

The therapeutic technic most appropriate for the patient will depend on a number of factors including his motivations and ego strength. The most accurate means of estimating the suitability of the approach is to observe the patient's reactions in the therapeutic situation as indicated by his verbal productions, behavior, dreams and the material brought up during the trance. Of crucial importance is the kind of relationship the patient is capable of establishing with the physician.

Since all therapeutic changes occur in the medium of an interpersonal relationship, it is important to estimate the kind of relationship the patient wants to establish immediately, the kind he can establish with help other than that which he desires, and, finally, the kind he will be able to establish in the future, in other words, his potentialities for productive relationships with people.

It is important at the start that the patient accept the

physician as a person in whom he can confide his difficulties. Unless the physician inspires some measure of confidence in the patient, little progress can be expected. The best way of doing this is to enter into a relationship with the patient on the latter's own terms provided these are within reason. Toward this end it is essential to understand the patient's operational system, the facades and defenses he utilizes, his frame of reference, so to speak, in order to convince the patient that the physician understands his language.

When an emotionally ill patient comes to see a physician, he usually has the expectation of having something done to him through some mysterious medical means. In part this is an outgrowth of the traditional attitude toward the doctor. In part it is because the patient's sense of confidence is crushed, and he feels helpless and hopeless. He is bound to regard the physician in the light of an omniscient authority who can guide him to paths of health and personal success. The sicker the person, the less faith he has in his own strength and the greater his tendency to collapse on the physician.

The physician must appraise the illness of the patient in order to approximate how directive and supportive he must be in the relationship. To shun a directive relationship at the start when the patient needs and demands this, may create such antagonisms and insecurities in the patient that therapy will be impossible. Because of his dependency, the patient will see no sense in a therapeutic situation in which he is expected to carry the bulk of the therapeutic work. Once the patient is convinced that the physician understands him and has his welfare at heart, it may be possible to impose on him greater responsibility for his own development.

Where the therapeutic approach is to be directive at all times, by virtue of the patient's limited motivations and ego strength, where a partial therapeutic goal is all that is desired, therapy will be expedited by the mantle of authority with which the patient automatically invests the physician.

The conduct of the hypnotic induction as well as of the therapeutic session is directive and authoritarian. Whenever the patient begins to minimize the dictates of the physician or to act hostile toward him, the sources of the need to devaluate and to attack are dealt with immediately in order to restore the superordinate and protective position of the physician.

It may be impossible to remove hostility in many instances, because the very nature of the authoritarian relationship prevents the individual from liberating himself from the yoke of authoritarianism that may be at the basis of his neurosis. The physician may try to set himself up as a new benevolent authority; but this will not influence the inner dynamics of the patient's personality. New directives, new ways of operation, although better than those the patient has followed most of his life, do not alter his self-structure. In relation to the physician he is still the child who has incorporated the mandates of the parent. He has been given no real opportunity to grow and to develop adult ego strength.

Any form of directive therapy has the disadvantage of keeping the patient on a dependency level longer than he should be. Where the aim in therapy is to make the patient self sufficient and capable of finding security within himself, a directive approach may inhibit this aim. In looking for support and security from the outside, from some person who will impose it or present it to him as a gift, the patient never develops the ability to take a stand in life and, through his own resources, become a stronger and more independent being.

A change in the conduct of the therapeutic session is thus essential at some point. By defining the therapeutic situation to the patient, an attempt is made to get him to participate more actively in the therapeutic work. The patient is expected to act through his own resources, to make his own decisions, to establish his own values and goals in line with his expanding insights. Only when he does this can he begin developing strengths within himself which will expand his ego and break his ties to authority.

However, the patient will resist desperately the effort on the part of the physician to assume a nonauthoritarian role. He will want to be told what to do. He will doubt his own capacities and choices. He will refuse to make decisions. A great upheaval may result with an exacerbation of the neurosis. Liberation of the self is always accompanied by fear and resistance.

Concurrent with the patient's desire for development there is always an irresistible impulse on his part to sabotage his progress. Resistances to cure are legion and manifest themselves in a variety of ways. They are caused by a fear of coming to grips with inner conflicts and strivings. They are conditioned by a refusal to relinquish vicarious gains fostered by the neurosis. They often are a product of the inability to acknowledge any real good in what is considered the normal pursuits of life.

Neurotic symptoms, debilitating as they are, serve a protective purpose in the mind of the patient. To give them up may threaten him with exposure to inconveniences far greater than he already suffers. Furthermore, the distortion in his sense of values induced by the neurosis may make normal values vapid and meaningless. Neurotic goals as for power, perfectionism, dependency, and detachment are so important to the patient that he will resent any effort to remove them.

It becomes apparent during therapy that the patient does not entirely want to get well. What he wants from the physician is a formula that will permit him to hold on to his neurosis and still escape suffering, that will allow him to be dependent and still strong within himself, that will let him detach himself from people and yet reap the fruits of good interpersonal relationships. He will actually resent efforts on the part of the physician to integrate him toward normal living. Consequently he will interpret therapy as an assault on his way of life. He will strive to protect himself by such devices as disarming the physician through artificial insight, by forced temporary flight into health, by praise of or great devotion to the doctor, by inhibitions in thinking, by fatigue or self devaluation, by suspicion or aggression.

During therapy the physician constantly must dissipate these resistances by interpreting to the patient their existence and purpose. Additionally, he must attack whatever values, protective and otherwise, the patient's neurosis has for him, and he must build up the incentives in the patient to enjoy normal goals.

Insight is the greatest incentive to change. Once the patient realizes how his life has been ruled by misconceptions and fears rooted in unconscious conflicts and in unfortunate experiences and conditionings, he will have the desire to approach people on different terms. He will want to attempt to dissociate the past from the present and to alter his neurotic patterns for more adaptive behavior in line with existing reality. He will begin to recognize why he resists growing up and refuses to make his own decisions.

The physician at this point may interpret to the patient the reasons for his self paralysis, and he may emphasize to the patient the need to make his own choices no matter how inappropriate these may be. The patient may be told that because of the fact that he never developed confidence in himself as an individual he has doubted his right to do things for himself and to experience himself as a decent, constructive human being. The insidious operation of his dependency may be demonstrated, and the patient may be shown how dependency has crippled his efforts toward self growth. He is warned that in his relationship with the physician he will expect the doctor to give him all the answers, and to make all decisions for him. Should the doctor do this, the patient will never develop strength in himself. He will continue to feel weak inside. The physician, therefore, wants to give the patient the opportunity to grow within himself by encouraging him to make his own decisions. The patient may be apprised of the fact that he will feel his decisions to be wrong; but even though he makes mistakes, the very fact that they are his own mistakes will teach him more than being told what to do at all times. The physician does not want to withold support from the patient, but he must do so now out of consideration for the patient's right to grow.

A definition of the nondirective nature of the treatment situation in this way will give the patient an incentive to take responsibility. It will not serve to liberate the patient completely. His neurotic attitudes and behavior patterns will continue in force. He will still exhibit toward the physician the same insecurity, submissiveness, fear and aggression he always has manifested toward authority. He will claim the same ineptitudes in dealing with life and people. He will ingratiate himself, or act destructive, or detach himself in his customary manner. But he will do these with a slight difference, with doubts that they are really necessary.

Because the therapist is a new kind of authority, the patient will experiment with this authority. He will act more assertive in therapy and make decisions about minor things, such as the topics for discussion. He will disagree with the physician albeit with trepidation. He will make plans and express choices. He will experience failures, but he will also have successes. And his inner strength will grow on the bedrock of his successes. He will develop new feelings of integrity and a new sense of self.

Ego change will thus develop within the therapeutic situation itself. It is contingent to a large extent on the permissiveness of the physician and his encouragement of the patient's activity and self expressiveness. The fact that the patient figures things out for himself during the treatment session eventually shows him that he is not at the mercy of destiny. Ultimately he comes to the conclusion that he can make decisions, not because he is told to, but because he has the right to do so. He feels equality with the physician and a growing sense of self respect. The fact that he can act assertive in therapy promotes projection of this feeling toward the extratherapeutic environment.

The conduct of the therapeutic session in this manner requires that the physician be so constituted that he permit the patient to feel equality. The personalities of some therapists are essentially so authoritarian that they will not be able to function on equal terms with the patient. They automatically will set themselves up as leaders making judgments, giving directives, and setting goals for the patient they expect him to follow. They may respond with hostility if challenged or abused by the patient. This is least apt to occur where the physician has been psychoanalyzed and can analyze the countertransference before it interferes with the treatment situation.

In Volume Two the principles outlined in this chapter are taken up in detail and illustrated with case material.

Since a knowledge of psychopathology is indispensable for best results in therapy, the next ten chapters have been devoted to a discussion of the dynamics involved in the most common disease syndromes. How hypnosis may help alter the pathology is merely indicated in each condition. In Volume Two an elaboration of the actual technic which may be employed is presented.

X

HYPNOSIS IN ANXIETY NEUROSIS

IN ANXIETY neurosis the individual is victimized by periodic attacks of nascent "free-flowing" anxiety which produce such symptoms as choking sensations, heart palpitations, numbness of the extremities, epigastric discomfort and a general sense of foreboding. In some instances, anxiety may be more or less localized in psychosomatic symptoms ("anxiety equivalents") like vertigo, increased perspiration, trembling, shivering, urticaria, anginoid pains, asthmatic-like attacks and gastrointestinal symptoms, without conscious feelings of apprehension.

Anxiety attacks may occur in the daytime or during sleep, from which the person may awaken with an expectation of imminent disaster. There is a tendency to associate attacks with the environmental situation accompanying the development of panic; whereupon the individual will strive to avoid similar situations in a vain attempt to circumvent anxiety. In nocturnal anxiety the person may try to avoid the horrors which sleep brings on by developing an intractable insomnia.

The emotion of anxiety is a manifestation of an inner disruptive process and indicates that the adaptive resources of the person have collapsed to a point where he is overwhelmed by catastrophic helplessness. Destructive as it is, anxiety tends to mobilize the physiologic and psychologic resources of the individual to help him cope with the situation of danger.

Because the sources of danger are usually unknown to the individual, he is virtually helpless in defending himself. As a general rule the mechanism of repression is utilized to keep anxiety provoking conflicts encapsulated. Flurries of anxiety are indicative of the inadequacy of the repressive defense, and phobic, compulsive, and other anxiety-binding mechanisms may be utilized, which, even if partially successful, constitute reinforcement for the weakened ego.

In some individuals no such subsidiary defenses develop, and bouts of anxiety assault the ego periodically as repression weakens. Why certain persons never elaborate a structuralized psychoneurotic condition, but rather continue to suffer from periodic attacks of anxiety over a period of many years is a question difficult to answer. There are some authorities who believe that a definite type of personality is present in the individual who continues to exhibit anxiety states. A delineation of the component personality traits present in such persons is unconvincing in so far as specificity of the reaction is concerned. Examination of some patients who maintain themselves in an anxiety neurosis for a long period of time shows that they are so intent upon fulfilling various conflictual drives and goals that they refuse to give up contradictory motivations which would result from the adoption of another type of psychoneurotic defense. Apparently rather than abandon the fulfillment of coveted goals and drives, they would rather pay the penalty of anxiety which serves as retaliatory punishment. In some cases a secondary gain element is exploited, and anxiety may come to signify for the individual an appeal for aid on the basis of his helplessness.

Most persons during their life are confronted with minor and temporary attacks of anxiety especially at times when they are overwhelmed by external difficulties. These attacks, however, are short lived and disappear upon resolution of the disturbing environmental circumstance. In anxiety neurosis, the individual is confronted by persistent attacks of anxiety which show no apparent relationship to fluctuations in his environment. Because no startling situational difficulties are apparent to the person, he is nonplussed by his attacks. This creates further feelings of helplessness, the victim reacting as if he were being assaulted from ambush.

The cause of the anxiety syndrome is usually residual in unconscious conflict or in a shattering of the individual's defenses which have habitually permitted him to maintain his security and to support his self esteem. Analysis reveals that the most potent source of anxiety is rooted in impulses and strivings of which the individual is so fearful that he has relegated them to the oblivion of repression. Such a tendency is usually found in persons with a hypertrophied conscience who react to the emergence of certain strivings within themselves as if they virtually will be abandoned or punished by a tyrannical parent who ceaselessly holds vigil over their actions.

The specific impulse which precipitates anxiety is more or less unique for the individual, and is determined by his particular experiences and conditionings in his relationship with his parents. Where he has been reared by excessively authoritarian parents and has been brought up to abide by standards of extreme submissiveness and ingratiation, he may regard any tendency toward self assertiveness as destructive on his part. Similarly where aggression or sexual curiosity occasion vigorous disciplinary measures, the person may feel obligated to repress hostile or sexual strivings even though later their expression may be culturally condoned.

The adjustment of the individual becomes conditional to the successful repression of hostile and sexual drives, as well to the abnegation of impulses toward self assertiveness. Since these strivings are overwhelmingly powerful at certain epochs in life, they may break through the repressive forces initiating anxiety.

Anxiety attacks are sometimes the product of failing character defenses, which, for one reason or another, are no longer functionally active. The dependent person thus may experience attacks of anxiety upon death of a parent or parental substitute. A compulsively ambitious individual can collapse in the event of a demotion or cut in salary. A person with strong strivings of arrogance may show anxiety when he realizes that he is merely mediocre in his accomplishments. A perfectionistic individual may become ill when he finds that it is impossible to perform without flaws in any new task or enterprise. A threat of closeness in interpersonal relationships in a detached person may produce anxiety. Being put into a dominant position where one operates on the basis of submissiveness and subordination, or being obliged to fulfill a subordinate role in an individual who has domineering tendencies are also capable of provoking attacks.

Another powerful source of anxiety is a blow to the self esteem of the individual. Whenever the self-image is seriously threatened so that the person is unable to marshal a compensatory reaction, he may respond with an attack of anxiety. The actual circumstance that shatters the individual's confidence in himself will, of course, depend upon his specific experiences, and upon the symbols which represent his ideas of self worth. Circumstances which cause him to feel evil, contemptible, destructive and incapable of loving or of being loved are most disastrous to the ego. Failure to fulfill vital goals and ideals, or a violation of these goals, are also potentially anxiety provoking.

In treating an anxiety neurosis, it is almost mandatory to determine the underlying cause. Being brought to awareness of what is going on in his unconscious gives the person the best chance of overcoming his anxiety. Hypnosis may be of signal help here.

A woman came to therapy because of persisting anxiety attacks over a period of six months. Her first attack occurred while she was sitting in a beauty parlor having her hair shampooed. At this time she became aware of a severe pressure on her chest which caused her to gasp for breath. She thought she was having a heart attack and she believed herself to be on the verge of death. Struggling out of the chair, she staggered to a window for air. After a few minutes the attack stopped. Thereafter she refused to enter a beauty parlor. Two weeks later, while in the subway, the same thing happened. As a result she began avoiding subways. From that time on anxiety attacks occurred regularly.

The patient was unaware of any cause for her anxiety. Married, with one child, she believed herself to be reasonably happy. She was unable to recall any provocation for her attacks in the beauty parlor or in the subway. During the therapeutic sessions she waited anxiously and expectantly for something dramatic to happen. She presented no spontaneous dream material, although she remembered dreaming constantly.

Under hypnosis, when asked to recall her dreams, she said, "It's a very funny thing, but since I've been having these attacks, I've been having the same kind of dreams. I've been having very, very peculiar dreams. I've been having dreams of a baby being put on a doorstep. Not only that, but of a man standing on the side and turning his back."

In associating she brought up, with considerable emotion, an experience that had occurred one month prior to the development of her anxiety. She had gone through her husband's pockets on this occasion and had found some condoms in them. Her first response was rage, then contrition. She was an educated woman, she told herself, a woman of the world. Such things happened all the time. She must be an understanding wife; some day she herself might get a crush on another man. She then would feel privileged to have an affair. So she encouraged her husband to talk, convincing him that she would not condemn him. In great relief he confided to her that he had been having an affair with one of her best friends. She was completely understanding and sympathetic. One month later she had her first anxiety attack.

The basis for her anxiety was that she felt resentful toward her husband and hostile toward her friend. Inwardly she felt devastatingly inferior. Her husband's philandering was a tremendous blow to her self esteem. However, she tried to keep these emotions from awareness.

At the beauty parlor, she recalled in a trance, she had noticed wrinkles around her eyes. Fear of growing old and losing her husband mobilized her insecurity. She believed herself unable any longer to swallow her pride, to hold down her resentment, or to condone the actions of her husband. She felt devalued and shamed. Because she imagined she could not compete with the woman who was taking her husband away from her, she was losing faith in herself. These thoughts had gone on mostly beneath awareness. On the surface she tried to crowd them out of her mind.

Her dream of a baby abandoned on a doorstep symbolized her sense of helplessness. The experience had evoked unconsciously the infantile fear of separation from the mother. Her husband in the dream was a symbol of her mother who, with back turned, was deserting her. The core of anxiety was separation from the mother with the fear of death that this entailed.

Bringing these facts to her attention, and permitting her to express her indignation and resentment, convinced her that she had the right to demand fidelity from her husband. Insisting on this right at the threat of separation, a reconciliation was effected with a new and better understanding between her husband and herself. Cessation of anxiety attacks followed.

Environmental manipulation, thus, may, in the event of an anxiety neurosis of recent duration, restore the individual to his previous functioning. He will still, of course, possess neurotic character patterns. Nevertheless, he will be able to function to a more satisfactory degree. Ventilation by the patient of his conflicts and fears may rid him of misconceptions which generate anxiety.

Where the patient's character defenses are more or less adequate, emphasis may be placed upon submerging anxiety through the fortification of those defenses that had previously protected the ego against danger. Hypnosis with reassurance, guidance, externalization of interests, socialization, occupational therapy, persuasion and re-education may be utilized in fulfillment of this goal.

Where anxiety attacks are related to deep seated conflicts in the personality structure, which have little relationship to inimical environmental difficulties, a hypnoanalytic approach is indicated. Here an attempt is made to discover the sources of anxiety, their meaning, and historical origin. The duration of therapy will be dependent upon the rigidity of personality and the extent to which the neurosis has been structuralized. The individual must be shown how his present day attitudes are distorted by anxieties which are rooted in past misconceptions and in unconscious conflict, and a reintegration to life and to people must be effected in the light of his new understanding.

XI

HYPNOSIS IN CONVERSION HYSTERIA

CONVERSION hysteria is a neurosis which classically responds rapidly to hypnotherapy. While hysterical symptoms can often be removed dramatically in relatively few hypnotic sessions, the personality constellation associated with this condition will require more prolonged psychotherapy along the lines indicated in the chapter on character disorders.

The conversion syndrome is found in persons who have an infantile attitude toward life, who are explosive in their reactions to stress and frustration, and who tend to act out their personal conflicts and demands. The world for the hysteric is a theater in which he dramatizes himself for the benefit of those around him whom he considers his audience. The histrionic performances are ingenious and utilize for their content prevailing attitudes and customs. It is for this reason that the forms of hysterical behavior of different epochs, though seemingly dissimilar, are actually of one fabric. Thus the religious dramatizations of the medieval hysteric, the prudish overacting of the Victorian, and the present day hysterical concern with health and hygiene are different only in so far as they utilize divergent symbols. The motivations underlying the behavior distortions are the same. Essentially there is a need to display oneself, and to gain recognition and sympathy from people, particularly authority.

The relationship the hysterical individual establishes with authority is aimed toward winning praise and admiration, and in this effort the person will press into service a host of technics and devices. The super-ego of the hysteric, though enlarged and punitive, prohibiting the expression of inner

220

needs and strivings, is remarkably plastic. The person, consequently, is extraordinarily suggestible, and when he establishes faith in an authoritative individual, he generally abides by the latter's mandates, even to the abandonment of symptoms which have served a defensive purpose. This explains why the hysterical patient is so susceptible to hypnotherapy. The hypnotist in the mind of the patient becomes a sort of deity, the embodiment of power and omniscience. The yielding of a symptom upon command is apparently motivated by a desire to derive security gratifications through compliance. The basic motif of life then is dependency with a need to gain security through the agency of a more powerful individual.

Another characteristic of the hysteric is that he tends to solve conflict through the mechanism of repression. Many of the symptoms he displays, like amnesia, paralysis or anesthesia, are conditioned by a need to reinforce the repressive mechanism. Repression is undoubtedly fostered by a punitive conscience that invokes anxiety, which, when analyzed, is equivalent to loss of love or to injury and mutilation at the hands of authority.

Repression, nevertheless, in most instances, does not suffice to prevent the expression of forbidden impulses. These take on disguised subversive forms manifesting themselves in peculiar dissociated states. There is an autonomous living through of impulses and attitudes which are isolated from the main stream of awareness, as in somnambulism, fugues and multiple personality. The dissociative tendency seems to be exaggerated in hysteria and serves the function of avoiding guilt feelings and anxiety.

The impulses which inspire repression and which strive for a dissociative vicarious form of gratification are usually of a sexual or of a hostile nature.

A tremendous amount of fear and guilt surrounds the sexual function in the hysteric. Unconsciously sexuality is conceived of as an abhorrent incestuous phenomenon, expression of which is equated with castration. Death wishes toward the parents may be coincidental. Masturbatory tendencies are often prominent, but masturbation, too, absorbs the taboo extended to all sexuality, and may be replaced by symptoms such as enuresis, tremors, spasms and various sensory disorders. Impotency, frigidity, dyspareunia and vaginismus are psychosomatic defenses which attempt to protect the individual from sexual involvement. A kaleidoscopic assortment of symptoms spring into being to serve the same purpose.

The origin of sexual fears and misconceptions is residual in a faulty solution of ambivalent attitudes toward the parents. Disturbed relationships with the parents and inimical environmental influences foster insecurities and fears that inhibit sexual maturation. The extent of taboo that invests the sexual instinct has a great deal to do with the manner in which the child handles his sexual drive. In some cultures, where children are allowed to play with each other without too much supervision, to explore each others genitals and even to have sexual relations, it may be expected that there will be a draining off of sexual tension. In our culture, masturbation, intercourse and genital exploration among children is more or less condemned. Consequently, sexuality is apt to become over-emphasized in the child's mind in both its positive and negative aspects. The child's sexual feelings are intensified, and he may develop sexual inclinations toward a parent or sibling in excess of what is to be expected.

Psychoanalytic studies of conversion hysteria bring out the fact that the individual never seems to have progressed beyond an infantile phase of sexuality, with incestuous wishes toward the parent of the opposite sex, fears of retaliatory genital damage, archaic notions of impregnation and birth, and impulses toward the acquisition of a male genital organ as a means of restoring strength and power. These notions persist in the unconscious of the individual and influence his behavior. Although repressed, they may reveal themselves in symptoms, which embrace both an expression of the infantile impulse as well as its denial.

A boy of thirteen was referred for the treatment of a nasal tic which consisted of sniffing followed by a wrinkling of the nose. With hypnoanalytic therapy it became obvious that his conflict involved a desire for an anal attack by a paternal figure which was countered by a fear of castration that such a passive relationship entailed. The sniffing symbolized a displacement of the anal incorporative impulse to the nose through which opening the patient fantasied absorbing a penis by sniffing. At the same time contraction of the nose represented a renunciation or rejection of the penis.

An adolescent girl presented a disturbing symptom of inability to chew food or to swallow. She had, as a consequence, lost thirty pounds in weight. Examination of the symptom disclosed that it was a defense against the impulse to bite off and to swallow her father's penis, which was in turn motivated by strivings for masculinity to overcome feelings of ineffectuality and lack of aggressiveness as a woman. In addition, the fellatio fantasy represented a pregnancy wish in terms of early ideas of oral impregnation.

The investigation of many conversion symptoms will, consequently, disclose that they are condensations representing repressed sexual desires, masturbatory wishes, infantile conceptions of pregnancy and birth, and the primitive acquisition of a male genital organ to replace a fantasied damaged genitality. At the same time a punitive activity may accompany the symptom which is often castrative in its meaning, as if the individual must mutilate himself for his impulses.

Premature ejaculation is a hysterical symptom which, when analyzed, is frequently found to be a regressive form of pleasure functioning embracing both masturbation and urinary activities. In the psyche of the individual, it often represents a form of sexual gratification equivalent to the mother's holding of the child's penis as he urinates. Enuresis, also, is a masturbatory equivalent, serving as a urinary outlet for sexual tension. Additionally, it may represent an aggressive attack on the parent. In a girl it may symbolize possessing a penis; while in a boy it may embrace the wish to function in a passive, dependent, castrated manner. Impotency likewise signifies a fear of as well as a desire for castration. Hysterical seizures, dream states, fugues, somnambulisms, spasms, tremors, tics, paresthesias, vomiting, anorexia, globus hystericus and other psychosomatic symptoms are frequently motivated by impulses which are distorted and expressed symbolically to disguise their sexual nature. Other hysterical symptoms, such as anesthesia, paralysis, amnesia, aphonia, and sundry inhibitions of cognitive, affective and conative activities, serve the purpose, more or less ineffectually, of keeping sexual strivings repressed.

The impulse of hostility may similarly be subjected to repression, following the same mechanisms as with the sexual impulse. Anesthesia, visual disturbances, aphonia, amnesia, fugues, somnambulisms, multiple personality, tics, tremors, choreiform movements, convulsions, and certain other psychosomatic manifestations may be expressions of the breaking through of hostility, with denial of the impulse, defense against it, as well as punishment for its symbolic fulfillment.

There is in hysteria, therefore, a disturbance involving the capacities of the individual to deal realistically with conflict.

A strong secondary gain element is almost always operative after the formation of symptoms. Here the ego exploits the symptom to further the individual's security pursuits. He may gain sympathy, financial compensation and freedom from offensive duties through his illness. This factor must always be kept in mind in therapy, and incentives to get well must be created to offset the benefits of continuance of the symptoms.

The question is often asked regarding the choice of organs or systems which are used to express and to defend oneself from inner strivings. This question will be dealt with more fully in the chapter on psychosomatic illness. In brief, constitutional factors in the form of an inherited weakness of an organ, conditionings and fixations in childhood as a result of overemphasis of certain functions, and identification with ailing parents or siblings are associated.

The treatment of conversion hysteria is dependent upon the motivations of the patient, his need for compliance to authority, and the role the existing symptoms play in his life adaptational scheme.

Symptom removal by authoritative suggestion is possible in some instances, particularly where the symptom produces great physical discomfort and interferes with the individual's social and economic adjustment. There are some symptoms which serve a minimal defensive purpose in binding anxiety. The inconvenience to the patient of such symptoms is an important incentive toward their abandonment. Where the symptom constitutes a plea for help, love and reassurance on the basis of helplessness, the hypnotist, by ordering cessation of symptoms, virtually assures the patient of support and love without his needing to utilize symptoms for this purpose.

Such symptoms as paralysis, aphonia, visual disorders, anesthesia, astasia-abasia and hysterical contractures may be removed in relatively few sessions with a strong authoritarian approach. One must not overestimate the permanency of the cure, however, since the original motivations which sponsored the symptom are not altered in the least, and a relapse is always possible. Consequently, wherever the physician can do so, the patient should be prepared for further therapy by explaining the purposeful nature of his symptom and its source in unconscious conflict. Symptom removal with active participation of the patient, used in the manner outlined in Volume Two, usually yields more per-

manent results than where one depends solely on hypnotic
commands.

Since hysteria often represents a reaction to unpleasant
circumstances which stimulate inner conflicts, a guidance
approach with hypnosis may be utilized, in appropriate cases,
to adjust the patient to environmental demands from which
he cannot escape, and to help him to modify existing remediable situational difficulties. Sometimes it is possible to
get a hysterical individual to make compromises with his
environment so that he will not be so inclined to over-react
to existing stresses. Here, too, an attempt must be made to
acquaint the person with the fact that his symptoms, though
inspired by external difficulties, are actually internally
sponsored. Once the patient accepts this fact, therapy along
analytic lines may be possible.

The treatment of hysteria through hypnotic symptom
removal and by guidance therapy are least successful where
the symptom serves the purpose of providing intense sub-
stitutive gratification for sexual and hostile impulses. Here
hypnoanalysis with analysis of the transference or with
desensitization and re-educational technics, as described in
Volume Two, will be found useful.

Difficulty will also be encountered where the symptom
tends to reinforce the repression of a traumatic memory or
conflict, as in amnesia. The extent of amnesia varies. It may
involve a single painful experience in the past, or it may
include a fairly wide segment of life. It may actually spread
to a point where the person loses his identity and forgets his
past completely. Amnesia serves the defensive purpose of
shielding the individual from anxiety. The intractibility of an
amnesia, consequently, is related to the amount of anxiety
bound down, and to the strength of the ego that is available
to cope with the liberated anxiety. The fear of being overcome by anxiety may be so great that an impenetrable block
to recall will exist despite all efforts to reintegrate the person
to his past memories. Indeed the fear of uncovering a mem-

ory may be so strong that the person will resist trance induction.

Where resistance to hypnosis is encountered, a light barbiturate narcosis, either oral or intravenous, may remove the block. A trance, once induced, is deepened, and a post-hypnotic suggestion is given the patient that he will hence-forth be responsive to hypnosis without narcosis.

Once a deep trance is obtained, the recovery of the memory may be achieved by a variety of technics detailed else-where[1] along lines of direct recall, delayed recall, dream induction, automatic writing, mirror gazing, and regression and revivification.

Regression is particularly adapted for the recall of for-gotten experiences. A woman of twenty-seven was brought in to therapy by her husband with the history that she had, since her marriage one month previously, experienced three brief attacks of total blindness. She had been examined by an eye specialist and no organic pathology could be dis-covered. When interviewed, the patient exhibited a placid, indifferent manner, and seemed not to be disturbed by her symptom, although the reason for her spells of blindness puzzled her. She was, she insisted, extremely devoted to her husband, and she was certain that there was nothing in the marital situation that could account for her illness. Her Rorschach test showed a typical hysterical record, but no inkling of her conflict could be discerned from the responses.

She confided that her first attack had occurred while she was in college seven years previously at which time her dormitory caught on fire. "I was awakened from bed by the smell of smoke. I got the other girls out of bed. I don't remember everything. I smelled something funny. I looked out in the hall. The front steps were on fire. I was perfectly calm as we got out. I kept good control. But then I went out of my head. It was snowing and I went blind for a few minutes."

Her second attack developed six weeks prior to her marriage while engaged. "I had a fight with my husband; that is, he was my boy friend then. It was about getting married. I was menstruating, I remember. When he left, I lay on my bed and cried. Then I had a vision of a ski tow and snow, and losing my engagement ring in the snow. I cried for my mother; then I couldn't see for a while."

Shortly after her marriage, she had her third attack of blindness. "We were home talking, when all of a sudden we got into an argument. I said to my husband, 'You don't respect me at all, do you,' and he said, 'Sometimes I don't.' After that I got an attack of blindness that lasted one-half to three quarters of an hour."

The fourth attack developed when the patient was at home alone. She had been reading a book, and as she approached a part of the book that dealt with a snow scene, she discovered that the print became blurred and that she could scarcely see. Following this her vision left her completely. This time she was not particularly upset, but went to sleep and awakened with full vision.

The last attack occurred shortly before coming to therapy. "I was visiting my husband's family with my husband. We were upstairs in our room when we got into a fight about his mother. He stormed out of the door and went downstairs. I got angry at her. Then I felt sick to my stomach, and I found that I couldn't see anything at all. This lasted about one and one-half hours."

The content of the patient's first few interviews involved the fact that as a child she had always felt that her mother preferred the other siblings to herself. Her fantasies concerned leaving home, getting married and having someone who would really love her. "I hate women and can't get along with them. I am very much in love with my husband, but I am sure that his mother does not like me. I feel with my mind that my husband loves me, but I doubt that anybody could love me." The patient then revealed the fact that she might be pregnant and she remarked that she wanted to have a child badly.

At the next visit the patient described three dreams which apparently had been inspired by her interview with me. The first dream was this: "I was trying to get a job so I could raise enough money to pay your fee. I got a job in a flower shop. The colors were vivid and beautiful." The second dream she described as follows: "I went home and told my parents I was going to have a baby. They raised perfect hell. My mother seemed to be very angry." The third dream was: "We were playing hockey. I could see ice and snow around. I was the goalie and I got hit by the puck in the head so hard that everything went black." When an attempt was made to get the patient to associate to her dreams, she blocked. She remarked that she looked forward to seeing me, since she believed I might be able to cure her spells of blindness. She wanted to have a child, and was not certain that her folks would actually object. Nothing came to her mind when she thought about playing hockey. When she was apprised of the fact that snow seemed to play an important part in her dreams and also in her episodes of blindness, she readily conceded this, although she was unable to understand its significance, other than that it was snowing at the time her dormitory caught fire when she had her first attack.

Under hypnosis, she revealed that, for some reason, she both feared her mother and felt hostile toward her. When an attempt was made to get her to associate to her attacks of blindness, she sobbed in a pitiful manner and was unable to verbalize her thoughts. Slowly she was inducted into a deep trance, and she was given the suggestion that she would gradually return to a time when she had experienced her first attack of blindness. After a pause, during which the patient sobbed convulsively, she said, "I am in a car with someone. I am eight years old. I am coming from my aunt's house. We go past the round house. Then it happened. It's at the railroad. There it is. The two trains; they hit each other. They explode. It scares me. It is horrible." Saying this the patient raised both hands up before her eyes and shrieked, "It must not, it must not happen." She was reassured and encouraged to continue. "There was snow on the ground. I can see it. They took him out of the train. He was burned. It was the first dead person I saw. Then I went home. I went home. The fire, it was our oven. It got on fire. Mother got burned. I thought about the man in the train. I got frightened and I couldn't see."

The patient's hysterical symptom of blindness served the purpose of reinforcing the repression of the traumatic scene of the man who was killed in a train wreck. Killing had become associated with hostile feelings toward her mother. In repressing the traumatic event, the symptom served as a means of denying her aggression toward her mother. Her hostility stemmed both from feelings of frustrated dependency, and from jealousy inspired by a desire for a closer relationship with her father. Her marriage inspired feelings of rejection which she related to her husband's cold attitude. This mobilized her hostility and revived her intense aggression toward her mother with the killing fantasy that this entailed. She then attempted to deny its existence by blinding herself to it through her hysterical eye symptom.

It must again be emphasized that while hysterical symptoms may be treated rapidly through short-term therapy, personality problems, which are associated with the hysterical disorder, are not so easily solved. They will require a considerable period of treatment along re-educational or psychoanalytic lines.

REFERENCE

[1] WOLBERG, L. R.: Hypnoanalysis. New York, Grune & Stratton, 1945, pp. 245-254.

XII

HYPNOSIS IN ANXIETY HYSTERIA

A NXIETY hysteria is a syndrome characterized chiefly by the development of phobias. It is allied to obsessional states in compulsion neurosis and to conversion hysteria. For clinical rather than pathologic reasons, it is treated as a distinct entity.

Unlike conversion hysteria, anxiety hysteria is usually unresponsive to symptom removal by hypnotic command. The psychopathology of the condition apparently does not lend itself to this form of approach.

Anxiety is the central problem in anxiety hysteria. Instead of being free-floating as in anxiety neurosis, the anxiety is controlled by the formation of phobic defenses. Phobia formation is a technic by which anxiety is objectified as an external danger, the individual adapting himself to this danger through avoidance and inhibition of function. Exposure to the situation which is being avoided creates anxiety. The patient usually realizes that his fear is groundless or ridiculous, but he cannot seem to do anything about it.

Although some phobias are developed accidentally through chance conditionings, and though others reflect attitudes and fears which the child has absorbed from the parent, the content of most phobias is determined by some unconscious impulse or conflict which it comes to represent symbolically. Thus fear of the dark may represent a fear of being alone and helpless, at its core constituting the same kind of desolation as early separation from the mother. Terror of animals often signifies a fear of being injured or destroyed by people, masking the individual's own aggressive tendencies. The deeper content of animal phobias may contain an underlying fear of castration. Fear of falling from high places may symbolize fear of, as well as desire for self destruction. Agoraphobia is frequently a cover for fear of a sexual attack, masking a wish for seduction. Claustrophobia and fear of being alone may represent a defense against masturbatory impulses. A touching phobia similarly is often related to apprehension in handling the genital organs, while a fear of contracting venereal disease may represent a desire for illicit intercourse.

Many phobias, consequently, are developed as a means of concealing or denying impulses so repulsive or dangerous that they cannot be openly expressed. The super-ego, while punitive, is still not sufficiently strong to keep inner strivings from obtruding themselves into awareness. The phobia serves to reinforce the repressive process by projecting these strivings, attaching them to relatively innocuous external situations. In this way the impulse is concealed and denied. For instance, strong hostility may be disowned and projected as a fear of dangerous animals who might hurt or devour the person. Impelling sexual drives may be converted into a fear of sexual attack on the part of other persons.

The inhibition of function associated with phobia formation is designed to evade the circumstance which, symbolically linked with the impulse, creates anxiety. It is here that the mechanism of anxiety hysteria is so closely allied to that of conversion hysteria in which there are also inhibitions involving sensory, motor and autonomic functions. While in anxiety hysteria the individual avoids facing dangerous self-created external situations, in conversion hysteria he avoids acknowledging activities that are symbolic of disowned inner impulses.

A number of phobias are the product of anxieties perpetuated through fear of gratifying character strivings conceived of as dangerous. For example, claustrophobia may sometimes represent a fear of being overwhelmed in a dependency situation. The character structure of this type of claustrophobiac shows, on the one hand, a tremendous need for dependency, and, on the other, overpowering fears of being mutilated or destroyed by the passivity that dependency entails. However, since the person must pursue dependency due to his helplessness, he is impelled to seek a dependent relationship. At the same time he projects his fear of being trapped to closed spaces and to confining situations. An individual with strivings of detachment may develop phobias of crowds or of being in close contact with people. A striving for compulsive independence may produce a fear of losing control, as fear of jumping out of open windows.

Another group of phobias is conditioned, not by inner conflict, but rather by chance associations. For instance, a child in crossing the street is struck by an automobile. Thereafter he may develop a fear of streets, or of crossing streets. A man in a car may accidentally kill a pedestrian, then refuse to drive because of panic while in the driver's seat. One must always suspect in such situations that problems exist which are not apparent on the surface, since the average individual will gradually desensitize himself to such traumatic situations. However, a large number of fears do develop fortuitously and do persist. An anxiety attack developing in a particular locality may produce a fear of this locality, even though it has no relationship to the source of anxiety. For example, a woman, hostile to her husband, may develop an anxiety attack on a subway while reading a newspaper account of a wife who slaughtered her husband. Thereafter she may avoid traveling in subways.

As a general rule phobias spread, involving increasingly diffuse situations which are more and more remotely related to the original situation. Thus a fear of being locked up in one's room can extend itself to a fear of being indoors and then to a fear of being under a roof. Unless the source of the phobia is checked, there is little likelihood that the phobia will vanish of its own accord.

A direct attack on a phobia is usually futile even when

strong injunctions are given the patient while he is in a deep trance. Pointing out the foolishness of the patient's fears also has little deterrent effect on their power. Since the person is unaware of the meaning of the phobia, his will and intelligence are of little help to him. Attempts to banish by hypnotic command even those fears that are conditioned through chance associations are usually of little avail. This may be demonstrated experimentally by exposing the individual to an electric shock, measuring his galvanic skin reflex which indicates his fear reaction. After a few shocks, the mere approach of the operator will elicit a galvanic reflex. When the subject is shown that the wires leading to the shocking apparatus are disconnected, and he understands that he cannot possibly receive a shock, the operator's approach to the apparatus will still produce a positive galvanic reflex. The entire reaction of fear seems to go on outside the realm of awareness.

It is to be expected, therefore, that phobic removal by hypnotic suggestion, as well as the mastery of fearsome situations through hypnotically reinforced will power, will result in limited success.

Hypnosis with psychobiologic therapy is nevertheless sometimes successful in anxiety hysteria, particularly with technics of persuasion, reconditioning, desensitization and re-education.

Through persuasive methods an attempt is made to build up the individual's self confidence and self esteem, encouraging him to engage in activities which will overcome his phobia. Unfortunately, although the patient is apt to make a better adjustment, and although he may learn to master his fears on the basis of positive benefits he derives from their conquest, he will still experience panic reactions, and he will have to force himself over and over again to face fear-provoking situations.

Associated with persuasive technics, technics of self

mastery through the medium of self hypnosis may be utilized. Here the individual fortifies himself to face a phobic situation by minimizing its fearful aspects, and by concentrating on the pleasure values incidental to the phobic pursuit. Persistent suggestions to gather courage and to master his fears may inspire sufficient fortitude to pull the person successfully through a situation he ordinarily would be unable to face. Needless to say this technic is palliative and results are temporary at best.

Fears that are conditioned through chance associations may, under hypnosis, occasionally be reconditioned by associating strong pleasure stimuli with the situation that inspires the phobia. For instance, if a person has experienced an anxiety attack while climbing stairs, and has associated stair climbing with anxiety, a dramatic technic may be utilized under hypnosis, during which he indulges in a pleasure pursuit at the very time he has to climb stairs. The patient is enjoined, in the trance, to climb an increasingly greater numbers of stairs.

Another means of treating phobias is by desensitization. Under hypnosis the patient is given suggestions to expose himself gradually to the terrifying situation. The aim in desensitization is to get the patient to master his fears by actually facing them. It is essential for the individual to force himself again and again into the phobic situation, in order that he may finally learn to control it. For example, if a person fears open spaces, or going outdoors, he can, on the first day, walk several steps from his house, and then return. On the second day he may increase the distance between himself and his house, and similarly on each following day until he is able to walk a considerable distance from his home. The hope is that the conquering of graduated doses of his fear will desensitize him to its influence.

Re-educational methods, utilizing psychobiologic or psychoanalytic approaches along with hypnosis, are far more rational than the aforegoing technics, since they deal with the causes of the phobia. The object is to understand the function of the phobia, and then to readjust the individual to its dynamic source.

Hypnoanalysis is often eminently successful in tracing the origin of a phobia. Where a fear has been produced by an incident so terror inspiring that it has been repressed, it may be possible to get the person to recall the original emotional experience under hypnosis and then to re-evaluate the situation in terms of his present day understanding. A helpful technic is to regress the person to a period prior to the development of the phobia, and then gradually to reorient him in his age level to later and later periods of life, until the original situation associated with the development of the phobia has been uncovered. Where the phobia is the product of character patterns that have originated early in life, it will be necessary to produce a more or less drastic reorganization of the personality through further therapy after the phobia has been analyzed and its sources determined.

A married woman of thirty, whose husband had become impotent, met a young man at a vacation resort who made sexual advances toward her. Upon returning home she began to experience tension and intestinal distress. On one occasion she developed an anxiety attack on the street during which she imagined she was being pursued by men who might attack her sexually. She developed an agoraphobia shortly thereafter. Prevailing upon her mother to live with her, she refused to leave her home unless accompanied by her parent. During hypnoanalysis it was clearly demonstrated to the patient that at the time she experienced her anxiety attack, she had felt sexually excited by the sight of a man who resembled the person she rebuffed at the resort. She became aware of the fact that her fear of the street concealed a desire to give herself sexually to the first man who approached her. Her need to have her mother around was to protect her from her impulses. These realizations relieved her of her phobia, but further treatment along analytic lines was required to correct her general timidity and her submissive tendencies.

Another woman of thirty applied for treatment complaining of a water phobia so extreme that it interfered with bathing. Even sight of a bathtub created panic. Her difficulty, though present since early childhood, had become increased after her marriage five years previously.

She remembered that during childhood she feared swimming in large bodies of water. As she grew older, the fear extended to ponds and swimming pools. However, by avoiding places where there was swimming, she was able to master her fear.

Upon marriage she gave up a lucrative newspaper position in order to devote herself to housework. Her fear of water became progressively more exaggerated. Following an anxiety attack in the bathtub, she became more and more depressed and guilt ridden.

Her sole objective in coming to therapy was to rid herself of her phobic symptom. So far as she knew she was getting along quite well with her husband and with people in general. She was aware of no problems except for the symptom which distracted her so that she felt she might lose her mind.

She was able to enter a deep trance and, upon suggestion to dream about her greatest fear, she dreamt of a large lake surrounded by mountains. It was then suggested that she would, the same evening, dream of the origin of her water phobia. At the next session she reported a fragment of a dream in which she and another person were standing near a body of water. Under hypnosis she recovered other elements of the dream which she had forgotten. She saw a child being pushed into the water from a raft by a person whose identity was unclear, but who seemed to be more like a man than a woman.

The technic of regression was next utilized, and the patient was urged to return to the time when she first became afraid of water. Gasping for breath, she relived a traumatic experience at the age of three during which she visualized herself drowning. "He pushed me, he pushed me," she expostulated, then broke down into spasmodic crying. The details of the experience could not be obtained at this time, nor could it be determined whether the experience was a real memory or a cover memory. A suggestion was made that she would gradually understand her problem better and better, and would, if the drowning experience were actually true, be able to recall it.

Upon awakening the patient was visibly shaken and upset, although she had a complete amnesia for the trance events. During the next few weeks she began to exhibit resistance to therapy which was coupled with resentment toward me. The first inkling she had of her resentment was when she began to criticize physicians as a group. Then she revealed irritation at my refusal to take more responsibility in planning her life routine. She intimated that in reading books on psychiatry, she had recently become interested in doing therapy herself. During hypnosis she gave vent to a tirade of abuse in which she pictured herself as a hapless depreciated person who could never achieve my stature.

In discussing her ambitions, she began to realize that she was extremely hostile toward her husband. In dreams she brought up intense competitiveness with him, which she felt obliged to forget because of the destructive feelings involved. Dreams of drowning followed verbalization of her hostility toward her husband.

Through various hypnoanalytic technics, it was possible to trace the origin of the patient's competitive feelings and to understand the meaning of her phobia. As a small child she was in rivalry with a brother two years her senior. Furious because she was unable to emulate her brother in his activities and achievements, she responded to her penis envy by acting in a hostile and destructive manner toward him. Her brother retaliated in kind. On one occasion, while bathing at a resort, she had become furious with her brother and had scratched him. The two children were separated by the father, but when they walked out on a small pier, the brother, in a fit of rage, pushed her into the water. Before her father fished her out, she had inhaled a considerable amount of water and was badly frightened.

Shortly after this experience, the patient became submissive and avoided arguments with her brother. She also developed a fear of swimming. She recalled an incident, under hypnosis, of her father trying to force her to go bathing while she resisted violently. Following this, she alleged, she had begun to experience panic whenever she gazed at a body of water. It was obvious that her fear of water was conditioned by a fear of her own aggressiveness. Any hostility that was generated by competitiveness was masked by surface compliance and diffidence. The existence of hostility, nevertheless, created a fear that she would be punished in some catastrophic manner. There was a prototype in the drowning experience, and the fear of water signified a conviction she would be injured for her hostility by drowning. So long as she avoided competitiveness with men, she was able to keep hostility at a minimum.

Her marriage, however, relegated her to an inferior role as a housewife, and created resentment toward her husband which she repressed. As hostility mounted, the fear of water became more intensified, almost as if she would again be subjected to a drowning experience. She attempted to cope with her anxiety by avoiding water.

As soon as the patient became aware of how her hostility and competitiveness toward me caused an exacerbation of her phobia, and when she became cognizant of the role she had played with her husband, she began to appreciate the significance of her symptom. Her phobia became less and less troublesome to her, and finally it disappeared completely. She was able to obtain a part time newspaper position, and to experience a new found happiness in her relations with her husband.

XIII

HYPNOSIS IN COMPULSION NEUROSIS

COMPULSION neurosis, or obsessive-compulsive neurosis as it is often called, is characterized by obsessive fears and thoughts with or without the presence of compulsive acts and rituals.

The obsessive ideas are accompanied by intense anxiety, involving chiefly fears of injuring oneself or others, fears of disease, and of death. There is sometimes an anxious preoccupation with sex and with toilet activities. Tension, insomnia, physical distress and other psychosomatic symptoms are present in greater or lesser degree.

The compulsive acts, which consist of illogical rituals, such as counting, pointing, touching, recitation of key words or phrases, or more complicated ceremonials, are performed for the purpose of neutralizing obsessive thoughts or impulses. The person realizes his performance is senseless. He may even be ashamed of it; yet he is forced to carry out the act under pressure of a compelling anxiety.

An analysis of the compulsive-obsessive reaction shows that it develops in a specific type of personality organization, which itself is a response to the same conflicts that produce the neurosis. The character structure of the obsessive-compulsive, being defensive in nature, protects the individual from his inner strivings and fears. When this organization fails in its defensive function, repressed impulses gain access to consciousness in the form of obsessions, which the individual then attempts to eliminate by compulsive acts.

The conflicts engendering compulsive character defenses are residual, to a large degree, in disturbed early conditionings and experiences in relationship with parents and other important adults.

Two types of parental handling may be discerned. In the first type, anal functions have been overemphasized in a positive sense, and the child coordinately has been overindulged and pampered. Out of this type of conditioning inordinate pleasures are vested in anal activities, the anal area becoming a chief pleasure zone. Indeed it may usurp the sexual zone as a source of pleasure, and toilet activities and desires for anal penetration may preoccupy the individual. Should the person respond to his impulses, he is usually rewarded by guilt feelings, which reflect social displeasure. He may attempt to repudiate his desires by "reaction formations" in which he tries to eliminate his craving for anal stimulation. This inspires tension and hostility with a desire to attack those forces which deny him gratification.

In the second type, the child has been subjected to vigorous toilet training and to excessive disciplines. Severely disciplinary parents, reflecting the cultural emphasis on meticulousness and overcleanliness, are precise in their requirements that the child be socialized and scrupulously toilet trained. This makes anal activities a battleground in the child's struggle with authority. The child seeks to maintain control and to express his assertiveness by regulating his own bowel movements; yet he feels he must yield fecal contents on command.

The anal function becomes tremendously overvalued. On the one hand, possession of fecal material becomes a sign of power and assertiveness. On the other hand, since the parents insist that excretory products be released regularly on the basis that he will become ill as a result of poisonous retentions, the individual develops an ambivalent attitude towards excretory products. They become imbued with foul, destructive and killing potentialities. These misconceptions concerning excretory substances may persist in the unconscious of the individual and may condition a number of attitudes. Being able to retain the fecal mass, or being able to soil at will thus may become signs of his own capacity to function independently, and may be associated in his mind with being a firm, independent individual who can do what he wants when he wants to do it. He may evince, as a consequence, a tremendous interest in feces at the same time that he expresses disgust for it.

At puberty, strong impulses motivate the person to express himself sexually. The individual as a result again comes into intense conflict with authority. He will then try to work out his relationship with authority in the same way that he did during the period of toilet training. Furthermore, the strong sexual drive at this time will light up his desire for anal pleasures. Anal activities may become a substitute for sexual activities, and homosexual fantasies or impulses may replace the heterosexual urge. The interest in anal functions inspires guilt and stimulates the person's defenses to neutralize his urge.

The first line of adjustment to the conflict that occurs in the compulsion neurotic in his struggle with authority is a compulsive character of stubbornness, orderliness, preciseness, meticulousness, and cleanliness. Apparently, the individual's anxiety is so intense that he attempts to adjust to the conflict of wanting to maintain his independence by arranging things in an orderly and precise manner. In this way he protects himself from attack. The person may become overly meticulous in everything he does. He must put everything in its proper place; he must say the correct thing at the right time. The dynamic basis for this lies in a fear of being caught off guard. In planning and figuring things out in utmost detail, he tries to evade being caught unprepared. Thus he avoids what he considers being domineered, overwhelmed and destroyed.

Another character trait that develops is obstinacy. In obstinacy the person seeks to preserve his intactness by refusing to yield anything. In being stubborn, he avoids personal invasion. In the same light miserliness, and the need to accumulate and to hold onto possessions, serve the purpose of keeping things within himself. There is a fear of being outgoing. In his intellectual pursuits, too, the obsessive lives a very rigid routinized life. He must plan everything in advance. In a physical sphere his muscles are tense. His oral and anal sphincters may be constricted and spastic, as if he must shut himself off from the world even here.

A person with this type of character organization is in constant fear of attack. Hostility is incessant and often overwhelming. Indeed hostility may become so intense that the only way he can control it is by detaching himself from people, by attacking them, or by "reaction formations" of meekness, ingratiation and submissiveness which mask his hostile impulses. Inwardly he burns with resentment, but since his hostility is equated in his mind with killing, and because the object toward whom he feels hostile is usually one on whom he is dependent, he must repress his emotion. Fears of killing and of being killed are almost universal in obsessive personalities. These fears are more or less conscious, frequently occurring as obsessions which haunt the individual so tenaciously that they cannot be shaken from his mind.

One patient, meek and submissive in the facade that he presented to the world, under hypnosis broke through with the following exhortation: "I want to kill my parents, because if I kill my parents that means that I will be let alone. Nobody will hurt me then. I will be strong; I will do what I want. Nobody is going to take me over; nobody is going to tell me what to do. So if I kill them, I'll be able to do what I want to do. I'll be able to marry and do what I want."

Another component of the obsessive-compulsive character is a strong dependency striving, the person feeling he can function only by being dependent upon someone else. In his dependency he has strong sadistic fantasies of destroying his host, because dependency implies that he will be domineered or emasculated. Yet he craves passivity. These ambivalent attitudes appear in the therapeutic relationship and account for much of the turmoil that develops during treatment. The obsessive person desires to be dependent, but when he feels himself getting close to a person, he fears he will have to give up his defenses, and that he will virtually be castrated. Being dependent means giving up his masculinity. Nevertheless he wants to be dependent, and he may have homosexual fantasies such as those voiced by one patient: "If I make myself a woman, then I will be able to be dependent. I will be able to be taken care of. I will be given things, and everything will be all right. But if I do that, I will lose my sense of strength, my aggressiveness, my power, everything that makes life worth while. I will be destroyed, so I must protect myself against that. I will kill anybody that tries to make me dependent. But if I get independent and strong, that really means that I will do what I'm afraid I'll have to do and that is that I'll have to kill everybody."

Anxiety in the obsessive-compulsive individual becomes intense, and often is dealt with by detachment. Since close contact with people arouses his anxiety, the person tries to avoid intrusion. Yet his dependency drives him to seek people with whom he can be dependent. He may conceive of the idea that the only way he can overcome his dependency is by killing; the only way he can express his sexual needs also, and avoid being injured by authority, is by killing.

In analyzing compulsive persons, one frequently encounters the idea that if he can maintain a detached attitude towards life, if he acts in an ingratiating, obsequious way, if he is orderly, and meticulous, and figures out everything in advance, if he does not permit any emotions to develop within him (since emotion is equated with hostility and killing) then everything will be under control. However, the person does develop feelings of closeness toward people in spite of himself, and when he does his defenses begin to crumble.

In compulsion neurosis there is also a marked damage to self expressiveness and self esteem. The security of the person swings from dependency desires with impulses for submission, passivity and homosexuality (passivity being equated in the unconscious with homosexuality) to a swing in the other direction towards self sufficiency with an attempt to maintain assertiveness at all costs. Unconsciously the latter is equated with murderous destructivensss. Consequently, hostile and destructive impulses may come to possess an intense pleasure value for the individual, but they are repressed because of the individual's fear of counterhostility.

Obsessive ideas which embrace his ambivalent drives then begin to torment the person. He tries to neutralize his obsessions by various technics, one of which is "isolation." Here the individual tries to divest his feelings from his intellect. The content of thought is dissociated from its deep emotional roots to protect the person from feeling.

Another technic that he utilizes is the phenomenon of "undoing." "Undoing" is a means of neutralizing and controlling obsessive fears. It operates on the basis of a magical principle, as if the person says, "If I do certain things, it will undo what has happened before." The most fantastic actions may be utilized for this purpose. One patient had a compulsion to count in threes. In analysis it was determined that counting to three neutralized an obsession to dispose of his parents. Three meant restoring his mother, father and himself. Many seemingly meaningless ceremonials and rituals may be utilized to eliminate obsessive fears or impulses. These become compulsive in nature, and unless the individual performs them in a routinized way, he is filled with anxiety.

The type of thinking present here is reminiscent of the thinking of children. It is probably the sort of magical

thinking utilized during the early phase of language formation, perhaps around the period when the most intense
conflicts occur in the obsessive-compulsive. The magical
thinking is apparently an attempt to undo destructive
tendencies, to counteract anal interests, as well as the fears
that these interests precipitate.

The treatment of compulsion neurosis is notoriously
difficult. This is because the relationship with the therapist is
of an extremely ambivalent nature. On the one hand, the
patient desires to be dependent on the therapist, and toward
this end he will employ varied technics like making himself
obsequious, ingratiating, and submissive. On the other hand,
in spite of the fact that he desires to be dependent, he will
resent dependency. He will express hostility toward the
therapist either openly or covertly. While on the surface he
may exhibit a great deal of deference, inwardly he is re-
bellious and is fired with much resentment. The dreams he
displays, related to the transference, demonstrate the intense
hostility he feels towards the therapist. The patient looks
upon his impulses for dependency and compliance as threats
to his independence and to his capacity to function by himself.

The battle with the therapist can go on for a long time
without the patient's being aware of how he seeks to make
himself dependent and at the same time to detach himself.
While he asks the therapist for help, he will stubbornly
oppose accepting the therapist's interpretations or suggestions. He will be tremendously demanding and desire to be
relieved of his symptoms, yet when attempts are made to
help him in a positive way, he will resist these, and then become hostile at the therapist for not helping him more. The
rigidity he displays during therapy is manifested in in-
tellectualizing what is going on. This serves as a defense
against his feelings. Many compulsive persons are capable of
learning the mechanism of their illness without this having
the slightest effect upon the intensity and severity of their

symptoms. Their tendencies to doubt make interpretations difficult. When they do accept interpretations, evincing a tremendous amount of interest in what goes on in their psyche, it is quite apparent that they do not feel what they intellectually accept. The "isolation" of the intellectual processes from the emotional content makes therapy extremely difficult.

The compulsive personality will attempt to disarm the therapist by obeying punctiliously every suggestion or command expressed or implied. While he may be responsive on the surface, inwardly he maintains a tremendous amount of scepticism about what goes on. One may attempt to change the patient's way of life by pointing out prevailing contradictions. Though the patient seems to have accepted and understood thoroughly the implications of his difficulties, and though he voices a desire for change, the way he acts outside the analytic situation indicates that he has not really absorbed the insight he verbalized. Sometimes the behavior of the patient is in a direction opposite to his intellectual understanding. Unconsciously the patient seeks to ridicule the therapist by contradicting his suggestions.

Compulsion neurosis does not respond to psychoanalytic therapy as well as do other neurotic syndromes. It can be treated, of course, by psychoanalytic methods, but the analyst must be extremely skilled in the handling of the transference, and he must have much fortitude to tolerate the vicissitudes that will come up in the course of treatment.

Frequently the most that can be done is to fortify the patient's failing defenses, and to get him to function with the personality makeup he had prior to the development of disabling symptoms. The complicating element is that the detachment, which is one of his primary defenses, may be the symptom the patient desires most to abandon. He seeks to live a better life, and he is thoroughly disgusted with his detachment. He understands that he is missing many of life's pleasures. When the patient realizes that yielding his detachment creates in him anxiety and great turmoil, and that he will have to return to his customary isolation from people, he may become depressed. In some instances desperation can even drive him to suicide.

Whenever possible, therefore, the physician must attempt not only to control the patient's symptoms, but to promote sufficient alteration in the character structure to permit a reasonable functioning with people in a close relationship situation. Where the patient has a motivation to gain normal satisfactions in life, and where he realizes that his detachment, obsequiousness, perfectionism, meticulousness, obstinacy and other character traits create difficulties with people and prevent enjoyment in living, he may then have the incentive to tolerate and to work through the anxieties incumbent upon giving up these traits.

The therapy of compulsion neurosis or compulsive-obsessive personality disorders must take into account the patient's dependency, the profoundly hostile impulses he has toward people, his need for detachment, the tendency to "isolate" intellect from feeling, and the magical frame of reference in which his ideas operate.

Among the most important tasks to be achieved in the therapy of this condition are demonstrating to the patient that his symptoms have a definite cause and that they stem from no magical source; that aggression is a normal impulse originating in hostile attitudes; that he can express a certain amount of hostility without destroying other people or injuring himself; that he can relate to a person without needing to make himself dependent or compliant.

Hypnosis is often valuable in achieving these objectives. Because the framework of compulsive thinking is magical, the compulsion neurotic very often is motivated towards receiving hypnotherapy. Secretly he hopes that hypnosis can, in some magical way, neutralize his obsessional concern with injury, with killing, with death and with sexuality. Where this is the sole motivation, hypnosis is bound to fail, since hypnosis will not effect a magical neutralization of impulses. Another motive the compulsion neurotic has for hypnosis is that the hypnotist reinforce his waning repressive powers. Inasmuch as his inner impulses and demands make him desire to break down his controls, he may feel that his will power, unless buttressed, will not keep in check the tumultuous emotions within. As a consequence, he will want the hypnotist to play a parental role giving him orders to lead a restrictive, rigid life. Under these circumstances, too, hypnosis is apt to fail. The individual, though he asks for this type of handling, will actually resist the hypnotic process, or hypnotic suggestions, or he will develop intense hostility towards the physician.

In the induction of hypnosis, certain problems occur in the obsessive-compulsive that are not encountered in other neuroses. The individual may be obstinate, so insistent upon exercising his will, and so resistive to accepting suggestions that he will be unable to enter a trance state. One means of circumventing this, is to couch suggestions in such a way that the patient himself feels that he is in control of the hypnotic process. Many patients will spontaneously ask that this be done; as a matter of fact, some compulsion neurotics come to therapy for the sole purpose of learning self hypnosis. There is an attempt here to reinforce a waning superego, to get strength from some outside agency which will enable them to control their inner conflicts and drives. Once the initial resistances which militate against assuming a trance state are overcome, the individual usually makes an excellent subject.

The patient thus may be quite resistive to hypnosis at the start, and one may gain the impression that it is impossible to hypnotize him; however, with properly phrased suggestions directed at making the patient believe he is in control of his own processes, he will eventually be able to enter a hypnotic state. Very often it is essential to spend a great deal of time in the first induction process to break through resistances. It is usually best to induct a compulsion neurotic as deeply as possible at the first trance. He will be caught off guard the first time, but thereafter will know what to expect and will mobilize his defenses better. A slow induction brought to a depth where the patient will be able to follow certain suggestions posthypnotically, convinces the patient that he has been in a trance and that he can follow suggestions effectively.

The particular type of therapy to be employed with hypnosis is determined by the patient's motivations and inner resources, and by the therapeutic goal. In my experience, a combination of psychobiologic and psychoanalytic technics is most effective. This involves a directive reeducational approach along psychoanalytic lines, avoiding a neurotic transference, and utilizing guidance, persuasion and reassurance whenever necessary.

At the start the patient is bewildered, tense, and torn by ambivalent strivings. He pleads for relief and often assumes that the physician is delinquent in his obligations when he fails to remove his symptoms. Furiously he may insist that he feels no better, that he has uncontrollable impulses to do damage to himself and others, that he is impelled to engage in sexual activities which repell him, that he is helpless in coping with his tension and panicky feelings. It is essential to explain to him that his symptoms and feelings have a meaning, that it is necessary to understand the causes creating his difficulties, and that it is possible to correct the causes. As a general rule the patient is skeptical about this explanation, since deep down he believes his difficulties are caused by some sort of evil magic. Only when he establishes some confidence in the physician is it possible to influence his superstitious nature.

Hypnosis serves to bring about a feeling of confidence in the physician more rapidly than any other available technic. In compulsion neurosis a deep trance is not essential. As a matter of fact the patient is so informed prior to trance induction, and he is told that a light trance, in which he experiences some feeling of relaxation, may be preferred to one in which he goes into a stuporous state. He is assured that suggestions penetrate to the deeper layers of mind even in a light trance.

As soon as the patient achieves as deep a trance as can be brought about without too great an effort and without inciting resistance, he is given reassuring and persuasive suggestions to the effect that he can get well, that others sicker than himself have been able to experience relief from their symptoms, and that, if he has the desire to recover, he will want to do what is essential in overcoming his difficulties.

One of the most important things he is to realize is that his symptoms are not the product of supernatural forces, but rather follow scientific laws of cause and effect. Understandably, because he is victimized by fear, tension and panicky feelings, which seemingly come from unknown sources, he has been unable hitherto to ascertain the meaning behind his symptoms. However, the reasons he suffers will become known to him as he begins to connect events in his environment with how he feels. Nothing in the universe happens by chance. If he hears a sound, he knows very well something has created the sound. Science has definitely shown that a causal relationship exists in the world.

The patient is usually reassured by such a talk, since he virtually feels himself to be at the mercy of wicked inscrutable forces over which he has no control. These forces are nightmarish in quality and give him the feeling of being manipulated by demons. It must be remembered that the compulsion neurotic thinks in terms of witchcraft. To be advised by a person he respects that a matter-of-fact cause lies behind his agony, gives him much solace. Accepting this explanation on faith, however, is not enough. It is essential to point out to him how, when he gets involved in specific environmental difficulties, his symptoms become exacerbated.

One patient was obsessed with the idea of the number "36", which he felt portended death. Wherever he went he could see the number "36".   On one occasion he read in the newspaper that a man aged 36 was indicted for murder; in another instance, he came across an ambulance with the license number "3636" on it; in a third circumstance he walked past a door on which there was a wreath with the house number "36" below it. All these events implied to him that things were being brought to his attention, that somehow he, himself, would either be killed or he would do the killing because his unlucky number was 36. Actually he was 36 years of age, but could see no connection.

After a lengthy explanation about the scientific causes for world phenomena, the patient was told that each day a person is confronted with thousands of experiences, and that, therefore, coincidences are common. Through coincidence it would be possible to find each day several instances which seemed to substantiate his deepest fears. If his fear was that people talked behind his back, he would always be able to notice a few people mumbling together. Actually they would not be talking about him, but because he was so sensitive, he would misinterpret their action as referring to himself. Any person sensitive about certain things will be very keenly attuned to looking for those things, and will probably, in the course of a day, find evidence that seems to bear out his concern. Natural forces rule the world; the idea that things are happening to him through some supernormal force is a residue of childish forms of thinking and feeling. Nothing actually could happen to him even if he did see the number "36" daily. This talk, coupled with persuasive injunctions to involve himself in more work and to socialize more with people, helped him to abandon his preoccupation.

An explanation of the dynamics of his disorder may be given the patient, geared to his intellectual capacities and couched in interpersonal rather than libidinal terms. This approach, utilizing concepts which he is intellectually capable of comprehending, gives him an explanation for his illness far more reasonable than the confused situation which he has customarily imagined to exist. Once he has begun to divest his thinking of its magical associations, he will be able to absorb deeper insights, and to utilize them in the direction of change.

A persuasive technic may be employed coordinately in hypnosis and in the waking state. The patient is first reassured about his obsessive fears and impulses. He is told that were he actually going to carry them into action, he would do so without tormenting himself. The chances are that he will not perpetrate any of the wicked deeds of which he is so frightened.

For instance, if he fears he may become violently dangerous and kill people, he may be shown that actually he expresses aggression far less freely than the average person. As a matter of fact, he probably fails to exhibit even ordinary amounts of assertive aggressiveness. He is encouraged to observe himself in his daily reactions with people, to see whether he is not restricting a show of aggressiveness.

A man of thirty-five, a broker by profession, developed an obsessive fear of injuring or stabbing his wife. This fear occurred shortly after his marriage and had become progressively more exaggerated until he found himself unable to look at knives or other potentially lethal objects. His tension and anxiety became so extreme that he was incapable of going to work several days out of each week. One of the fantasies that occupied his mind was sneaking up on his wife and killing her by smothering her with feces. This thought terrified him to a point where he insisted upon sleeping in a separate room.

Utilizing the above described technic, the patient was told in a light trance that the first task was to make him aware of his deeper emotions. He had already seen a number of psychiatrists and had intellectual insight into the dynamics of his condition. Indeed he could recite tracts from Freud which described some of his reactions exactly as he felt them. Because of the mechanism of "isolation," however, he was unable to react deeply to his insight. After explaining to him that one of his problems was the expression of aggressiveness, which was abnormal in that he felt obliged to keep hidden any show of anger, he was told that he had developed great fears of exhibiting even normal aggressiveness, since this in his mind was equivalent with destroying everything and anybody.

If it were true that he might kill his wife, it would explain why he had a desire to watch everything that he did, why he had to be certain there were no pointed instruments around which he might inadvertently use. If it were true that in relaxing his vigilance he might lose control over his destructiveness, it would explain why he had to keep thinking about his fear so incessantly. Nevertheless, he could be assured that even if he were to take his mind off worrying about killing, nothing would happen. He would find that he had been needlessly concerned with defenses which actually had little usefulness. The reason for this was that the basic premise was wrong. He would kill or hurt no one in actual reality. He was then told that gradually he would feel better and more self confident. He would feel more self assured and stronger. He was asked to watch himself to see what actually happened in his life situation that stirred up his feelings.

Not long after this the patient reported an incident in which he had wanted to become angry at somebody who had done him an injury, but he could not bring himself to express anger. He was given an explanation, both on waking and hypnotic levels, that what had happened was sufficient to make anyone feel resentful, that being resentful was normal and permissible at times. Because of his own particular problems, however, even ordinary amounts of resentment were associated with such fears that he might do injury that he had to repress this feeling. Were he to explode from time to time like anyone else, and give vent to the resentment, he would get rid of much tension. He would then prevent his resentment from piling up on him to a point where he believed he would explode and hurt someone. Such a situation was to be expected. The patient was then given an example of steam in a boiler. If a boiler with water were sealed and put over a fire, steam would accumulate. If no outlet for the steam were provided, eventually the pressure would become so extreme that the boiler would explode. It was the same way with a powerful emotion like resentment. If no outlets for resentment were found, eventually resentment would pile up and become overwhelming until the person felt like exploding. Actually, normal resentments were part of living, and everybody to some extent experienced and expressed resentment. The job of living involved the ability to express resentment in such a way that the person felt he was justified in standing up for his rights.

The patient responded to this explanation with the statement that if he allowed himself to express any resentment, he was certain something terrible would happen; he might even lose control completely and kill his wife. In a trance, he was encouraged to release resentment, nevertheless, whenever the situation justified it, if only to release energy so that it would not accumulate. It did not necessarily mean that he had to "bop" somebody over the head with a chair when he got resentful; it meant that he could take a stand when he felt justified in doing so. That was expected of him; people would respect him more, and he would respect himself more. When the time came, he would be able to express his resentment; and this would result in his injuring nobody. These suggestions were repeated on both waking and hypnotic levels, and he was enjoined to practice diverting his thoughts from his preoccupation with killing. He was also encouraged to be with people more in order to get away from being by himself. Were he to divert his mind, he would begin to feel better and more assured.

Within the next week the patient started putting these suggestions into practice. His brother-in-law had come to live with him, and he had gotten into an argument with the man. He thought his brother-in-law should do some shopping; but the latter was a "lazy lout" and just did not want to do any work at all. He was very angry with his brother-in-law and with his own wife who took sides against him. However, remembering my statement, he decided to insist on his rights. He berated his brother-in-law and his wife. That evening he had a headache, and then the thoughts of killing suddenly disappeared. For four days there were no thoughts of killing, and then they returned in full force. "But, you know," he said, "I really saw something this time. I think it's because I get very angry at my wife, and I get so angry that I can't control myself, and then I'm afraid that I might hurt her." He repeated that as naively as if he had never been analyzed at all. It was somewhat like a revelation for him to feel what he knew intellectually. He related two dreams. The first was that he was angry with his wife and his brother-in-law, and waved his fist at them in displeasure. The second dream was that he was with his mother. He did something clumsy, including dropping a glass. The glass broke and his mother then became infuriated with him. The scene shifted and he saw his wife in a state of rage. She left him and then married somebody else. He stormed angrily at his wife, but she would not come back to him.

As he associated, he began to talk about how dependent he had been on his mother; how his mother had refused to permit him to be aggressive or to argue with her; how he had to give in to his mother all the time; how he was forced to be a good boy and act as an example of good breeding. When asked whether he had ever felt angry with his mother, he said, "No, I never felt mad at mother. Well, isn't it abnormal that I didn't feel mad at her?" At this point he was able to piece together a number of facts, namely that he could not feel aggressive toward his mother because he might be abandoned by her, and that he could not feel anger toward his wife for fear she would leave him too.

The fact that he could actually express his anger and that no retaliatory disaster occurred such as he had envisaged was the first step in a recreated attitude toward people in general. With the gradual release of his ability to be aggressive, his killing fantasies disappeared.

One of the tendencies of the compulsion neurotic is an impulse to keep tormenting himself with his fears and anxieties. A masochistic element undoubtedly exists here. It is sometimes helpful to point out to the patient, while he is in a trance, that occupying his mind with frightening ideas stirs up tension and physical symptoms. The patient is told that the mind is closely linked to all the organs in his body. Upsetting ideas can thus upset all of the bodily organs. More perniciously, irritating the mind with frightening and uncomfortable thoughts may delay mental healing. It is like a person with a sore on his arm. The itchiness of the sore makes the person want to scratch it. However, scratching removes the epithelium and prevents healing.

The patient is told that suggestions will be given him to switch the type of thinking that preoccupies him. This may not be successful at first, but it will begin to work after a while. What is necessary is that he begin to direct thoughts away from concern with his obsessions to some other group of thoughts, no matter what they may be. This could be some activity, or hobby, or some period in life when his happiness was greatest. The patient is warned about the difficulty of controlling his thinking at first. He will be tempted to tease himself with his fears, to torture himself, just like picking at an irritating sore. Surely the sore may be provoking. It itches, and the person wants to scratch it; but as long as he does, healing will be delayed. It is the same with irritating ideas. Even though these are provoking, it is necessary purposefully to divert thoughts into some other channel. This persuasive approach, though superficial, often helps the patient exercise some control over his obsessions which tend to preoccupy him to distraction.

A word is necessary concerning dependency in the compulsion neurotic. Because of the patient's desires for dependency, and because of the difficulty in controlling a neurotic transference, it may be best not to permit the patient to come too frequently for treatments. Should treatment sessions be too concentrated, the patient may become inordinate in his demands on the therapist on the basis that he cannot function by himself. Therapy once weekly is ample in most cases, and an effort is made to terminate treatment as soon as the patient is able to function without symptoms. Often a nondirective approach is possible in the terminal phases of therapy, helping the patient to make decisions for himself. Analysis of the patient's dependency may also be necessary. Insofar as hypnosis is concerned, once the patient begins to change his attitude toward his illness and to lose his symptoms, hypnosis may be abandoned for psychotherapy in the waking state.

It is very helpful to give a Rorschach test to compulsion neurotics to see whether any elements of schizophrenia are present. Some compulsion neurotics are very close to schizophrenia, and in such instances the therapist should be chary of offering analytic interpretations. Rather, one should be reassuring, manipulating the individual's environment so that he can function as well as possible with his existing personality equipment. The prognosis here is not too favorable, but a great deal can be done for the patient when therapy is oriented along lines such as used in schizophrenia. Should a psychoanalytic approach be applied is such cases, the chances are that the therapist will be rewarded with a therapeutic failure. The ego is too weak to handle the anxiety released by analysis. Sometimes a compulsion neurotic of this type develops a psychotic-like excited episode. Shock therapy may be expedient here.

The prognosis in compulsion neurosis will depend upon the severity of the condition and the amount of ego strength that remains. It will also depend upon the length of time the patient has been ill. In some instances, compulsive-obsessive patterns appear to be of relatively recent duration, the patient having functioned fairly well in his relationships with people, the compulsive difficulty having developed as a result of external pressures and problems to which the patient could not adjust. Under these circumstances the prognosis is much more favorable than in instances where the compulsive illness has been with the individual ever since puberty.

XIV

HYPNOSIS IN TRAUMATIC NEUROSIS

HYPNOSIS is one of the most effective agents in the therapy of the traumatic neuroses. During the last war it was utilized with great success in many of the acute combat reactions.[1-8] The psychopathology of traumatic neurosis apparently makes it remarkably susceptible to the hypnotic method.

Traumatic neurosis is due to a violent episode of a physical or emotional nature obtruding itself in the life of the person. Under civilian conditions the usual causes are transportation and industrial accidents. In military life the causes are contingent on the stresses of war.

As a general rule the traumatic stimulus acts on an individual whose adaptive resources are being taxed to an extreme. He is then unable to cope with the added stress imposed on him by the inimical event. Traumatic neurosis, thus, is not the result of a single catastrophic circumstance, but rather is the end product of a number of harsh situations to which the individual has reacted adversely.

Everyone has his breaking point, and may be overwhelmed by a disastrous situation with which he is powerless to cope. Customary controls and defenses being ineffectual, these may be abandoned for regressive modes of adaptation which are, of course, inadequate to deal with the situation. However, in the average individual, recovery takes place shortly after the traumatic stimulus ceases.

Where the individual's adaptive resources are crushed and where his sense of mastery is destroyed, he may resign himself to feelings of helplessness even when the catastrophic event is over. He will, therefore, be unable to cope with life in an aggressive and assertive manner, and the original reaction to the traumatic incident will persist.

The traumatic situation acts upon the individual in two ways; first, the person responds to the experience as a symbol, mobilizing variegated defenses against it in line with his previous technics of adaptation; second, he reacts to the incident with a number of symptoms that constitute what is known as the "traumatic syndrome."

Kardiner and Spiegel[8] contend that the traumatic syndrome is a distinct entity upon which is superimposed a variety of neurotic reactions characteristic of the individual's habitual responses to anxiety. The symptoms of the syndrome are irritability, temper outbursts, increased sensitivity to stimuli, anxiety dreams, feelings of helplessness and an altered conception of the self and the outside world. The individual displays a reluctance to talk about his accident or a complete amnesia of the event involved.

One of the most characteristic symptoms of a traumatic neurosis is a disturbance in sleep. This may consist of outright insomnia, or of a type of sleep that is interrupted by dreams of a terrifying stereotyped nature. The dreams may be the most prominent feature of the illness, and in them one frequently sees repeated the original traumatic experience, or the repetition of a scene in which the person is being injured or destroyed.

A severely traumatic incident in precipitating anxiety may bring into play latent defenses such as phobic, hysterical and compulsive symptoms which have in the past constituted methods of adaptation to stress situations. Frequently the traumatic event is interpreted as castration or as a loss of parental love, and it accordingly invokes appropriate defensive and propitiatory mechanisms.

Consequently, the traumatic syndrome does not appear in pure culture, but rather is accompanied by a variety of psychoneurotic disorders including neurasthenia, anxiety neurosis, anxiety hysteria, conversion hysteria and psychosomatic illness. The symptom picture may involve a state of tension with emotional instability, affective lability, and motor restlessness. There may be anxiety manifestations with or without phobias, exhaustion and fatigue symptoms. The most frequent psychosomatic disorders affect the gastrointestinal, cardiac and respiratory systems. There may be hysterical, motor and sensory symptoms with paralysis, spasticity, tics, tremors, gait disturbances, anesthesias, blindness, deafness, or dissociative episodes accompanied by amnesia, somnambulism, fugues, cataleptic or epileptoid reactions. Headaches are often prominent. Sometimes traumatic neuroses merge into reactions which resemble psychotic states. Confusional syndromes range from mild disorientation to delirium and stupor. In instances where the individual is unable to organize his defenses and to establish some control, he may proceed to hypomania, manic-depressive psychosis, paranoid reaction or schizophrenia.

While severely traumatic experiences are possible in a highly industrialized society, or may occur as the result of natural disasters like floods and storms, the most consistently catastrophic situations prevail in times of war. The two World Wars, waged on a scale and under conditions hitherto unknown, and, in addition, involving large "civilian" armies and noncombatant populations, induced a high incidence of nervous disorders. During these two periods psychiatry learned many of its most valuable lessons; hypnosis, as an effective short-term therapeutic method, underwent a renaissance. These lessons can be applied to peacetime traumatic neurosis, but to understand the technics developed and the underlying principles it would be well to examine in some detail the problems which emerged under wartime conditions and how they were treated.

There has been a tendency to credit war neurosis to cowardice and malingering. Actually there is no relation to these conditions. War neurosis is a reaction designed to cope with overwhelming anxiety. The end result may be devastating to the adjustment of the individual, particularly where there is regression and disorientation, but in all instances the neurosis serves the economic function of disposing of anxiety which is violently disruptive to the psychobiologic equilibrium.

War imposes a number of hardships on the individual which may sensitize him to a traumatic neurosis. Wrested from his customary security props and thrown into a regimented order, many inductees were apt to show tension and anxiety. As part of a fighting unit, the individual is expected to comply and to obey orders of his superiors without question. He must suppress his own personal opinions and his feelings of indignation. The majority of persons are able to make an adjustment, but those whose character structures enjoin them to resist authority, or who view a subordinate role as a blow to their self esteem, are apt to react in a disturbed manner.

Another potentially disorganizing element of military life, particularly to independent and detached persons, is the lack of privacy and the intimacy with which one is thrown into contact with his fellow soldiers. In addition to this the person is forced to forego many gratifications he has come to regard as vital. Loss of freedom, separation from loved ones, and sexual abstinence are among the more common deprivations. The reaction to deprivation will depend upon the ability of the individual to tolerate frustration. Where the character structure is such that deprivation is regarded as a blow to security and self esteem, the conditions of military life will produce much hostility. The effect of separation from loved ones will depend upon how dependent the individual is. In persons whose security is maintained largely by clinging compulsively to others, separation from a love object may plunge them into helplessness and anxiety.

It is not correct to say that all persons who were neurotic in civilian life tended to collapse under war conditions. There are certain neurotic individuals who thrive under circumstances of war. A neurotic need to submerge oneself in work, sacrifice and suffering, to exhibit fealty to a leader, and to expose oneself to danger may make the individual an intrepid soldier. As a general rule, nevertheless, the more unstable the individual has been in civilian life, the greater the likelihood of a neurotic breakdown when he is exposed to inimical war conditions.

Secure and stable persons are most capable of tolerating stress. However, experience in World War II has shown that men who have no manifest neurotic problems can develop a neurosis if the strain is sufficiently severe.[1] Fatigue, unhygienic conditions, sleeplessness, overexertion, exposure to bombardment under conditions from which there is no escape or retaliatory action, may eventually undermine a relatively healthy individual. Needless to say, those persons who have personality defects will over-react to hardship. Early unresolved fears of injury and mutilation may be revived which tend to overwhelm the person.

War gives impetus to aggressive and sadistic impulses which are customarily repressed in civilized living. Under battle circumstances the individual may be unable to make retribution to his conscience for his destructiveness. In spite of the sanction society has placed on killing during wartime, the person may respond with guilt and fears of counter-hostility. The problem of the handling of hostility has always been extremely vital in warfare. Hostility toward the enemy is, of course, essential to arouse fighting attitudes. The individual's ability to express hostility toward the enemy is dependent to a large extent on how he handles hostility in everyday life. Where the superego is not so severe as to prohibit the expression of hostility, the person may be able to maintain a fighting spirit against the enemy provided his faith in the state remains high. The individual who fears hostility may be overwhelmed when he realizes he must kill or be killed. He will, in spite of social condonation, be unable to repress his guilt over killing.

Another problem that occurs during war involves the conflict that rages between self preservation and standards of patriotism, loyalty and a desire to be part of the war effort. The fear of death is a powerful emotion, and because fear is apt to motivate the person toward flight, with implications of cowardice in this desire, the person may physiologically respond with panic. The confusion of fear with cowardice paralyzes him and contributes to his anxiety.

The soldier, consequently, is exposed to many conflicts which sensitize him to stress. One of the first signs of an incipient breakdown is a disturbance in sleep. Insomnia and terror dreams are associated. There is often a fear of sleep or of the dark, and momentary episodes of panic occur with mild confusion. Tension creates moodiness, seclusiveness, irritability, episodes of rage or depression, and motor restlessness which the soldier may attempt to overcome by overindulgence in drink.

While army life is associated with hardships incidental to regimentation, separation from loved ones, and subordination of personal interests to interests of the state, the most traumatic situation is the actual threat to life. Particularly insidious are unexpected catastrophes which the person does not anticipate and for which he is totally unprepared. With the advent of the precipitating factor, the predisposed soldier will collapse, showing the usual symptoms of traumatic neurosis.

War neuroses, then are motivated by the desire to escape from an intolerable situation in real life to one made more tolerable by a neurosis. The extent to which the individual can resist neurotic collapse will depend upon the elasticity of his defensive structure, the relative intactness of his ego, and his ability to dispose of tension and anxiety in socially acceptable ways.

Knowledge of the dynamics of war neurosis made certain preventive measures possible in World War II. Where the soldier had had effective training that made him feel he could defend himself under all circumstances, where he was shown that he had adequate weapons of attack, where he had confidence in his leaders, and where he had obtained sufficient indoctrination and morale building, he was best prepared to resist a breakdown. An important element in prevention was group identification. Cooperation with others was essential, and the individual had to be made to feel that he was part of a team, with enough of an idea of the battle situation and the planned strategy so that he would not be caught by surprise. The incidence of war neuroses is proportionate to shattered morale and to feelings of isolation from fellow soldiers. An organized body of men fighting for a cause they consider just can best overcome war stress and hardship.

The treatment of the soldier with acute battle exhaustion depended upon whether he was or was not to be returned to duty. The sequel of all battles are reactions of fear and great fatigue. Only later are these reactions organized into actual neuroses. Experience in the last war has shown that evacuation and a too reassuring attitude encouraged collapse. Unless the individual anticipated going back to the front in spite of his reactions, he might develop neurotic illness to avoid duty.

Combat exhaustion, if treated early, did not necessarily result in neurosis. Early therapy consisted of sedation, rest, good food and assignment to noncombat duty at the clearing station. It was assumed that the soldier would be returned to the front. Where there was reluctance to return to battle duty, appeals to patriotism, courage, and "not letting one's buddies down" often built up the person's morale and determination. Encouragement to verbalize fear and disgust was vital, since the soldier in this way released tension, and discovered that others shared in his anxieties. The value of respecting the soldier's "gripe" in building morale has long been recognized. The role of the leader is important, too, and an intrepid commanding officer has always been of great service. It is amazing how often a change of attitude on the part of the individual can prevent neurotic collapse. Treatment, in peace as it was in war, should be started as soon as possible since delay permits the neurosis to become more highly organized and allows the secondary gain element to take hold.

In treating war neurosis in the incipient stages, where sleep disturbances and states of tension existed, a breakdown could often be averted by adequate periods of rest during the daytime, by the use of hypnotics, such as seconal and veronal, and by the person's being permitted to sleep in a dimly lit room. Many soldiers in the incipient stages showed terror of the dark and of being alone. They were given, therefore, some assurance on this account.

Where sedation therapy failed to resolve the disorder, the soldier was sent to an evacuation hospital, from where, if his condition warranted it, he was sent to the rear echelon hospital. The immediate treatment consisted of rest, good food and quiet. The soldier continued under military discipline. Psychotherapy was in the form of persuasion, suggestion and appeals to go back and try again. A simple explanation of anxiety was given to the patient along with assurances about the universality of fear reactions. The soldier was made to feel that there was nothing unusual in his breakdown and that he could learn to control his fear. Individuals who had not developed too severe reactions could occasionally be helped to return to combat. In some instances pressure was exerted by stressing the fact that release from the fight is dishonorable, that it is the soldier's duty to finish the job for the sake of his loved ones and for his companions.

Where the patient had a well defined traumatic neurosis, hypnotherapy was often remarkably effective. Hypnosis was utilized for purposes of symptom removal and as a means of controlling insomnia and tension along the lines detailed in Volume Two. Though palliative, these measures often reassured the patient and restored to him a sense of control and mastery.

Under hypnosis it is possible to intensify, to diminish, or to remove a symptom, to transfer it to another part of the body, and, finally, to demonstrate to the patient that he can do the same things through his own suggestions. This frequently removes feelings of helplessness. Kardiner and Spiegel[9] illustrate this method, as used in war, with excellent case material.

In instances where anxiety is extreme one may utilize an "uncovering" type of technic. Here hypnosis and narcosynthesis are of signal help. The recovery of amnesias, and the reliving of the traumatic scene in action or verbalization have markedly ameliorative or curative effects on acute traumatic neuroses.

While hypnosis and narcosynthesis accomplish approximately the same results, the emotions accompanying hypnotherapy are much more vivid, and the carthartic effect consequently greater, than with narcosynthesis. There are other advantages to hypnosis. The induction of a trancelike state, once the patient has been hypnotized, is brought about easily without the complication of injections and without post-therapeutic somnolence. Additionally, hypnotic suggestions are capable of demonstrating to the patient his ability to gain mastery of his functions. Details of the "uncovering" hypnotic technic are outlined in Volume Two under the heading "Hypnoanalytic Desensitization."

Where it is essential to remove an amnesia, the patient is encouraged under hypnosis or narcosynthesis, to talk about the events immediately preceding the traumatic episode, and to lead into the episode slowly, reliving the scene as if it were happening again. Frequently the patient will approach the scene and then block, or he may actually awaken. Repeated trance inductions often break through this resistance. Also it will be noted that the abreactive effect will increase as the patient describes the episode repeatedly. Apparently the powerful emotions which are bound down are subject to greater repression than the actual memories of the event.

In the treating of postwar neuroses of traumatic origin Hadfield's original technic is still useful.[10] The patient is hypnotized and instructed that when the physician places his fingers on the patient's forehead, the latter will picture before him the experiences that caused his breakdown. This usually produces a vivid recollection of the traumatic event with emotions of fear, rage, despair and helplessness. The patient often spontaneously relives the traumatic scene with a tremendous cathartic effect. If he hesitates, he must be encouraged to describe the scenes before him in detail. This is the first step in therapy and must be repeated for a number of sessions until the restored memory is complete. The second step is the utilization of hypnosis to readjust the patient to the traumatic experience. The experience must be worked through, over and over again, until the patient accepts it during hypnosis and remembers it upon awakening. Persuasive suggestions are furthermore given him, directed at increasing assurance and self confidence. After this the emotional relationship to the physician is analyzed at a conscious level to prevent continuance of the dependency tie.

Horsley[11] mentions that where the ordinary injunctions to recall a traumatic scene fail, several reinforcing methods can be tried. The first has to do with commanding the patient to remember, insisting that he will not leave the room until his memory is complete. The second method is that of soothing, coaxing and encouraging the patient, telling him he is about to remember battle scenes that will remind him of his experiences. The patient may, if this is unsuccessful, be told that although he does not remember the experience during hypnosis, he will remember it upon awakening. He may also be instructed to recall it in a dream the next day.

Various hypnoanalytic procedures, such as dramatization,

regression and revivification, play therapy, automatic writing and mirror gazing, may be utilized to recover an obstinate amnesia. The reaction of patients to the recall of repressed experiences varies. Some patients act out the traumatic scene, getting out of bed, charging about the room, ducking to avoid mortar shells and approaching tanks. Other patients live through the traumatic episode without getting out of bed. Some individuals collapse with anxiety, and they should be reassured and encouraged to go on. Where the patient voices hostility, he should be given an opportunity to express his grievances and dislikes, and clarification of his feelings of injustice may afford him considerable relief.

It must be remembered that the object in therapy is to dissipate feelings of helplessness and of being menaced by a hostile world. The sense of mastery and the ability to adjust oneself to life must be restored. It is necessary to proceed with therapy as rapidly as possible to prevent an organization of the condition into a chronic psychoneurosis. Follow-up therapy is essential with integration of the material brought up during the trance on a waking level. Re-educational therapy utilizing psychoanalytic insight may be required in those cases where anxieties relating to war stress have precipitated hysterical, phobic, compulsive and other reactions characteristic of the ways the patient has dealt with anxiety in civilian life.

In chronic traumatic neuroses, treatment is difficult, due to the high degree of organization that has taken place, and because of the strong secondary gain element involving monetary compensation and dependency. Hypnosis with a re-educational approach employing psychoanalytic insight is often useful. The recovery of amnesias should always be attempted, but even where successful will probably not influence the outcome. An incentive must be created in the patient to function free of symptoms even at the expense of forfeiting disability compensations, which in comparison to emotional health may be shown to be diminutive indeed.

REFERENCES

1 SLATER, E., AND SARGANT, W.: Acute war neuroses. Lancet *2:* 1, 1940.

2 SALMON, T. W.: Care and Treatment of Mental Disease and War Neurosis in the British Army. New York, Nat. Comm. of Mental Hygiene, 1917.

3 BROSIN, H. W.: Panic states and their treatment. Am. J. Psychiat. *100:* 58, 1943.

4 KUBIE, L. S.: The emergency care and treatment of the acute war neuroses. In Manual of Military Neuropsychiatry (Ed. by H. C. Solomon and P. I. Yakovlev). Philadelphia, W. B. Saunders, 1944, p. 541.

5 GRINKER, R. R., AND SPIEGEL, J. P.: Brief psychotherapy in war neuroses. Psychosom. Med. *6:* 125, 1944.

6 FISHER, C.: Hypnosis in treatment of neuroses due to war and to other causes. War. Med. *4:* 565–76, 1943.

7 KARTCHNER, F. D., AND KORNER, I. N.: The use of hypnosis in the treatment of acute combat reactions. Am. J. Psychiat. *103:* 630–636, 1947.

8 KARDINER, A., AND SPIEGEL, H.: War Stress and Neurotic Illness. New York, Paul B. Hoeber, Inc., 1947.

9 Ibid, pp. 83–94.

10 HADFIELD, J. A.: Functional Nerve Disease (Ed. by Crichton-Miller). London, 1920.

11 HORSLEY, J. S.: Narco-analysis. London, Oxford Univ. Press, 1943, p. 12.

XV

HYPNOSIS IN PSYCHOSOMATIC CONDITIONS

For many years it has been recognized that the internal viscera are responsive to the emotions of elation, tension, anxiety and rage. This notion, first scientifically confirmed by Cannon,[1-3] has been corroborated by a host of other investigators who have emphasized the close relationship that exists between mental and physical processes. Illustrative is the work of Faulkner[4] who demonstrated that esophageal spasm occurred when there were thoughts of insecurity and frustration, and that esophageal relaxation developed when there were thoughts of a pleasant nature.

That unconscious conflict may cause physical abnormalities is a well recognized fact, confirmed by clinical as well as experimental data.[5-8] Neurophysiologic studies indicate that the autonomic nervous system is represented in the brain, and that disorders of the higher psychic functions may provoke widespread vegetative changes, such as disturbances in circulation, respiration, temperature and water balance.[9] Most commonly productive of psychosomatic manifestations are anxiety, hostility and a generalized state of tension.

A certain degree of tension is a usual concomitant of living. It is a manifestation of disturbed homeostasis, the product of unfulfilled physiologic and biologic needs which excite the organism toward goal directed activities to restore homeostasis. Under normal conditions tension causes the individual to mobilize his physical and psychologic resources toward overcoming obstacles in the path of gratification of fundamental needs.

Tension excitations reach the central nervous system at various levels of integration: visceral, somatic and psychic.

Visceral symptoms result from stimulation of the hypothalamus and subthalamus with resulting changes in the smooth muscles and glands. Somatic stimulation increases the tonus and the potential power of the skeletal musculature. These effects prepare the organism for action in its contest with the environment. The psychic apparatus is stimulated by way of the cortico-hypothalamic pathways. Under average conditions, excitations arising from disturbed homeostasis are psychically perceived. The conscious appreciation of the state of unrest fosters an integration of adaptive behavior patterns and their effective application toward gratification of needs in line with past successful conditioned patterns of response. Restored homeostatic equilibrium dissipates the tension state.

In many neurotic persons, on the other hand, there is faulty passage of excitations to cortical levels, and, therefore, failure of what should be the consequent marshalling of resources and defenses toward restoring equilibrium. This is due to an extraordinarily severe repressive mechanism. Inimical experiences in the individual's relationship with past authoritative personages often result in a hypertrophied conscience that initiates anxiety and guilt feelings whenever basic impulses and needs are expressed. The child may, as a result, come to regard self assertiveness, sexual curiosity, and the display of aggression as prohibitive strivings. He will then feel that he has no right to gratify personal needs and demands. Their very penetration into consciousness serves to stimulate anxiety. Where the ego is thus menaced by biologic needs, the individual may attempt to organize his life so as to avoid their expression. His biologic impulses will, nevertheless, continue to strive for release, stirring up tension. Repression, however, blocks awareness of unpropitiated needs. The result is the virtual obliteration of the psychic apparatus as an adaptive tool.

In addition to the danger that invests the expression and

even appreciation of biologic impulses, the neurotic person suffers from a distorted sense of values that makes the normal pursuits of living vapid and meaningless. The past relationships of the person with his parents were so disturbed that he had to elaborate character patterns, such as inordinate dependencies, power strivings, masochistic impulses, submissiveness, detachment, and compulsive perfectionism, to gain for him a vicarious security fulfillment. Life becomes an arena in which there is ceaseless quest for spurious goals which become so overvalued that average pursuits in comparison are pallid indeed. Interpersonal relationships lose their normal meaning, and biologic goals are subordinated to those which fulfill neurotic character strivings.

The neurotic individual, consequently, will feel himself menaced by his needs and he will respond to these with anxiety. Psychosomatic manifestations that result are a somatic expression of his expectation of injury.

The average individual is capable of substituting compensatory gratifications for those needs which circumstances make it impossible for him to fulfill. The neurotic person, on the other hand, may look upon frustration of his drives as a sign that he is being subjugated by the world. Hostility is the usual consequence. As a complicating factor, hostility is often regarded as dangerous and is repressed. While the psychic apparatus is shielded from hostility by repressions, there is no such barrier to the deeper neurovegetative connections. Drainage of hostility through autonomic channels may produce such syndromes as cardio-vascular neuroses,[10–12] migraine,[13–16] epileptiform seizures,[17–19] laryngitis,[20] peptic ulcer,[21] and even the common cold.[22]

Thus the neurotic individual has a psychic and physical apparatus which is constantly in an uproar. He feels himself unable to satisfy security needs, self esteem, and strivings for love and companionship. He is confronted with feelings of helplessness, with ideas of being unloved and unlovable, with convictions of worthlessness and contemptibility. He is subject to inordinate tension, anxiety and hostility. As a result his vegetative nervous system is subjected to incessant bombardment, and he has to assume a perpetual state of psychologic emergency to maintain his crumbling defenses. He is at the mercy of the slightest adverse environmental circumstance. A harsh word, a cold glance, a head cold, or a trifling inconvenience may suffice to upset his delicate balance tumbling him into the depths of distress.

The organic instability of neurotic individuals can be demonstrated experimentally.[23–24] Massive autonomic stimulation affects practically every organ and tissue of the body. A wide variety of symptoms result, among which are spasticity of the smooth musculature, a disturbance in glandular secretions, contraction or dilatation of the vascular bed, increased tonus of the striated musculature with muscle spasm, tics and general "neuromuscular hypertension." A disturbance of the biochemical equilibrium of the body may provoke changes such as are seen in the allergic diseases.

CLINICAL MANIFESTATIONS

The most common psychosomatic ailments are gastrointestinal disorders, such as peptic ulcer, "dyspepsia," gastritis, constipation, and diarrhea; cardiovascular disorders, like pseudoangina, tachycardia, palpitation, arrhythmia, and essential hypertension; muscular and joint pains; asthenia; genitourinary disorders like impotence, premature ejaculation, frigidity, dyspareunia, enuresis and other urinary ailments; skin disorders and allergic conditions.

Tension, anxiety and hostility thus may upset the entire parasympathetic and sympathetic nervous systems. There is nothing specific about the organs influenced. However, an organ which is constitutionally defective is most likely to break down, much as violent strain will cause a rupture of a chain at its weakest link. Some evidence exists of a constitutional factor in determining weakness of organs, and this factor has been brought out by Thacker,[25] Robinson and Brucer,[26] Draper[27] and Sachase.[28] A constitutional element explains why irreversible changes develop in some organs even with stress over a short period.

While the severely neurotic individual is subject to psychosomatic illness even under so-called normal conditions, presumably well adjusted persons may exhibit somatization reactions to violent situations of stress. This was brought out in sharp focus during the last war.

In contradistinction to diffuse nonsymbolic somatization responses, there are certain psychosomatic reactions which seem to express emotional attitudes and impulses through specific organ systems.

Psychosomatic responses here serve as a method of solving conflict and correspond to the general characterologic makeup of the individual. Alexander[29] has divided conflict solution into three elemental tendencies; the wish to receive, the wish to eliminate, and the wish to retain. The wish to to receive is characteristic of persons who have a desire to be loved and protected, and who try to attain security by the unconscious wish to be fed. These persons develop gastric symptoms, like peptic ulcer, as an expression of tension. The next group has, in addition to receptive wishes, the desire to give as a form of restitution. Giving is often symbolized by bowel elimination, and the most common resulting symptom is diarrhea which, in addition, is a means of expressing aggression. Other manifestations are mucous and spastic colitis. The third group is characterized by an inhibition in giving out anything because of a fear of losing one's intactness. The basic conviction is that since one expects nothing from others, he need give nothing in return. This is symbolized by anal retention, and here one may encounter the symptom of constipation.

The factor of personality type in the choice of symptoms is

still relatively unexplored. Dunbar[30] believes that there is a definite correlation. She contends that hypertension is apt to develop in persons with a compulsive character who have few outspoken neurotic symptoms. Syndromes associated with dyspnea and palpitation appear in patients who show phobias and prominent conversion mechanisms. Patients who are prone to get into accidents have a character structure similar to the hypertensive, revolving around submission to authority along with great hostility. But unlike the hypertensive they resolve this conflict by inhibition. Fracture patients, among those who are accident prone, express their conflicts in action. On the other hand, some authorities like Saul[31] believe that attempts to correlate definite characterologic defenses with specific psychosomatic syndromes have not yielded uniform results.

There are a number of psychosomatic diseases that resemble conversion hysteria in that the malfunctioning organ serves a symbolic purpose. In certain individuals, expression of basic wishes and fears, gaining neither cognitive nor conative outlet, is sought through an organ or organ system. For instance, the intake of food may be equated with the receiving of affection and love. Biting and chewing have a destructive quality and may come to signify a means of expressing aggression. Hostile tendencies are indicated by teeth gnashing and grinding during sleep. Loss of appetite may signify an actual or psychologic loss of a love object, as in fasting rituals with depressive attacks. Anorexia may also be the product of an association of eating with attacking or destroying. Furthermore, infantile fantasies of oral impregnation may be reflected in a stubborn dietary abstemiousness (anorexia nervosa) which may proceed to the point of actual starvation. Vomiting may have the symbolic quality of ejecting evil impulses and attitudes. Globus hystericus often signifies incorporation of a dreaded but coveted object like the penis. Gastric neuroses are frequently discovered to be an appeal for succor and support. The desire for infantile dependence may stimulate the stomach to overactivity with eventual ulcer formation. Eliminative functions may also be associated with aggression, possessiveness, defiance, disgust, yielding and giving. Emotional attitudes can thus be reflected in disturbances of elimination, in the form of diarrhea and colitis. Some authorities believe that these conditions are also reactions to guilt in the patient for grasping and dependent attitudes. Constipation may be a reaction to a realization that one can expect nothing from others and must for security hold onto things within himself. It may also be a form of hostile defiance. The respiratory system lends itself to emotional conflict. Weiss[32] and French and Alexander[33] contend that the basis of the asthmatic attack is a profound dependence on the mother with need for security, shelter and protection.

What determines the choice of organ in psychosomatic illness is an important question. In hysterical somatization reactions it was indicated that the organ was chosen for its symbolic significance in representing important unconscious attitudes and strivings. Weiss and English[6] suggest that the organ is most likely to be one whose function was in the ascendency at the time of the most traumatic period of life. Thus where anxiety developed during the period of toilet training, the bowel and bladder functions may be used as organs through which anxiety and hostility are expressed. Diarrhea and enuresis may here come to symbolize aggression. Constipation and urinary retention may stand for a recalcitrant defense of one's intactness.

In some instances the individual identifies with an ailing parent or sibling, and utilizes a similar disturbed organ or function.[34] In other cases the psychosomatic disorder is brought about by suggestion in somewhat the same manner as organ disturbances may be produced by hypnotic suggestions. Dunbar[35] cites the case of a girl who developed a severe generalized urticaria because of the statement by her lover that he liked to see welts over her body.

A secondary gain element is very prominent in psychosomatic illness. An appeal for sympathy, love, freedom from responsibility, and for monetary compensation may cause an exacerbation and persistence of complaints. It must be understood, however, that the desire to exploit symptoms is not primarily responsible for ill health; it is purely a secondary factor.

Treatment of Psychosomatic Conditions

Hypnosis lends itself admirably to the treatment of many forms of psychosomatic disorder. Where somatic symptoms have a symbolic meaning, simple symptom removal by authoritative suggestion is often remarkably successful. This is especially the case in an individual with a hysterical makeup, in whom the symptom serves a symbolic function as well as a means of pleading for help, love and reassurance. The hypnotic situation here seems to fulfill an important need in the patient, and compliance with the physician's command to abandon a symptom is often automatic. There are many limitations to this type of therapy, since effects are treated rather than causes. Character disturbances are influenced minimally even though an abatement of symptoms has been brought about.

Simple symptom removal is usually ineffective where the psychosomatic disorder is the consequence of a diffuse autonomic drainage of tension, anxiety and hostility. Furthermore, where the symptom represents an important defense against anxiety, simple suggestions are insufficient. For instance, where impotency or frigidity represent a defense against acknowledging one's sexual needs, or reflect a fear of relating oneself intimately to another person, the removal of the symptom may be interpreted by the patient as potentially dangerous. He will consequently resist suggestions along lines of symptom removal.

Hypnosis, utilized as a means of persuasion and guidance, may permit the patient to organize his life around his defects and liabilities, to avoid situations that arouse conflict and hostility, and to attain, at least in part, a sublimation of his basic needs. This approach is, of course, more scientific than simple symptom removal because it deals with the causative emotions themselves, attempting to control their severity. The object here is to build up ego strength to a point where it can handle damaging emotions more rationally, as well as to improve interpersonal relationships so that hostility and other disturbing emotions are not constantly being generated. In many instances, hypnosis used with such psychobiologic therapies liberates the individual from the vicious cycle of his neurosis, facilitates externalization of interests, increases self confidence, and provides a means of discharging emotions by way of motor channels instead of internalizing them with drainage through the autonomic system.

Another approach to the problem of psychosomatic illness is desensitizing the patient to the effects of his emotions by exposing him under hypnosis to situations in which he can tolerate graduated doses of anxiety and hostility. Dramatic technics in which scenes are re-enacted that provoke the patient's psychosomatic symptoms teach the patient the dynamics of his illness and permit him to master provocative emotions. For instance, if symptoms of gastric distress have been found to be associated with hostility stirred up by a competitive relationship, demonstrations to the patient, by means of an experimental neurosis, may show him how he develops and represses hostility. During hypnosis dramatized scenes may also be suggested in which the patient is capable of expressing hostility without fear of counter-aggression.

The technic of creating an experimental neurosis to produce or to exaggerate the patient's complaint is a most convincing demonstration to him of the validity of the physician's interpretations regarding the dynamics of his disorder.
Such demonstrations have a potent effect in modifying disturbed character patterns.

Hypnosis with confession and ventilation may be useful
in certain types of psychosomatic illness. Where a patient
represses certain impulses on the basis of a fear of estrange-
ment from an authoritative person on whom he is dependent,
a somatization response may result. French[36] believes that
psychogenic asthma is brought about by this mechanism.
In asthma, when confession of impulses to the mother or
mother substitute occurs, with reassurance on her part to
the effect that the person will not be rejected, considerable
relief is consequent. Hypnosis may aid in uncovering forbidden impulses, as well as in facilitating their expression.
The physician encourages the patient to talk, and then
reassures him that there will be no retaliatory rejection.

Determining the meaning of the patient's psychosomatic
illness in terms of its historical development is successful in
removing some symptoms, particularly of a hysterical
character. Recall in the hypnotic state either at adult or
regressed levels, may result in the recovery of traumatic
memories and experiences associated with the original development of the illness. It is essential to remember that while
a symptom may be relieved, the basic personality structure
is not influenced by this technic.

Where the character structure is very neurotic, an analysis
of the individual's interpersonal relationships in operation
may be the only way of removing his physical illness. Here
a hypnoanalytic approach may be used, with analysis of the
transference or re-education utilizing analytic insight. The
discovery by the patient of his unconscious compulsive
drives, the uncovering of the genetic origins of these drives,

the inevitable liberation of submerged anxiety and hostility lead to a new phase of independence and to bettered relationships with people. The changing of the patient's sense of values, and the ability to pursue biologic and social goals previously repressed, serve to remove sources of tension. The uncovering of anxieties rooted in unconscious conflict helps reintegrate the patient to a present shorn of the fears related to his past.

The treatment of any neurotic condition, including a psychosomatic disorder, is understandably never complete until the individual is rehabilitated in his attitudes toward people. Of course, the patient may be made comfortable and may be relatively well adjusted with the fulfillment of the partial goal of symptom removal. However, the sources of his difficulty remain uninfluenced, and a relapse is always possible.

The best way of achieving the goal of rehabilitation is through an analytic technic. Hypnoanalysis is most effective here. Before this technic can be utilized, it is important that the patient be motivated to inquire into the sources of his problem.

As a general rule a patient with a psychosomatic illness is driven to seek relief because of the inconvenience or discomfort brought about by his symptoms. He expects the physician to give him medications or some form of dramatic nonmedicinal help. He can see little connection between his symptoms and his problems with people. Unless the patient is brought around to an understanding that his symptoms are not fortuitous, that they have a meaning and origin, little progress can be expected. In therapy the patient must be shown that there is a causal relation between his symptoms and existing difficulties in his dealings with life. The circumstances under which symptoms become exaggerated are investigated with the object of determining failure in his interpersonal functioning. Once a pattern is discerned, its significance and origin are explored. Finally, the patient is encouraged to put into action his retrained attitudes toward life and people.

This process may be illustrated by the hypnoanalysis, involving analysis of the transference, in a patient with a migrainous headache who was insistent at the first visit that I prescribe sedatives for him. The patient was told: "The prescription that I'm going to give you will be much better than medicine. It is going to be a prescription that may take possibly a little time; but this thing did not develop last week. What I am going to ask you to do is to connect up for me your headache and any fears or conflicts or problems that exist in your life. Once you do this, your headaches will have the best chance of disappearing, because you will then be able to take the steps necessary to correct the cause. If I fail to give you medicine, it is because medicine does not help the kind of problem you have. You must be patient and work this thing out with me. Relief will then come."

The patient was somewhat dismayed at my reaction, and he retorted: "But I don't see any real connection between the headache and what I'm doing. Sure, I wish I had a better job, and I wish that maybe I could get more sleep, but everybody has that. I don't have anything worse than anybody else. I'd like to have some more money. I'd like to be able to travel and see this and that, but I'm not any more dissatisfied than most of the people that I know. So even though you say that maybe there is some connection, I don't see it."

An attempt was made to show the patient that the most important difficulties in a person's life need not be conscious, that problems might exist of which he was not aware, and that we would try to work out those problems if he would cooperate with me.

The patient was obviously skeptical even though he promised to cooperate. No discernible change in his attitude was noted in the next few sessions except that he became less and less expressive and sat in his chair expectantly, as if he believed something important might happen to him soon. Hypnosis was started and the patient turned out to be a good subject.

Under hypnosis a suggestion was made to the effect that he would experience posthypnotically a hypersensitivity of his right hand, even though he did not remember that such a command had been given him. Upon awakening he complained of tenderness in his hand, but he was unable to understand why this was so. He was puzzled that a suggestion made to him in the trance could influence him in this manner. At the next session, he was told, prior to the trance, that I would suggest to his unconscious mind that his left hand become numb when he awakened from hypnosis. He was amazed that my prediction was correct. The opportunity was then taken to explain to him how the unconscious may influence any organ in the body. Fears and conflicts, he was assured, could reflect themselves in disturbances of the various organs, including headaches. It was possible that his headaches might be so determined. I urged him to observe the things that might cause his next headache.

At the next visit he remarked that he had had a headache. He said, "I can see no reason why I had the headache. I suppose I could tell you what happened during the day. I went to work, and everything went along pretty well. I did my job as well as anybody there, and I went home and I expected to go bowling with a friend. Now this friend called me up, and we were supposed to go out on the date. He said, 'Supposing I meet you at eight o'clock.' And right at that point my wife, who had been coming down with a head cold, says to me, 'Why don't you postpone your going out until later on, after the kids are in bed or tomorrow?' And she did have a terrible cold. So I told my friend we'd go out the next day. I didn't want the kids to get the cold, so I put the kids to bed and then I sat on my wife's bed. She was sniffling, and I began getting an awful headache right at that point. And there was no reason for it." When asked whether he might have resented the fact that he had to stay home and put the children to bed, he remarked, "No, why should I? The kids would have gotten a cold. I could have bowled the next day; there's no reason why I should." The patient was assured that perhaps there was no cause for the headache that we could see at this time, but that it was necessary to continue observing the circumstances under which his headache developed.

One week later the patient reported a severe migrainous attack. "Again I had an awful headache. Things went around. I had a bunch of junk last night, and it was probably what I ate." When asked to talk about the events that had occurred, he said, "We went over to call on some people we know. They are nice people, but I don't care very much for them. But my wife thinks that because he is my superior at work we've got to cultivate them; and I suppose if I really want to go along, get ahead in my job, that I might as well try to be friends with him. So I went over there, and I sat there, and we drank a while and we talked. They're terrible bores. I really don't like being with them. Then it started; an awful headache."

When asked whether he resented making the visit, the patient replied, "Sure, I didn't want to be there. I just resented being there." He was then reminded that he had presented two instances in which his wife had asked him to comply and that in each case a headache followed. "Yes," he admitted, "I don't know; maybe you've got something."

That he had made a connection was evidenced by his reaction to his next headache. He said, "By George, you know what happened? My wife asked me to stay at home again and I didn't want to, and while I was talking, I got a headache." Almost excitedly he continued, "When I look back, I can see the headache just comes like that. There have been innumerable times when automatically I feel as if I have to do what my wife asks me to do, that I can't say no. I say she is a reasonable person and a nice person, and I get a bad headache every time. Now, why should that be?"

Under hypnosis an experimental conflict was created in which the patient imagined himself in a situation with his wife where she insisted that he go shopping for groceries when he really wanted to go to a bowling match. He complied with her request nevertheless. He was told when he awoke he would feel exactly as if he had executed her command, but he would not recall the situation suggested to him. Upon awakening the patient had amnesia for the trance events. He complained of an excruciating headache for which he was unable to account. He was rehypnotized, and the nature of the experiment and the meaning of his headache was explained to him in terms of resentment at having done something against his wish.

At this point real analytic work began, since the patient was able to concede the fact that his headache had a source in what was happening to him in his daily life. A motivation to inquire into the source had been created. He was told, "So you do see a connection between your life situation and what has happened to you? Now, that's a rather interesting situation isn't it? Here you notice that things happen at home; you've never been aware of them before. A headache occurs when your wife suggests something that you resent or that makes an imposition on you. Supposing we start inquiring into that, and supposing you, yourself, begin to figure out for yourself, with my help, what goes on here." He retorted, "Well, can't you do that for me? Can't you tell me why?" This explanation was given: "If I told you, it wouldn't do you any good, because if you figure things out for yourself, the insight will stick."

The therapeutic situation was clarified by pointing out that now he was convinced that the headache was not mysterious, but had an origin in certain attitudes. He would want to figure things out more in detail, and his inner strength would increase if he figured things out for himself. The purpose behind these remarks was to motivate him toward accepting a more nondirective type of relationship with me.

When it was ascertained that he understood the need for more activity, the technic of free association under hypnosis was described to him. He readily agreed to try this technic, and decided to lie on the couch for this purpose. After several sessions during which he discussed certain resentments toward people which had bothered him, he expostulated in an irritable way that nothing seemed to be happening. "I just can't seem to figure things out. I can't seem to make any sense out of what I'm saying or why I lie down here. I can't possibly arrive at the reasons why these things go on inside of me. Now why don't you tell me? Why don't you tell me what's going on, and why do I get these headaches?"

Emphasis was again placed on the need to work things out for himself. "But I'm trying to," he replied, "and nothing happens. All right, I'll try." At this point he began to complain of a beginning headache and he started rubbing his forehead. "I can't see how my wife is responsible here because nothing has happened. I've had several awful headaches in the last couple of days and I can't see the sense in it. As he talked he became critical of the technic of free association. He then revealed a dream of fleeing from a dangerous man who had plugs in his ears. He associated the ear plugs with a stethescope. He remarked, "This man, he had a stethescope, and he was chasing me, and I didn't want to do what he wanted me to do, and I felt he was going to hurt me and so I ran." In reply, I said, "Is it possible that you are doing something now that you don't want to do?" "No," he re-torted, "I want to get well. I want to do what you say. I want to do everything you say, even though I feel that it's not exactly what I want to do. I want to do everything you say." The reply was this: "Well, it seems apparent that you are developing toward me the same type of feelings that you have toward your wife. Here you feel I'm forcing you to do something you really don't want to do. Aren't you doing exactly with me what you do with your wife? Aren't you complying with me, and doing free association, and trying to figure things out for yourself, when you would really like to sit up and have me tell you what to do?"

At the next session the patient reported a dream. "There is a baby, a tiny baby in the arms of its mother. The mother is stuffing a nipple of a baby bottle down the child's throat. The child yowls and screams and shakes his head, and as he shakes his head, he bangs it against the wall." The patient then exclaimed, "I have a terrible headache, one of the worst headaches I've had." It was pointed out that the banging of the baby's head in the dream might symbolize a headache. The patient acquiesced that his head felt as if he were banging it against a wall. Free association in the waking and hypnotic states yielded little except complaints about his misery and his difficulty in thinking clearly.

In the trance state the patient was regressed and he was asked to return to the first time when he had experienced a headache in childhood. The period to which he returned was when he was six years of age. His mother had put him in a baby swing. He had wanted to play in the open with the other children, but his mother refused to permit him to do so. He screamed in rage, but he was forced to sit in the swing. He then developed a headache.

He was returned to an adult level and it was brought to his attention that there was an association, in his early memory, between his headache and his mother forcing him to do something he did not want to do. He admitted this and he agreed to explore the matter further. Upon awakening he remarked, "I remember a dream I had. It was about myself as a child. I was in the park and mother held me in a swing when I wanted to play around with the other kids. I got an awful headache."

Following this the patient spent several sessions in violent abuse of his mother. She had overprotected him, he insisted, and she demanded compliance as a reward for her love. He felt powerless to resist her demands. He recalled many episodes of having to swallow his pride, and having to conform with his mother's commands without revolt. The aftermath of each of these episodes was a violent headache. The patient was then able to connect his past relations with his wife with this pattern, and he could also see that he had developed the same kind of attitude toward me in complying with my suggestion that he utilize an analytic technic and do free association. He could see that he entered automatically into a type of relatedness with people in which he did what was expected of him without questioning its propriety. The result was always a headache.

Soon afterward the patient began to express open revolt toward his wife's demands. He could see that in feeling hostile toward her, he was beginning to challenge his need to comply. Headaches became less and less pronounced. In the therapeutic relationship, too, he became more openly aggressive.

The next step in therapy was showing him that his compliance and passivity were the products of his own doing. In his relations with me he was always exceedingly formal, even obsequious at times. He was extremely punctual about his appointments. On one occasion he came in a few minutes late. He was profoundly apologetic about this and spent some time trying to convince me that he had no resistance. This gave me the opportunity to point out to him that he seemed to need to do what was expected. It was possible that he maneuvered himself into a role in which he had to act compliantly, perhaps even forcing people to act in a domineering way to him.

The patient accepted this interpretation and later reported that he had observed himself with his wife. While she did domineer him, he actually did maneuver her into a position where she took a protective role. He seemed to feel so helpless within himself that he automatically believed he had no right to resist her requests. I then brought to his attention the fact that he might see these things, but that nothing would happen unless he did something constructive about them.

With some trepidation the patient began to act more forceful with his wife. He made decisions and assumed a more and more dominant position in the household. He discovered that he could disagree with his wife, and resist demands he believed to be unreasonable, and that she adjusted to his new attitude toward her. Indeed she seemed more contented in many ways. Life began to assume an entirely different aspect. He had tested himself and found he did not have to be compliant nor submissive. He did not have to sacrifice his integrity and his sense of self. With this reoriented attitude, his attacks of headache disappeared completely.

In utilizing a psychoanalytic approach, it is always necessary to be on guard. Often the somatic disturbance represents the most acceptable avenue available to the patient for the discharge of anxiety and hostility. Because his ego has been unable to handle these emotions on a conscious level, he has utilized the mechanism of repression. Where this mechanism is threatened without a coordinate strengthening of the ego, where the person becomes prematurely aware of his deep unacceptable conflicts and strivings, there is definite danger of precipitating a crisis. The patient may exhibit such intense anxiety that he will invoke other mechanisms to bind this emotion. He may, for instance, develop hysterical or compulsive symptoms, or he may display characterologic defenses. Failing to control anxiety may allow it to get so out of hand as even to shatter the ego to the point of psychosis. These may also be the consequences of removal of psychosomatic symptoms by authoritative hypnotic suggestions.

Keeping this possibility in mind, the physician must always work toward a strengthening of the ego to enable it to handle basic impulses without resorting to neurotic defenses. Didactic training and practical experience in the handling of patients with emotional problems will teach the physician how and when to make interpretations toward the inculcation of insight.

REFERENCES

[1] CANNON, W. B.: Bodily Changes in Pain, Hunger, Fear and Rage, ed. 2. New York, Appleton-Century, 1936.

[2] ——: The role of emotion in disease. Ann. Int. Med. *9:* 1453–1465, 1936.

[3] ——: The Wisdom of the Body. New York, W. W. Norton, 1939.

[4] FAULKNER, W. B.: The effect of the emotions upon diaphragmatic function. Psychosom. Med. *2:* 139–140, 1940.

[5] DUNBAR, H. F.: Emotions and Bodily Changes, ed. 2. New York, Columbia Univ. Press, 1938.

[6] WEISS, E. and ENGLISH, O. S.: Psychosomatic Medicine. Philadelphia and London, W. B. Saunders, 1943, p. 1.

[7] ALEXANDER, F. AND CO-WORKERS: The influence of psychologic factors on gastro-intestinal disturbances: A symposium. Psychoanal. Quart. *3:* 501, 1934.

[8] WOLBERG, L. R.: Hypnotic experiments in psychosomatic medicine. Psychosom. Med. *9:* 337–342, 1947.

[9] GELLHORN, E.: Autonomic Regulations. New York, Interscience Publ., Inc., 1943.

[10] MENNINGER, K. A., AND MENNINGER, W. C.: Psychoanalytic observations in cardiac disorders. Am. Heart J. *11:* 20–21, 1936.

[11] DUNBAR, H. F.: op. cit., reference 5.

[12] MILLER, M. L., AND McLEAN, H. U.: Status of emotions in palpation and extra-systoles with note on "effort syndrome." Psychoanal. Quart. *10:* 545–560, 1941.

[13] KNOPF, O.: Preliminary report on personality studies in 30 migraine patients. J. Nerv. & Ment. Dis. *82:* 270–286, 400–415, 1935.

[14] SLIGHT, D.: Migraine. Canad. M. A. J. *35:* 268–273, 1936.

[15] FROMM-REICHMAN, F.: Contributions to the psychogenesis of migraine. Psychoanal. Rev. *24:* 26–33, 1937.

[16] WOLBERG, L. R.: Psychosomatic correlations in migraine: report of a case. Psychiat. Quart. *19:* 60–70, 1945.

[19] KARDINER, A.: The Bioanalysis of the Epileptic Reaction. Albany, Psychoanal. Quart. Press, 1932.

[18] BARTEMEIER, L. H.: Some observations on convulsive disorders in children. Am. J. Orthopsychiat. *2:* 260–267, 1932.

[19] JELLIFFE, S. E.: Dynamic concepts and the epileptic attack. Am. J. Psychiat. *92:* 565–574, 1935.

[20] WILSON, G. W.: Report of a case of acute laryngitis occurring as a conversion symptom during analysis. Psychoanal. Rev. *21:* 408–414, 1934.

[21] SZASZ, T. S., ET AL.: The role of hostility in the pathogenesis of peptic ulcer. Psychosom. Med. *9:* 331–336, 1947.

[22] SAUL, L. J.: Psychogenic factors in the etiology of the common cold and related symptoms. Int. J. Psychoanal. *19:* 451–470, 1938.

[23] McFARLAND, R. A., AND BARACH, A. L.: The response of psychoneurotics to variations in oxygen tension. Am. J. Psychiat. *93:* 1316–1341, 1937.

[24] JACOBSON, E.: The physiological conception and treatment of certain common "psychoneuroses." Am. J. Psychiat. *98:* 219–226, 1941.

[25] THACKER, E. A.: Comparative study of normal and abnormal blood pressures among university students, including cold pressor test. Am. Heart J. *20:* 89, 1940.

[26] ROBINSON, S. C., AND BRUCER, M.: Body build and hypertension. Arch. Int. Med. *66:* 393, 1940.

[27] DRAPER, G.: Human Constitution. Baltimore, Williams & Wilkins, 1928.

[28] SACHASE, H.: Heredity of allergic diseases, especially of hay fever. Ztschr. f. menschl. Vererb. *22:* 165, 1938.

[29] ALEXANDER, F.: The influence of psychological factors on gastro-intestinal disturbances: a symposium. I. general principles, objectives and preliminary results. Psychoanal. Quart. *3:* 508, 1934.

[30] DUNBAR, H. F.: Character and symptom formation. Psychoanal. Quart. *8:* 18–47, 1939.

[31] SAUL, L. J.: Physiological effects of emotional tension. In Personality and the Behavior Disorders (edited by J. McV. Hunt), vol. I, New York, Ronald Press, 1944. p. 280.

[32] WEISS, E.: Psychoanalyse einer Falles von nervosem Asthma. Internat. Ztschr. f. Psychoanal. *8:* 440–455, 1922.

[33] FRENCH, T. M., ALEXANDER, F., ET AL.: Psychogenic factors in bronchial asthma, Parts I and II. Psychosom. Med. Monogr. *1:* No. 4; *2:* Nos. 1 and 2, 1941.

[34] DEUTSCH, F.: Social service and psychosomatic medicine. News Letter of the Amer. Ass'n. Psychiat. Soc. Workers *11:* 6, No. 4, 1942.

[35] DUNBAR, H. F.: Psychosomatic history and techniques of examination. Am. J. Psychiat. *95:* 1290, 1939.

[36] FRENCH, T. M.: Brief psychotherapy in bronchial asthma. Psychosomatic medicine. Proceedings of the second brief psychotherapy council, Chicago, Ill., Jan. 1944, under the auspices of the Institute for Psychoanalysis, 43 East Ohio Street, Chicago, Ill.

XVI

HYPNOSIS IN CHARACTER DISORDERS

The treatment of character disorders by hypnosis is no less difficult than by traditional methods of psychotherapy. Time itself is an element in the treatment, since the disturbance is deeply structuralized and involves extensive areas of the personality. It is doubtful whether hypnosis is capable of reducing the time element required to reorganize the obdurate habit and behavior patterns that are present in most forms of this condition. Hypnosis, nevertheless, can help in the management of some types of character disorders, and may bring success where otherwise failure might have resulted.

There is much misunderstanding as to what actually constitutes a character disorder. Some psychiatrists are inclined to limit this diagnosis to conditions in which the individual is severely handcapped in his relations with people, with the world, and with himself, and in which there are few overt neurotic symptoms. Actually there is a close correlation between character disorders and psychoneuroses. All neurotic states are associated with a widespread involvement of the character structure,[1,2] while character disturbances are coincident with psychic, somatic and visceral symptoms such as are found in psychoneuroses.

Whether to classify a patient as psychoneurotic or as suffering from a character problem will depend on the presenting complaints. Most patients are acutely aware of their symptoms, particularly anxiety, and they are peculiarly oblivious to problems in interpersonal relationships and in self evaluation. Other patients, especially those who have psychologic or psychiatric knowledge, are more aware of character problems and minimize their neurotic symptoms.

Difficulties in the hypnotic treatment of character disorders stem from the fact that the patient does not understand the seriousness of his condition and is inclined to expect that hypnosis will, in relatively few sessions, cure his condition or fulfill his neurotic expectations. For example, he may yearn for perfectionism and feel frustrated by his mediocrity. Hypnosis to him is the magical means to superior performance. He may be inordinately dependent and expect that hypnosis will make him self sufficient. He may harbor within himself grandiose strivings, and wish to be made invincible and omniscient through the instrumentality of the trance state. On the other hand, he may recognize the irrationality of his impulses, and he may expect that hypnosis will force him into emotional health.

Character disturbances, whether they involve dependency, detachment, aggression, profound self devaluation, or other defects in the machinery by which the individual relates himself to others, are deep seated and tenacious. As conditioned modes of response, they have been elaborated in the earliest adjustment of the ego to pressures from the external world and to strivings from within. A review of the development of character strivings and their operation in promoting psychopathology is helpful in understanding the complications that present themselves in therapy.

The mother-child relationship may be regarded as the womb of character formation, since it is in this experience that the individual develops his first attitudes toward the world. The relationship serves as a medium in which the child gratifies his vital needs for nutrition, sucking pleasures, sensory stimulation, love and response. The extent to which the needs of the child are denied or gratified, the deprivation or security that he feels in his contact with his mother, acts as a core for his future relationships with people. His conceptualization of the world as either menacing or bountiful, and his idea of people as potentially inimical or friendly, are also conditioned by this experience.

As the child recognizes the importance of his mother in supplying his demands, he develops a tremendous need for her love and approval. Positive demonstrations of her affection insure his security, and enhance his self esteem. A gratified, emotionally satisfied child will develop a self structure that is capable of dealing aggressively and realistically with his environment. A child who is subjected to undue deprivations or rejection will evolve a self that is easily shattered by vicissitudes, that is insecure and must cloak itself constantly with various defenses.

The biologic helplessness of the infant and his extreme dependency on the adults around him for all forms of gratification make it mandatory for him to adapt himself to existing environmental prohibitions and injunctions in order to win love and support from the parent. There is consequently an incorporation of prevailing parental values and attitudes. Concepts of right and wrong, good and bad, imparted to the child by the parent, are accretions of the culture which the parents transmit through disciplines. The forms of conditioning to which the child is exposed, and his reaction tendencies later on, will, therefore, conform more or less to cultural standards. Parents, of course, have personal idiosyncrasies that vary to some extent from the accepted cultural norm. The child may, therefore, develop certain standards, values and reaction tendencies that are at variance with the norm.

Character drives which adapt the average individual to a culture are usually accepted as normal. What makes a character drive pathologic is its lack of real adaptive purpose, or the fact that it becomes overvalued and so surcharged with security virtues that failure of its functioning precipitates anxiety. A pathologic character trend is compulsive in nature and the individual must pursue it at all times, for only in its successful exploitation can he feel secure and enjoy a modicum of self esteem.

Pathologic character traits are, as has been indicated,

usually the product of unfortunate experiences and conditionings with early authoritative figures. For instance, where the parents are rejecting or overdisciplinary, and where the child realizes that his acceptance is based upon complete submission to authoritative demands, he may develop a compulsive need to repress his strivings for independence. Accordingly, he may also develop character drives which revolve around a need to submit to strong authority, in order to win love and to escape punishment.

Other character traits issue out of specific experiences with the parent. Where the latter is perfectionistic and ambitious, there may be tendencies in the child toward perfectionism and superiority in order to win approval. Where the parent has been cruel and punitive, a masochistic attitude may develop and the individual may believe that subjection of himself to punishment and self abasement are essential for purposes of security.

Pathologic character traits create difficulties in interpersonal relationships. The individual makes such demands on himself and others that he is constantly frustrated in his contacts with people. Concurrently there is a lowered self regard which gives rise to symptoms of a defensive nature, to various inhibitions, to perfectionistic and grandiose strivings. The disturbance in interpersonal relations fostered by the operation of compulsive character drives is enhanced by the existing low self esteem. The undermined person who feels contemptuous toward himself is bound to have contemptuous attitudes toward others. He may project his own attitudes of unworthiness toward others, crediting them with destructive designs on him. He may isolate himself from people and be resentful that others do not seek his acquaintance. He may have an exorbitant need for affection, yet feel so unworthy that it is impossible for him to accept love. This is also because an intimate relationship is a potential source of criticism and even injury. Hostile feelings are almost inevitable and are projected in the form of paranoid reactions or turned inward producing psychosomatic and depressive tendencies.

As a means of defending himself from other people, barriers are set up against close interpersonal relationships. This leads to general inhibitions and to timidity. The individual with low self esteem may feel obliged to cling compulsively to others for strength, utilizing self depreciation as a technic to prove he is worthy of consideration. On the other hand, he may attempt overcompensation by exploiting superiority strivings with compulsive drives for dominance, mastery and power. Impulses toward perfectionism tend toward efforts to be unassailable in all fields of endeavor.

The technics the individual utilizes to master devaluated self esteem may actually come in conflict with his security drives, producing anxiety and symptom formation. One of the most confounding features of character disorders is that a number of ambivalent drives coexist which create much conflict and confusion. For example, the person may be inordinately dependent and his pattern of life may be oriented around clinging to others. Yet his self esteem and strivings for independence may make such a pattern a source of danger. He will feel that while he needs to be dependent, he may be trapped in a dependency relationship. The conviction of being trapped may cause him to externalize his fears in phobias related to closed places or confining situations which symbolize his terror of being hemmed in. A person with a need for detachment, born out of a conviction that all people are dangerous and untrustworthy, may evolve various neurotic defenses and avoid closeness in interpersonal relationships by such phobias as fear of handshaking. A strongly dependent person, hostile because the magical figure on whom he leans fails to provide adequate bounties, may develop fears of killing this figure, and may attempt to escape his fears by various compulsive rituals which neutralize the hostile wish. Thus ambivalent strivings can produce anxiety with a generation of symptoms.

The clashing of conflictual strivings often causes a feeling of hopelessness which may be covered up by a resigned, stoical attitude toward life. Attitudes of discontentment and discouragement prevail, regardless of material circumstances, and depression is almost inevitable. Because neurotic character drives are compulsive and must be maintained at all times for security reasons, they wield a profound influence over the person. This makes him vulnerable, since it is manifestly impossible for him to maintain his character defenses at all times.

Another source of frustration is the fact that neurotic character drives are so overvalued that basic biologic and social needs become unimportant in comparison. The individual will shy away from values and goals that are accepted as normal by the average individual. Even the creature comforts of life may be relegated to neglect in comparison with such impulses as perfectionism or power or dependency. The result of this diversion in biologic aims is a disturbance in homeostasis with generation of tension.[3]

Failure of operation of a compulsive character drive is catastrophic to the individual, reducing him to a state of helplessness. The resulting anxiety may stimulate the ego into elaboration of varied defenses to restore equilibrium. A common defense is the exploitation of other character drives that have hitherto been latent because they were invested with less security values than the dominant character trait. For instance, if the individual's self esteem is shattered by failure in operation of a perfectionistic trend, he may attempt to gain security by plunging himself into a dependency relationship, parasitically gaining through his host recognition and glory. Because the capacity to utilize coexisting character defenses is usually limited, anxiety is inevitable.

It will thus be evident that the compulsiveness of neurotic character traits, and their involvement with needs for security and self esteem, make therapy a long and difficult procedure. The patient will want to overcome the consequences of his character disorder, and to remove the frustrations and anxieties that are inevitable in his disturbed interpersonal relationships, but he will obstinately cling to the very character drives that produce his difficulty.

In hypnotic therapy it is most important to understand what it is the patient desires from treatment. Should he seek hypnosis spontaneously, it is likely that he believes hypnosis will fulfill what life has failed to do, or else that hypnosis will break up a striving he recognizes as irrational, but which he is unable to control through his own efforts. Therapy is bound to be unsuccessful, since the motivation for hypnosis is neurotic in itself.

For instance, the patient who possesses a neurotic dependency drive, and who is experiencing symptoms because dependency is not availing him the gratifications he desires, may seek to utilize hypnosis as a means of reinforcing his dependency by pandering to his desire to cling to a parental figure for strength and sustenance. The power-driven individual might resist actively the relinquishment of his control and consciously or unconsciously defy the physician to put him into a trance. The failure of the physician to hypnotize the patient will serve only to mobilize the latter's scorn, and to drive him away from treatment. The detached individual, whose adjustment to life is founded on a need to maintain a chasm between himself and others, may become so terrified by the intimacy of the hypnotic relationship that he will utterly refuse to permit himself to cooperate. Or, if hypnosis is successful, panic and anxiety may cause him to abandon therapy. Under these circumstances, even though the hypnotic induction is successful, therapeutic failure is possible.

Before hypnosis is attempted, it is essential to understand

the motivations of the patient as fully as possible, and to clarify for the patient what hypnosis will and will not do. As an example we may take the case of a patient who has the problem of detachment from people caused by fear of being overwhelmed and injured. The immediate complaint for which he seeks treatment is impotency, which prevents him from marrying a young woman with whom he is presumably in love. He desires hypnosis because he believes it will make him potent. Any attempt to use hypnosis for this purpose is apt to fail because the impotency is a means of reinforcing his detachment which is being threatened by the young woman in question.

It is necessary, therefore, before hypnosis is started, to evaluate the patient's symptoms and his expectations from therapy, to acquaint him with what can reasonably be done for him and wherein his expectations may be exorbitant.

In the case of the man cited above, he may be told that it is first necessary to study his problem carefully to see what is behind his impotency. Once the physician ascertains the fact that the symptom of impotency is related to the deeper character problem of detachment, the patient may be given an explanation of his symptom in terms he can understand. He may be told, for instance, that for one reason or another he has developed a fear of closeness to people. Because he feels threatened, he tends to detach himself. So long as he was successful in doing this, he felt safe; however, he has been understandably lonesome and frustrated. His finding a young woman and his desire for marriage are in line with his need for love and companionship. Yet this need conflicts with the fear that he will be hurt in a close relationship. His impotency is, therefore, in all possibility, a means of avoiding being injured. It is necessary, then, to investigate the manner in which he fears hurt.

Hypnosis, he may be informed, will not act as a bludgeon to force him to do something he unconsciously interprets as harmful to himself. It will not magically remove his impotency. Nevertheless, it can help him in one of two ways. First, it may aid him to return to a detached attitude toward people, abandoning his desire for marriage. This may be disappointing, but it will permit him the same kind of stability he had before his involvement with the young woman. Second, he can attempt to work through this fear of people which actually causes his detachment.

Persuasive hypnosis may, in the first instance, reinforce the defense of detachment and help alleviate disappointment and depression at having to give up a biologic need. Utilized in a re-educational or analytic manner, hypnosis, in the second instance, may permit him to overcome the character disturbance that produces his impotency. Which of these two methods should best be utilized will depend on the willingness of the patient to undergo prolonged therapy as well as his available ego strength.

In some cases, hypnosis may seemingly be successful in combating certain symptoms without the formality of having to work through the character difficulty. However, such successes must be accepted cautiously, since they will usually be found to be incomplete. For instance, an artist came to therapy because of an inability to concentrate on his painting. A talented worker, he had reached a stalemate in the painting of a canvas for which he had received a commission. As time went on he became increasingly anxious at his inability to complete his assignment. A posthypnotic suggestion was given to him to the effect that he would be able to paint creatively the next day, and would by this effort be convinced that he could overcome his block. The patient accepted the suggestion and he was delighted with the completed result. However, he confided that he had become extremely resentful as he painted, having an impulse to smudge over the canvas. Analysis revealed that while he had followed the posthypnotic suggestion, he interpreted it as succumbing to an inability on his part to resist direction from authority. This for him virtually amounted to self annihilation. His inability to proceed with the painting was apparently a form of resistance against the authority who had given him the commission.

The therapy of many character disorders is difficult because of what has been called the "negative therapeutic reaction." The patient almost always utilizes his relationship with the physician as a focus for his various character drives. He may subject the doctor to attitudes of contempt and ridicule. He may seek to vanquish, provoke, and to hurt him in subtle ways. He may slavishly subject himself to ingratiating or masochistic tactics to win the tribute, affection and support he believes he deserves. Feelings of self devaluation and hopelessness will permeate his outlook and lead him to anticipate failure in therapy. In spite of the fact that the individual may be talented and outwardly successful, the inner image of himself is depleted and contemptible. Often self devaluation acts as a potent block to treatment.[4] One even gets the impression that the patient utilizes the facade of helplessness to avoid making any effort to get well.

Because of the vulnerability of the relationship with the physician, interpretations are apt to be regarded by the patient as a blow to his self esteem, initiating depression, rage or anxiety. They are evidence to the patient that the physician does not approve of him. He is apt to intellectualize the entire therapeutic process, using it either as resistance or as a means of fortifying himself against change. Despite all logic, the patient strives to wedge the physician into the framework of his distorted attitudes toward life. He exhibits great feelings of rejection and of distrust, and at the slightest challenge his defenses crumble, leaving him in a state of collapse and despair. He then exhibits a psychic rigidity that refuses to yield to reason or entreaty.

The same difficulties will be encountered in hypnoanalysis

as in psychoanalysis based upon the immature relationship of the patient to the physician. The patient will interpret the hypnotic process in accordance with his deep character patterns. For example, suggestions made to a patient with compulsive strivings for independence may be interpreted as an attempt by the physician to enslave the patient and to rob him of his free will and capacities for independent action. In such cases suggestions often are resisted by amnesia, or, if the patient feels powerless to resist suggestions, an anxiety attack may occur. In some cases a strong paranoid reaction may be precipitated which damages for a while the relationship with the physician.

The instability of this relationship can interfere with the hypnotic process, and the patient will successfully resist suggestions that he believes are against his interests. The resistance such patients show is astonishing. Even in somnambulistic trances, the patient may refuse to cooperate, and he may react with rage or depression that can persist for days after hypnosis.

The aim in hypnotic therapy must be toward a solidification of the interpersonal relationship. This process is expedited where the patient does not feel forced to comply with demands he believes are against his interests. Analytic probing and interpretation of unconscious material should be assiduously avoided until the patient is able to accept interpretations outside the framework of his immature ways of thinking.

The treatment of character disorders requires time and patience. In some instances the hypnotic process may expedite therapy by reinforcing the positive values of a close interpersonal relationship. Inevitably, however, the patient will respond to the physician with the full range of his disturbed character patterns. Until the patient is capable of understanding that many of his attitudes toward the physician have no basis in reality, but are rather an outgrowth of interpersonal difficulties, deep interpretive therapy must be delayed. Attempts are first made to establish a positive transference without analyzing its source. Hostile feelings toward the physician and other irrational impulses which interfere with a good relationship must be dealt with actively. It may be necessary to confine the entire treatment hour to current problems, shying away from historical material. Only when the patient's relationship with the physician becomes more congenial will it be possible for him to benefit from attempts to connect historical material with his present difficulties.

During the course of treatment, the patient will seemingly modify his attitudes toward the physician, but in this alteration the physician must search for areas of resistance. For instance, a submissive, ingratiating attitude, which is a cover for a fear of abandonment, may, upon interpretation, be replaced by an apparently sincere attempt to search for and to analyze inner problems. The physician may, if he observes the patient closely, detect in this attitude a fraudulent attempt to gain security by complying with what the patient feels is expected of him. While the patient appears to be analyzing his problem, his real motive is to gain security by adjusting himself to what he considers are the demands of the physician. In this way the process of analysis itself becomes a means of indulging his neurosis.

In analyzing resistances, their sources in infantile attitudes and conditionings usually become apparent. It is essential to bring the patient to a realization of how the machinery with which he reacts to the world is rooted in early conceptions and misconceptions about life. The interpretation of character strivings does not suffice to change their nature, for they are the only way the patient knows of adjusting.

A breakdown of character strivings often brings out in sharp focus the repressed needs and impulses from which the strivings issue. When the patient becomes cognizant of the conflicts which produce his destructive interpersonal attitudes, he has the best chance of taking active steps toward their modification.

It many instances, particularly where lack of time prevails, the only thing that can be accomplished is to adjust the person to his neurosis in as expedient a manner as possible. Environmental manipulation may be necessary to take pressures off the patient, and he may be shown, through various psychobiologic technics, how to adjust himself to his existing situation and how to obtain a maximum of pleasure and security from it. For instance, if the patient has a strong striving for perfectionism which drives him incessantly, involving him in projects he cannot handle with his intellectual and physical equipment, he may be shown how he can confine himself to a project which he can master proficiently. Whereas the scope of his operations may be limited, he can indulge his perfectionistic strivings in a circumscribed way, gaining in this some measure of gratification. If he is inordinately dependent, he may be shown that he can maintain his integrity in spite of the fact that he has to lean on authority. If he has a power impulse, avenues for its exercise through competition may be provided for him. This approach, of course, merely panders to the patient's neurosis, but it may be the only practical thing that can be done for the time being, and, in many cases, it will make the patient's life immeasurably more tolerable.

Whenever possible, the patient, through re-educational approaches utilizing psychoanalytic insight, should be acquainted with the nature, genesis, and dynamic significance of his character trends. He should be encouraged to observe how his strivings and defenses operate in everyday life situations, and he should be shown ways in which he can change his attitudes toward people. This directive approach, may, at some point, have to be altered toward a more nondirective technic particularly when the patient is better capable of mastering his own problems. Character disorders require perseverence in handling, since relapses are the rule.

While character trends can be classified in such categories as dependency, power strivings, and detachment, they are always interrelated and the fusion makes for a picture that is quite unique for each individual. Behavior is not the static product of a group of isolated trends, but rather is an integrate of the combination. The product of this intermingling differs from the sum total of the component trends. That is, if the person is compulsively modest, is fired by perfectionism, is unconsciously arrogant and aggressive, some of these trends will tend to neutralize and some to reinforce each other. Nevertheless, for treatment purposes, character disorders may be regarded in terms of the most dominant trend.

DEPENDENCY REACTIONS

The treatment of dependency reactions is complicated by the peculiar relationship the individual establishes with all authoritative persons. The latter are invested with godlike qualities, and the patient makes insatiable demands on them for gratifications of every conceivable sort. The peculiar overvaluation of authority is based on a feeling of helplessness that is inevitably present in dependent people. This leads them to seek an omnipotent figure who must cater to their demands. Whenever this figure falters in the least, security is cancelled and aggression results which may take on a paranoid form. Consequently there is a blind admiration for strength, and a contempt for any weakness, in the authority.

Hostility is a usual consequence of this form of adaptation, and it results from two sources; first, dissatisfaction with the amount and quality of the bounties derived from the authority; and, second, resentment at giving up one's independence and drive for self growth. Because the expression of hostility is regarded as a threat to the dependency situation, rage is repressed and converted into psychic and somatic symptoms. Physical suffering is often utilized as a weapon of aggression against the authority, and the individual may derive from it masochistic gratification.

The treatment of extreme dependency reactions poses special problems. Dependent persons are often brought to the physician for therapy not because they, themselves, feel a need for change, but rather because parents, marital partner, or friends insist that something be done for the patient. Visits to the physician, in such cases, are made merely as a favor extended by the patient to the concerned person. The patient expects that no change will occur, and he will thus be resistant to any effort that is made to get him to participate in the treatment process. The limit of his cooperativeness is to expose himself to the physician during the allotted hour.

With defective motivations such as this, little progress can be expected. The patient will be particularly resentful to interpretations which he regards as criticisms of himself. He will be antagonistic to the implication that there is something wrong with him. He may respond with bewilderment, aggression, or with pseudoconformity, behind which lies much resentment. He will show every resistance and defense he can marshal without incurring too great displeasure on the part of authorities around him. Months and even years of therapy may effect little alteration in the inner dynamics of the personality.

So long as the patient maintains his infantile motivations for coming to therapy, no change will be possible. The sole hope lies in convincing the patient that in the physician he has a friend who will not try to influence him against his will, who understands and sympathizes with the way he feels. The struggle with the physician will stop when the patient senses that the doctor is a person who does not challenge his scheme of life, but rather seeks to participate in it.

The only real way of aiding the patient is in helping him to establish a relationship with the physician which will take a more mature form than his previous interpersonal relationships. Unfortunately this is easier said than done because the dependent individual will utilize the physician in the same way that he uses all authorities—as a means to security and as a prop to his self esteem.

There is much in the relationship the patient seeks to establish with the physician which resembles the infant's attitude towards the parents. The patient does not seem to be interested in developing resources within himself. Rather, he desires to maneuver the physician into a position where he can receive constant favors of various sorts. He will abide by any rules of therapy in order to obtain his aim. He will even seemingly absorb insight. It is most disconcerting, however, to learn that assimilated insights are extremely superficial, and that the patient is less interested in knowing what is wrong with him than in perpetuating the child-parent relationship. He seems actually incapable of reasoning logically, and there is an almost psychotic quality to the persistence with which he demands that the physician support him or give him direction.

Interpretations of the patient's dependency are usually regarded by him as chastisement. He will assume that any attempt to put responsibility on his own shoulders is a form of ill will expressed toward him by the physician. He will demonstrate reactions of disappointment, rage, anxiety and depression, and he will repeat these reactions in spite of lip service to the effect that he is getting well.

In treating a dependency reaction, it is essential to recognize that aggression is inevitable in the course of therapy. The demands of dependent people are so insatiable that it is impossible to live up to their expectations. Only when the patient begins to experience himself as a person with aggressiveness, assertiveness and independence, will he be able to function with any degree of well-being. This goal, unfortunately, may in some instances never be achieved.

Hypnosis would seem to play into the patient's neurotic need for a magical helper. The dependent person is usually quite suggestible to trance induction unless there is coordinately present a tremendous fear of injury in the dependent relationship. Where the motivation in therapy is exclusively to supply dependency demands, hypnosis is bound to terminate in failure. The hypnotic relationship will gratify for a while the patient's desires for an omniscient authority. A suspension of symptoms will then, in all likelihood, occur, and in conformity with the demands of the hypnotist, the patient will abandon many of his neurotic aims and objectives to assure himself of the doctor's good will.

The physician must remember that symptom relief on the basis of propitiation of the patient's dependency needs is extremely temporary. It is essential in all cases to strive for a therapeutic approach in which the individual learns to accept responsibility for his own development. Self growth is obtained chiefly through achievement. It is necessary to get the patient to become more self sufficient and more capable of functioning through his own resources.

When it is decided to modify the therapeutic approach in line with this aim, a definition of the treatment situation will be required. The physician may show the patient that he makes persistent efforts to be dependent because he feels so helpless in himself. However, the very act of his becoming dependent infantilizes him; he cannot develop a stature that will enable him to be healthy and assertive.

There are some individuals whose self structure has been so crushed as a result of inimical experiences, that they will resist the attempt at making the therapeutic situation nondirective. Here the therapeutic program must be organized around a partial therapeutic goal. The physician must resign himself towards creating a modicum of security within the patient, educating him to function with his dependency strivings to the least detriment to himself.

To minimize his becoming dependent upon the physician, it may be essential to avoid hypnosis after the first few sessions. When it becomes apparent that it will be impossible to work along nondirective or analytic lines, and that the patient merely seeks to make himself dependent on the physician, visits may be cut down to once weekly, the patient being encouraged to establish relationships with other persons and to engage himself in various outside activities. He may be urged to affiliate himself with some group to which he can contribute his energies.

As much pressure as the patient will bear must be imposed upon him to make his own choices and decisions. It is to be expected that the patient will resent this vigorously, accusing the physician of refusing to accept responsibility in the therapeutic situation. Should this occur, the physician may explain to the patient that, were he to pander to the patient's demands for support and make decisions for him, this would tend to infantilize the patient, and make him more dependent and more unable to develop to a point where he can fulfill himself productively and creatively. An attempt should be made to show the patient why he has never been able to develop feelings of assertiveness and the proper self esteem. He must earnestly be instructed that the physician does not wish to shirk responsibility, but actually withholds directiveness out of respect for the patient's right to develop. Although the patient may still resent the physician's intent, he will understand more and more that unless he begins to make his own decisions, he will never get to a point where he is strong within himself. Security is fostered in proportion to the person's ability to develop resources capable of mediating his needs through his own positive efforts. Should the physician be too supportive of the patient, the patient will never be able to take those steps which will enable him to grow.

Many patients who seemingly are fixated on a dependent level can, with repeated interpretations of this sort, finally begin to accept themselves as persons who have the right to make their own choices and to develop their own values. Persistence, however, is the keynote. In therapy the patient will exploit every opportunity to force the physician from a nondirective to a directive role. Nevertheless, when the patient sees that the physician has his own welfare at heart, he will, if he has the slightest spark of self esteem, be able to develop more independence and assertiveness. The shift in therapy from a directive to a nondirective aim calls for considerable skill, and must be tempered to the patient's insight and ego strength. Unless such a shift is made at some time, psychotherapy will probably be interminable, and the patient will continue on a dependent level requiring the ever-presence of the physician as a condition to his security.

DETACHED REACTIONS

The treatment of persons with a character problem of detachment also presents many difficulties. Such persons are usually motivated to seek therapy because their detachment interferes with their livelihood or capacity to achieve social or sexual gratification. Often anxiety, which has developed from the individual's effort to emerge from his detachment, is the complaint for which the patient wants help.

The type of therapy employed will depend upon the function of detachment in the life adjustment of the individual. It will also depend on the ego strength of the patient and his capacity to tolerate the anxieties incumbent upon relating himself intimately to other persons.

Detachment may be a means elaborated by the individual to protect himself from intense dependency strivings. A close relationship poses dangers of being overwhelmed, for in it the patient may envisage a complete giving up of his independence. Detachment may also be a technic of avoiding injury or mutilation which the patient believes inevitable to his coming close to a person. Finally, it may be a method by which the patient protects himself from fears of attacking and destroying others. In treating the patient, therefore, the dynamic significance of detachment must be kept in mind, and efforts must be made to modify the cause if possible.

One way of estimating the capacity of the patient's existing ego to tolerate interpersonal relationships is through the Rorschach test, especially noting his reaction to the color cards. If forms disintegrate and bizarre responses develop, there probably are dangers in utilizing an analytic approach or in encouraging too intimate contacts with people. The best way of estimating ego strength is, of course, the patient's actual response to the therapeutic situation, and his dreams, fantasies and conscious feelings mobilized by the transference.

Where the patient's ego is so weak that it must fortify itself against shattering, and where there is little practical possibility of modifying its strength, therapy along psychobiologic lines may help the patient to reinforce his character defenses and to modify to some extent his detachment in line with a more comfortable adaptation. Where the ego strength will permit of close interpersonal relationships, a re-educational form of therapy utilizing psychoanalytic insight may result in a real alteration in the character structure.

In treating detached patients one must anticipate that there will be difficulty for a long time in establishing a close relationship. Hypnosis may sometimes shorten this period materially, since in the trance the patient, willy-nilly, finds himself in close contact with the physician. This tends to mobilize his fears of injury and inspires detachment. As his conflicts come to the surface, they can be clarified. Much active work will be required in detecting and dissolving resistances to insight. The detached patient often has a tendency to intellectualize the entire therapeutic process.

He will particularly shy away from expressing his feelings, since he will conceive of them as dangerous.

Great hostility is bound to arise which may be disconcerting to the patient, but the physician must realize that hostility is a defense against closeness in interpersonal relationships. It is extremely important that the therapist be as permissive to the patient's outbursts as possible. The patient will probably attempt to provoke the physician into expression of counteraggression to justify his retreat from people as untrustworthy, and withdrawal from the world as potentially menacing.

The trance state is helpful in encouraging the patient to participate in social activities, in competitive games and sports. Commanding, restrictive directions should be avoided. With encouragement detached people begin to integrate themselves with others. In groups they drift cautiously from the periphery to the center as they realize that they will not actually be injured in a close interpersonal relationship. Group therapy is often most rewarding in detached schizoid individuals.

A common reaction in the therapy of detached persons is anxiety, which is manifested by disturbing nightmarish dreams or by actual anxiety attacks. The reaction will usually be found when the patient experiences for the first time real closeness or love toward the physician. These emotions terrorize him and cause him to fear injury or destruction of an indefinable nature. It is essential to deal with this reaction when it occurs, and to give the patient as much support as is necessary. Sometimes detached patients whose defenses have been crumbling go into a clinging dependent attitude when they realize the full weight of their helplessness. A supportive type of therapy should be given them here, in the effort to provide them with an experience of not being rejected or injured in a dependent relationship. Analysis of the intense inferiority feelings may be required, should the patient bring up appropriate material. Crushed assertiveness rooted in sibling rivalry is commonly encountered.

POWER REACTIONS

Another type of character disorder is one in which power impulses predominate. In this condition all that seems to matter in life is forcefulness and strength. The feelings and rights of other people are disregarded. There is a blind admiration for everything invincible. The person is contemptuous of softness and tenderness, and self esteem is seemingly dependent on the ability to be dominant. In some persons the need to control is expressed in terms of intellect. Such individuals appear to have the fantastic notion that they can control the world by will regardless of how difficult or perverse the situation may be.

As in dependency, the dynamic force behind the power impulse is a profound sense of helplessness and an inability to cope with life with the individual's available resources. A motive behind the power drive is to coerce people to yield to one's will, to provide bounties for him of various sorts. Genetically the type of thinking that occurs in the individual with this character organization resembles that of the child at the stage of eruption of the teeth, when he becomes cognizant of his growing powers of observation and ambulation. Strivings for mastery occur at this period, and great rage is precipitated when there is any interference with the child's demands or impulses. He utilizes aggression as a tool to coerce the parents to give in to his will.

The treatment of the power driven individual is oriented around a building up of frustration tolerance, an increasing of the capacity to withstand tension, and a gaining of security through his own resources. A re-educational approach along psychobiologic lines utilizing hypnosis may be effective in permitting the individual to develop inner restraints capable of exercising control of his impulses. It is essential to be firmer in this type of disorder than in either dependency or detached reactions. The patient must be shown that there are limits beyond which he cannot go, and that he must face responsibility. Whenever possible the patient should be acquainted with the dynamic significance of his power drive, and he should be encouraged to make efforts toward the expansion of his inner resources.

Where dependency and power drives are fused, therapy must be directed toward correcting the core of selflessness, through re-educational and analytic approaches, which make for trends of compulsive submissiveness and dominancy. The individual here functions in a dual manner, seeking to suck security from stronger people by clinging to them helplessly, or wresting security from them by force and aggression. Therapy is useless unless it results in a strengthening of the ego which will enable the person to function under his own power.

Narcissistic Reactions

In treating the character disorder of excessive narcissism, much difficulty will be experienced. Persons with this problem seem to have such a need for personal admiration that they conceive of therapy as a means of making themselves more worthy of praise.

Unlike the mature person who gains security from cooperative endeavors in attitudes of altruism and sympathy, the narcissistic person concentrates most interest on himself. His self love may actually become structured into grandiose strivings, omnipotent impulses and megalomania. Although the image of the individual appears to be bloated, analysis readily reveals how helpless and impoverished he actually feels. There is danger here of precipitating psychotic depression or excitement in presenting insights prematurely. The shock-absorbing capacity of the ego must always be weighed, and interpretations should be made in proportion

to the available ego strength. In markedly immature individuals, little development may be expected other than a
somewhat better environmental adaptation through guidance
technics.

"Anal" Personality

A type of character disorder often found in our culture is
that of a self-entrenched and detached attitude that has
been called an "anal" personality. The core of this personality
is one of great distrust. This motivates the fear of being overwhelmed, and produces great suspiciousness and a desire to
preserve oneself by warding off all intrusions through the
building up of an impenetrable wall between oneself and
others. The individual seems to want to take things in, but
to give little up. Associated are impulses of stinginess,
orderliness, cleanliness, obstinacy and sadism.

The function of most of these traits is to preserve the wall
that protects the person from others. Cleanliness becomes
a means of warding off contacts with the outside world.
Orderliness is a technic that keeps things in place so that
the individual may not be caught unaware. Obstinacy is a
technic of fighting off overwhelming power by negativism.
Sadism stems from a feeling of weakness within oneself,
and from the necessity to deal with others in kind through
domination and force. One of the motivants of homosexuality, which often appears in this type of personality, is a
fear of people of the opposite sex who are not to be trusted
because they are different from oneself and hence potentially
evil. Intimacy with persons who are more familiar because
they have the same sexual organs is less threatening. Homosexuality also represents a means of destroying others, of
making oneself passive and dependent, and of gaining power.
Love is conceived of as dangerous; indeed any outgoing
feelings are dangerous.

There is much to indicate, in this personality disorder, that difficulties in relationships to parents occurred at the stage of social and toilet training, at which time intolerable frustrations were imposed on the child. During this period of development, the ego expands, and the child experiences a desire for mastery and dominance. He is exposed, however, to parental disciplines which challenge his claims for mastery. The child may strive to cling to his sense of power by conforming as little as possible to demands made on him. Toilet training usually becomes the arena in which he proves he can gain mastery over his parents. An ambivalent attitude exists in that he also realizes that by conforming to the demands of his parents in establishing habits of cleanliness, he will obtain their love and support. Nevertheless, his desire for power and mastery conflicts with this aim and creates impulses to retain fecal material or to soil. It is probably for this reason that excretory activities become so overvalued and constitute symbols of danger and destructiveness in dream and fantasy life. Punishment inflicted by others and self punishment may actually be symbolized by anal punishment. The intense hostility that is generated in this condition may be projected outward in a paranoid reaction. An obsessive-compulsive neurosis is also common. Understandably, therefore, the patient, for a long while, will regard therapy as a personal encroachment.

Patients with this type of problem tend to intellectualize the therapeutic process. This serves as a defense against feeling. Often all that can be done for the patient is to give him as much insight as he can tolerate, in this way cooperating with his need to intellectualize therapy. Interpretations should deal with the more superficial character defenses rather than with the deep hostile and sexual content. They should be made in a reassuring manner. A persuasive, re-educational approach as outlined in the chapter on compulsion neurosis is usually best, although in some cases an analytic technic is possible. Hypnosis may be resisted vigorously by the patient; however, if his active participation is sought, and if he is enjoined to accept or to reject suggestions according to his own desires, it is possible to secure a fairly good trance. Once hypnosis is induced, therapy can proceed along psychobiologic or analytic lines, depending on the goals toward which therapy is directed.

PSYCHOPATHIC PERSONALITY

The treatment of the heterogeneous disorder which has been given the loose term "psychopathic personality" is facilitated to a marked degree by the employment of hypnosis. The psychopath seems to be in search of an invincible authority with whom he can identify, and who in turn can reinforce his diminutive sense of restraint. Hypnosis conducted in an authoritarian manner places the physician in a position so strong that the individual feels powerless to resist his suggestions.

Psychopathic personality is not a specific diagnostic entity. It is rather composed of a group of disorders so diverse that they cannot be included among recognized diagnostic categories. These disorders have in common the fact that the individual deviates in a pathologic way from the cultural norm. Primarily he is unable to function in his relationships with people. He is at odds with the disciplines of society and with the prevailing moral code. His behavior is governed by his immediate emotional needs, and he shies away from shackling his current demands to reality restrictions. He will brook neither interference nor frustration and, like a child, he reacts with aggression when his pleasure whims are denied.

Psychopathic personality is thus a state of emotional infantilism. The inability to face responsibility, the sacrifice of prudence for immediate gratifications, and the failure to organize behavior in line with a purposeful pursuit of biologic and social goals all speak for an immature kind of personality integration. Intellectually the individual may be brilliant, but he is so easily side-tracked that his talents are fruitless. Boredom and lack of perseverence make success impossible. His efforts become disorganized and unsustained. His goals are fantastic and beyond realistic achievement. Failure fills him with rage, and he attempts to compensate by the use of force, by pathologic lying, or by the assumption of dramatic roles that symbolize his childish notions of great achievement.

Because he is ruled by egocentric needs, he is in perpetual conflict with the dictates of society. His personality lacks moral, ethical and esthetic qualities. Beneath his narcissism and grandiosity lies a deep sense of self devaluation and a feeling that he is unloved and unlovable. The psychopath actually feels alone and isolated, and he seeks to have his own way and to preserve his sense of self by striking out blindly. External pressures have little lasting influence on his demands for pleasure fulfillment. Unable to handle frustration, he makes recourse to such tension-relieving mechanisms as alcohol, drugs, sexual overindulgence and unmitigated pleasure strivings. His ego is so loosely organized that conflict or frustration may produce shattering, with the development of psychotic excitement, depression, and hallucinatory and delusional episodes.

Most psychologic studies of the psychopath reveal a defect in the conscience or superego that interferes with a sense of personal and social obligation. Yet the conscience need not be defective in the sense that it does not exist. Rather it may exert an uneven and vicarious influence on behavior, permitting the indulgence of impulses at one time, and punishing the individual for his indulgence at another. In some psychopaths, analysis reveals an inordinately severe superego, and the person's symptoms represent a rebellion against its harshness.

Among the main psychopathic tendencies are irresponsibility, nomadism, thirst for adventure and excitement, perverse sexual attitudes, alcoholism, drug addiction, emotional instability and immaturity, poverty of sentiment, inability to profit by experience, lack of feeling for others, and an inability to inhibit aggressive and sexual impulses and to conform with social demands and the dictates of sober judgment. Although the psychopath usually avoids neurosis by acting out his conflicts in behavior, episodes of excitement are common.

Most authorities agree that the treatment of psychopathic personality is most difficult. All therapies, including psychoanalysis, have yielded meager results. In many cases the only thing that can be accomplished is manipulation of the environment to eliminate as many temptations as possible which stimulate the psychopath into expressing his vicarious impulses.

If a psychopathic individual can establish a relationship to a person, the latter may be able, as a kind but firm authority, to supervise the patient's actions. Hypnosis can reinforce this authoritative relationship. Because the attitude toward authority is so ambivalent, one might speculate that the psychopath would be resistive to hypnosis. In practice this is not the case. Psychopaths are easily hypnotized with a proper technic. The physician can, by adroit suggestions, act as a repressive moral force and as a pillar of support, to whom the patient can turn for guidance when temptation threatens his judgment. Direct advice in the hypnotic state is usually more acceptable to the patient than in the waking state, and suggestions may be couched in such terms as to convince the patient that he is actually wiser and happier for resisting certain activities which, on the basis of past experience, are bound to result disastrously. On the basis of a guidance relationship, the patient may be taught the wisdom of postponing immediate gratifications for those which, in the long run, will prove more lasting and wholesome. He is taught the prudence of tolerating frustration, and the need to feel a sense of responsibility and consideration for the rights of others. Not that these lessons will be accepted or acted on, but constant repetition sometimes helps the patient realize that it is to his best interests, in the long run, to observe social amenities and to exercise self control.

Experience demonstrates that it is possible to modify to some extent the immature explosive reactions of the psychopath by an extensive training program, particularly in cooperative group work where the individual participates as a member toward a common objective. Adequate group identifications are lacking in the psychopath, and the realization that ego satisfactions can accrue from group experiences, may create a chink in the defensive armor. In cases where the psychopath comes in conflict with the law, and where incarceration is necessary, a program organized around building up whatever assets the individual possesses, particularly in a group setting, may, in some instances, bring success. In young psychopaths, vocational schools that teach the individual a trade may contribute to his self esteem and provide him with a means of diverting his energies into a profitable channel.

In a challenging book, Lindner[5] advocates the use of hypnoanalysis in the treatment of criminal psychopathy. Whereas the resistances may be so great as to preclude the use of an orthodox psychoanalysis, Lindner feels that the resistances can be successfully circumvented through hypnoanalysis, and he cites as evidence excellent results in a number treated by this method. Lindner, in his work, contends that the dynamic motivant of psychopathic behavior is an unresolved Oedipus situation or castration-anxiety, the compulsive criminal act being a disguised parricidal striving.

My own experience with psychopaths has not convinced me that an analytic understanding of the genetic determinants, or the knowledge of the symbolic significance of psychopathic behavior patterns, has very much of a curative effect. On the other hand, a guidance approach aided by re-education along psychobiologic lines has proven itself of value, particularly when utilized with hypnosis.

REFERENCES

[1] HORNEY, K.: New Ways in Psychoanalysis. New York, W. W. Norton, 1939.

[2] ——: The Neurotic Personality of Our Time. New York, W. W. Norton, 1937.

[3] WOLBERG, L. R.: Tension states in the neuroses. Psychiat. Quart. *17:* 685–694, 1943.

[4] ——: The problem of self-esteem in psychotherapy. New York State J. Med. *43:* 1415–1419, 1943.

[5] LINDNER, R. M.: Rebel Without A Cause: The hypnoanalysis of a criminal psychopath. New York, Grune & Stratton, 1944.

XVII

HYPNOSIS IN ALCOHOLISM

DRINKING is one of the most universal of all human habits. However, relatively few drinkers become alcoholics in the true sense of the word. Alcohol is consumed for a variety of reasons; chiefly for its narcotizing effect on the higher brain centers. Alcoholic beverages momentarily alleviate tension, bolster self confidence and provide the "lift" which tides the individual over uncomfortable situations and difficulties.

It is precisely for these reasons that alcohol becomes a "crutch" for the person with an emotional problem. It subdues anxiety in anxiety states; it permits the individual to master his phobias in anxiety hysteria; it deadens obsessive fears in compulsion neurosis; it brings surcease from distress in psychosomatic illness. Alcohol thus serves as a vehicle of escape from suffering. Whatever positive values it has for the individual here, these are secondary to relief from symptoms.

Alcohol is also commonly used by persons with diffuse character problems. Where there is a fear of people, a few drinks lessen the sense of menace. Alcohol dissipates surface hostility and makes the individual more congenial, permitting him to open up to others. Consequently, it helps appease loneliness and feelings of isolation. In those with a great sense of inferiority, alcohol fosters a spurious courageousness and strength. It covers up a deep devaluated self esteem, initiating compensatory boastfulness and confabulations that may border on "pseudologia phantastica." Where the individual's conscience is pathologically punitive, the deadening effect of alcohol allows the expression of basic impulses and needs. Many of the stimulating effects of drink are the product of removal of superego inhibitions. This permits persons who have a craving for perverse sexual satisfactions, and who are blocked by powerful guilt feelings, to express their curiosities and cravings.

While alcoholic overindulgence is sponsored by numerous neurotic and characterologic disorders, a consistently unique personality "type," who for want of a better term we can call the "essential alcoholic," shows the following characteristics: undue sensitiveness, inability to tolerate frustration, marked dependency impulses, feelings of isolation, devaluated self esteem, tendencies toward masochistic self destructiveness, profound unconscious hostility, narcissism, repressed grandiose ambitions, and overt or latent homosexuality. There is a compulsive yearning for sympathy and love. In men there are strivings for passivity with an unconscious desire for and fear of castration as a means of achieving a dependent feminine role in life. In women there may be a repudiation of femininity with strivings for a penis, which symbolizes mastery and dominance. The defense against homosexual impulses may assume a typical paranoidal quality.

The history of many alcoholics discloses that they have been overprotected as children, and that dependency was never really resolved. A deeper analysis frequently reveals that the individual suffered a trauma in the period of weaning, or that he never obtained adequate sucking pleasures in feeding. The oral frustrations experienced seem to make the mouth and upper gastrointestinal tract a most important zone. This is borne out by the dreams of the alcoholic, which may be seen to involve sucking or feeding activities.

Where a child has an extremely domineering or overprotective parent, he may never develop the incentive to grow up. An anxious, guilt-ridden mother, particularly, is unable to permit the child to master the frustrations of weaning. He will consequently become too dependent on the mother for gratifications long beyond the point when he should have begun to function on his own. At the same time, he will fear growing up because he believes he does not have the equipment to do things for himself. He will then be unable to develop the aggressiveness that is, in our culture, equated with masculinity. Inwardly he will feel that if he is dependent upon his mother, he must be like a girl. Even though he functions in a heterosexual capacity, deep down he doubts his manhood. Being dependent, he needs a protector to give him things, and in relationship to that protector he adopts a passive role. His associated fear of castration often precipitates attitudes toward his father as the possessor of power and strength. His desires for intactness bring out an impulse to identify with his father. In fantasy he believes that if he absorbs the penis of his father this will restore his damaged genitality. A homosexual element thus begins to operate insidiously. Even though he functions on a heterosexual level, the alcoholic has strivings for homosexuality. Usually he repudiates homosexuality, although, under the influence of alcohol, this tendency sometimes asserts itself. A denial of homosexuality in the form of a projective mechanism may be implemented thus:

"I am alone and helpless. I want to be taken care of like a woman. If I am helpless and passive, someone will take care of me like a woman. But then I will have to give up my claims for independence and masculinity. I will be castrated. I fear castration. I am not a woman. I do not want to have intercourse with a man. But men tempt me. They want to have intercourse with me. Men want to hurt me. They are against me. They hate me. I hate men because they do this to me." This denial results in a paranoidal state. The triad of alcoholism, homosexuality, and paranoia, is often found operating as a whole. In certain alcoholic psychoses, like acute hallucinosis, the paranoid mechanism comes out in almost pure culture.

In female alcoholics the dynamics are somewhat similar. There are, for the same reasons as in the male, deep cravings for oral gratification and satiation. There is associated also a homosexual desire which takes the form of wanting to be absorbed into the mother or to incorporate her breast. Active homosexual fantasies may occur, since penis envy complicates the picture, and the person may strive to flee from passivity by functioning as a man. Homosexuality here also may be projected and repudiated in a paranoidal form.

It is not surprising, therefore, that many alcoholics never have resolved their physical and emotional ties with their mothers. Should the male alcoholic break away from home and marry, he usually finds a maternal woman with whom he can become dependent. So long as the dependency need is supplied, the person may make marginal adjustment. Should the object on whom he is dependent leave him, he will respond with depression, with gastrointestinal distress, and with cravings for food or for alcohol. More importantly, the very dependency that he seeks creates conflicts which result in his rejecting the love object. For instance, his dependency demands may become insatiable, and when they are not gratified, he will react with hostility. Furthermore, as has been indicated, dependency is dangerous because it implies passivity and is equated with castration. The person will then repudiate the individual with whom he has established a relationship, and he will go out in search of a new idealized love object. His life is usually a series of involvements with people, men or women, toward whom he expresses a filial attitude. There is a repetition of his ambivalent pattern with frustration and depression.

Alcohol serves as a way of deadening his despair. But there are positive virtues too. A state of satiety induces pleasant relaxation. Psychoanalytic studies show that this state symbolizes to the alcoholic the nirvana such as the infant presumably experiences when, after having suckled milk, he relaxes at peace with the world. A feeling of "goodness" is coupled with elation and with a sense of omnipotence which nothing else seems to be able to duplicate, except, perhaps, benzedrine and narcotic drugs.

In both the anxiety drinker and the "essential alcoholic," therefore, alcohol serves a vital adjustment purpose. Unfortunately, alcohol in the excessive quantities in which it is used is a poison which eventually has a destructive effect on the person. Because alcohol depresses all mental and psychologic functions, it blunts critical judgment. The individual may get himself into business and social difficulties as a result. Alcohol also has an obliterative effect on repression. In the intoxicated state the person will be confronted with the upsurge of impulses which he repudiates in the sober state, and he may be unable to refrain from expressing these urges. Consequently, he may find himself in serious trouble. For example, a release of sexual and hostile drives may create tremendous complications for him later on. As drinking continues, inhibitions become increasingly relaxed, and a progressive deterioration occurs involving the person's morals and standards. The capacity for social adaptation is destroyed, and self esteem becomes vitiated. The individual becomes more and more isolated from his friends, and he seeks companionship in saloons and bars, where, in an alcoholic haze, he indulges in vainglorious boasting, maudlin sentimentality, and a pitiful appeal for understanding and love.

While drinking removes surface hostility and promotes camaraderie and congeniality, an increased concentration of alcohol deadens superego restraints and encourages a release of destructiveness and aggression toward people and property. The sadistic attitudes of the alcoholic are associated with strong masochistic tendencies. One need merely observe the suffering and contrition of the alcoholic during his "hangover" periods to appreciate that there is fulfillment here of a need to punish himself.

As drinking proceeds over a period of years the tolerance of the drinker is reduced. Bodily tissues become sensitized to alcohol, and the person seems less and less able to handle himself with composure. There is evidence that an allergy to alcohol develops, and that some constitutional element makes certain persons less tolerant of drink than others.

The point at which the drinker becomes a confirmed alcoholic varies. Arbitrarily a person may be considered an alcoholic when he needs alcohol habitually in order to function, or when he requires it as a chief source of pleasure. At first the alcoholic is able to control the amount and time of his drinking. However, alcohol ultimately robs him of the ability to master even nominal amounts of tension which become more and more intolerable until sobriety itself is tantamount with suffering.

In the "essential alcoholic" drinking has so many unpleasant consequences that these would more than seem to compensate for pleasures derived from the habit. In spite of the fact that the individual realizes that his drinking is a detriment to himself and his family, it may occupy so important a part in his psychic economy that no amount of argument or cajolery can dissuade him from the practice. There are many alcoholic individuals who suffer intensely from guilt following bouts of drinking, realizing that they are harming themselves and bringing shame to their families through a habit which they, themselves, eventually come to despise. Yet they seem powerless to control their craving.

When the average alcoholic applies for therapy, the physician is usually confronted with the expressed or secret hope that the patient will learn to drink normally and to "hold his liquor like anyone else." While this may be possible in the anxiety drinker following abatement of his neurosis, it is not true in the case of the real alcoholic.

Although there are some persons who believe that the alcoholic can be cured by weaning him gradually from the bottle, and who are of the opinion he may learn to engage in social drinking without exceeding his capacity, experience has shown that success is possible only where alcohol is completely and absolutely eliminated from the individual's regime. The object in therapy is complete elimination of all alcoholic beverages, including wine and beer.

The treatment of alcoholism does not simply involve removing the desire for alcohol; it involves also restoration of the patient to some kind of adaptational equilibrium. Without such restoration the person will become pathologically depressed, and his tension will drive him to drink no matter what pressures are put on him.

In the anxiety drinker, any attempt to force or to shame the person into sobriety will interfere with the therapeutic relationship. The patient should be made to feel that he need not apologize for his drinking desires. He should be shown that alcohol provides him with an escape, and that he will require liquor so long as his more fundamental problems remain. The danger of his continued drinking may be pointed out to him merely to create the incentive to overcome his neurosis. He may be informed that while the physician does not approve of the patient's drinking, he will not order him to stop. When the patient believes he is ready to give up alcohol, the physician will help him to do so. The therapeutic program should be organized around the treatment of the underlying neurotic or character problem. A sympathetic attitude toward the patient's need for alcohol is always appreciated by the patient. However, the physician must insist that the patient come in sober for his sessions.

While a psychoanalytic approach is useful in the anxiety drinker, it is usually futile in the "essential alcoholic." The ego of such persons is so immature that the capacity to integrate and to utilize insight in a constructive manner is impaired. In analysis the alcoholic will dig out fascinating dynamic structures, but this effort will have little influence on his drinking. In many cases the physician must be satisfied with a partial therapeutic objective of weaning the patient from alcohol, permitting him to adjust to life with his immature character organization in as adaptive and nondestructive a manner as possible.

The greatest difficulty will be experienced in the handling of those alcoholics who do not wish to stop drinking, and who apply for therapy under coercion of parents, mate or friends. Exposure to therapy is merely a device to retain the good will of the people dear to the patient. Treatment here will usually be unsuccessful, the patient utilizing the physician as a referee who is expected to arbitrate between himself and his family. Sessions are spent lamenting his plight or presenting himself as a misunderstood and abused person who is completely justified in his drinking.

Such alcoholics are best treated in an institution where they cannot obtain drink. The usual reaction to hospitalization is indignation and promises to refrain from drinking if released. When such release is not forthcoming, the person will make an exemplary adjustment, creating such an appearance of normality that one may be tempted to discharge him prematurely. One difficulty here is the attitude of relatives who will be goaded by the patient to secure his release. In the hospital, psychotherapy may be started and an attempt may be made to get the patient interested in hobbies, crafts, or an occupation which will engage his energies. Psychobiologic therapy of a guidance and persuasive sort is useful to help the patient discover and utilize his assets and talents. A period of one to two years of hospitalization may be required, and before the patient is discharged, his environment should be manipulated to assure a minimum of stress.

Where hospitalization is impossible, certain forceful measures may be required, particularly in the alcoholic who has no motivation whatsoever to abandon liquor. The best time to start therapy is when the patient is in an acute alcoholic episode. At this time he is given the usual detoxification therapy of insulin, sugar and vitamins. The contact with the patient here will serve a psychotherapeutic purpose in promoting a close relationship. The physician, utilizing the remorse and self condemnation of the patient during the "hangover" period, may enjoin him to give up alcohol on the basis that it is a poison which will eventually destroy him. To offset depression and to give the patient a sense of well-being, benzedrine sulfate may be utilized. Ten milligrams are taken by mouth twice daily, after breakfast and after lunch. A good diet supplemented with vitamin B is essential, and a sedative, like seconal, may be prescribed at nighttime in the event of insomnia.

The next phase of therapy is a coercive one in which an attempt is made to bring the patient to a point where he refuses to drink or is unable to drink. Cajolery and appeals to reason are usually futile. Sometimes a belittling and challenging manner mobilize in the patient a need to prove that he has the "guts" to master the craving for alcohol. This, however, cannot be depended on. Once the patient verbalizes a desire to stop drinking, conditioned reflex therapy may be started. The patient should be under some sort of supervision during this period.

In the event the patient is deeply hypnotizable—as are many alcoholics—he is, in the trance state, reminded that alcohol is a poison and that it will ultimately damage him. He can get "on the wagon" if he so desires, and he can learn how to be happy and adjusted without needing to drink. As soon as the patient verbalizes a desire to give up alcohol, he is told that strong suggestions will fortify his ability to abandon the drinking urge.

When the patient is able to follow posthypnotic suggestions, conditioned reflex therapy is started. The first suggestion deals with substituting some oral satisfaction for the alcoholic craving. He may be told: "When you awaken, you will have an uncontrollable desire to drink. You will find that all your thoughts are concerned with wanting to drink. At the same time you will realize that drink is like poison, that it will destroy your health and your mind. In spite of this realization, the craving for a drink will be strong. You will notice on the desk near you a bottle of malted milk tablets. You will reach for a tablet and put it in your mouth. As soon as you do this, the craving for drink will immediately leave you. You will be filled with a sense of pleasure and relaxation. You may have no recollection of the suggestions I have just given you, but you will follow them nevertheless."

A successful performance of this posthypnotic suggestion is repeated several times, and the patient is instructed that any kind of candy may be substituted for the malted milk tablet.

Following this, suggestions are given to the patient to fantasy or to dream about the worst thing and the best thing that can happen to a person. In the trance, the patient may be requested to observe himself in the orchestra of a theater, watching a play. As he observes the drawn curtain, he will notice a man (or woman, in the event the patient is a female) peering behind the curtain, with an agonized, fearful expression on his face. The patient will wonder what it is the man is watching, and he will realize that the man has noticed something that creates fear and shock. When the physician counts from one to five, the patient will see the curtain swing open suddenly, and he will then observe the scene which has frightened the man on the stage. Similar suggestions referring to a contented expression on the man's face, indicating that he has observed the most wonderful thing that can happen to a person, will give the physician clues as to how the patient symbolizes happiness.

The patient is then given the suggestion: "From today on, you will want to give up the drinking habit completely. You will experience a tremendous distaste for alcohol in any form —whiskey, gin, scotch, wine, beer or any other form of alcoholic beverage. Your craving for alcohol will become less and less. You realize that you have become allergic to alcohol, and that alcohol constitutes a poison for you. You must give up drinking entirely, and I am going to help you achieve this objective. From now on, whenever you have the urge to drink, it will be possible for you to control this urge by taking a malted milk tablet or a piece of candy. Much as you were able to control the craving for drink last time by appeasing your craving with a malted milk tablet, you will be able to do it again indefinitely. Do you understand me?"

Immediately thereafter the patient is given a suggestion that he will have a dream in which he observes, sees or feels something so revolting that it turns his stomach and causes him to want to vomit. As soon as the patient relates this dream, he is told, "From now on, whenever you have the urge to drink, you will be able to appease that urge by taking a malted milk tablet or a piece of candy. Should the urge to drink continue, you will begin feeling nauseated, but you will be able to remove this feeling of nausea by resolving not to drink. Should you, under any circumstances, be offered a drink, you will be able to refuse with the simple statement that you would like to have plain soda or ginger ale. In the event the craving for drink becomes so great that not even the nausea controls it, and should you begin to reach for a drink, under any circumstances, you will have the same sensations as in the dream. Drinking any kind of alcoholic beverage will do the same thing as what happened in the dream. Your stomach will tighten up, you will begin to feel violently ill, and, should you manage to get any alcohol down, you will immediately vomit it up. These suggestions will continue in force from this time on, and they will get stronger and stronger until you have resolved completely that it is foolish and unnecessary to drink. Remember that when you reach for a drink, you will feel just like the man felt on the stage, who was so fearful and upset. If you manage to control the urge to drink, you will feel like the man who was so extremely happy."

These suggestions must be repeated several times, and it must be ascertained that the patient understands them thoroughly. Following this the patient is told that even though he does not remember having been given these suggestions, they will continue in force. Should he ever recall that the suggestions had been made to him, this will not destroy their power to influence him. Finally he is told that when he awakens, he will find a small glass of whiskey on the desk near him. He will have an urge to drink the whiskey, and as soon as this happens, he will put into practice what he has just learned. He is then awakened and his reaction to the suggestions observed. Should there be any hesitation in executing the suggestions, he is rehypnotized and the suggestions are repeated until he is capable of following them automatically.

Reinforcement of the conditioning process is essential and, at the beginning, should be executed once daily if possible. Following this, suggestions are reinforced once weekly, until the patient has been sober for three months. Thereafter, reinforcement is essential at least twice monthly.

Where deep hypnosis is not possible, conditioned reflex therapy by hypodermic injection of emetine hydrochloride may be considered.[1-6] It is assumed that the physician is technically skilled in administering conditioned reflex therapy with drugs, since the technic is somewhat more complicated than one might imagine. The practical difficulties in instituting this form of conditioned reflex treatment make hospitalization advisable. However, there are relatively few sanitariums that are available for this purpose.

Coincidental with conditioned reflex therapy, an attempt must be made to establish a relationship with the alcoholic. Should the patient become dependent on the physician, the latter may utilize the dependency relationship to reinforce the patient's desire to abstain from drink and to motivate him towards utilizing his assets to best advantage. Interest in hobbies and recreations should be stimulated. The patient should also be urged to join a group like "Alcoholics Anonymous."

The group approach, such as is utilized by the "Alcoholics Anonymous" organization, is a most effective one. Here the person is forced to admit that he is an alcoholic, that he needs help and that he wishes to do something about his condition. He is enjoined to realize that because of his own powerlessness in managing his drinking, his life has gotten out of control. He is encouraged to feel that a Power greater than himself can restore him to health, and he is advised to turn himself over to this Power in his quest for security. He is furthermore encouraged to make a searching moral inventory of himself, admitting his faults to others in the group, as well as to God. He must be willing to make amends to those persons that he has in any way harmed. At the same time he is shown that he may have overemphasized his bad points.

In this type of approach the alcoholic is never actually urged to say he will stop drinking entirely. Rather he is informed that each day he will tell himself that he will remain dry, with God's help, for twenty-four hours. At the end of the day he may take an inventory of himself to see if he did anything which was not constructive or was intolerant, resentful, jealous, spiteful or unkind.

The meetings are extremely useful, since the patient finds companionship with others who share similar emotional problems. Furthermore, when the patient feels tempted to drink, he is able to telephone one of his friends and make an appointment to talk things over. An important part of the therapy is his helping other alcoholics who are in the grip of their drinking habit. The fact that the workers in the movement are ex-alcoholics enables them to display an enormous amount of tolerance, and to convince the patient that he, too, can do what others have done. It goes without saying that only an alcoholic really understands the drinker. An identification is thus expedited.

The psychodynamics behind the successes scored by groups like "Alcoholics Anonymous" involve the fact that the individual gains security and unity with a new mother figure,

which the organization symbolizes to him. The organization
becomes the idealized giver of things. He is capable of identifying with others and he feels himself to be an integral part
of the group. The organization, in bringing him close to other
more helpless drinkers, appeases his inner grandiosity. Vicariously the alcoholic mothers himself by taking care of others.
Should he abide by all of the precepts of the organization,
he may accept the omnipotence of a God figure, amalgamat-
ing himself with Him.

Many alcoholics stop drinking when they feel that their
dependency is appeased by an alliance with God. The religious cure of alcoholism is dynamically based on the drinker's
conviction that if he lives up to God's expectations and stays
sober, he will be given bounties and beneficences, if not now,
then in the hereafter. God becomes the ideal parent who is
all wise, all supporting, and all forgiving. The alcoholic is
unable to challenge this new parental figure, or to test his
omnipotence or weakness, as he can with a flesh and blood
person. His hostility is consequently held in check. When
a drinker "gets religion," he may therefore overcome his
alcoholic habit.

The treatment of the alcoholic who spontaneously applies
to the physician for help, while difficult, does not present so
many problems as does the person who is maneuvered into
therapy through the agency of another concerned individual.
In treating the patient here the following steps may be kept
in mind. First, a relationship is started with the patient with
the object of developing a positive transference. Second, an
effort is made to build up the patient's self esteem. Third,
his interests are externalized and outlets provided for his
aggression. Fourth, he is taught to handle frustration and
deprivation. Fifth, he is encouraged to stop drinking. Sixth,
he is urged to make social contacts with individuals and
groups.

The first aim is to get the patient to substitute a dependency relationship on the physician for his alcoholic habit. The alcoholic seeks and needs this type of relationship. When he accepts the physician and has confidence in him, the latter will then be able to utilize this relationship more forcefully to break the drinking habit. It is essential, therefore, to make the alcoholic feel that he is accepted on his own level, drunk or sober. The patient may be told that the physician wants to help him, but that he is not going to act as a policeman and force him to give up drink if he believes it is so vital for his adjustment. He is informed that the physician realizes that alcohol plays a major role in his life. Drinking does not make him a bad person. If he has the desire for alcohol, it is because of a sequence of conditionings and experiences that have happened to him which he can now overcome.

It may be difficult to convince the patient that the physician is interested in him, and he will often test the physician's good faith by indulging in repeated heavy bouts of drinking. Should the physician fall into this trap and become embittered with the patient, the relationship will terminate. One must remember that the patient habitually tries to wring out of the environment a good parental figure who will supply him with unqualified love and support. It is essential at first then to get the patient to accept the physician in this role.

Hypnosis facilitates the positive transference and makes the patient feel that something concrete is being done for him. During the trance, no effort is made to explore the dynamics or sources of the patient's problem. Rather a state of relaxation is secured, and a persuasive talk is given the patient to the effect that he will soon be able to feel better, to grow stronger and to be more determined to enjoy life on a more wholesome level. Towards this end he will want to do everything that is in his best interests. Should he, himself, decide that alcohol is undermining his health and depriving him of happiness, he will then have the desire to do what is necessary to substitute for this habit something more fundamental and satisfying. Suggestions related to the expansion of his assets and toward externalization of his interests are then proposed. The patient is also assured that the physician will make every effort to see him whenever he really requires help. In the event an emergency arises, he need not hesitate telephoning the physician.

Any existing remediable elements in the patient's environment which may be creating conflict for the patient should be straightened out, with the aid of a social worker if necessary. In spite of his expressed optimism, the patient is unable to handle frustration, and any objective source of difficulty may suffice to promote tension which will produce a craving for drink. An inquiry into the patient's daily routine and habits may be expedient. Often one finds a gross defect in the person's diet. Alcoholic overindulgence is coincident with a depletion in dietary intake and with vitamin deficiency. The prescription of a well-balanced diet with sufficient calories and with supplementary B vitamin is of great help. The patient should also be encouraged to appease his hunger whenever he feels a need for food. Hitherto he has propitiated hunger pains by drinking alcohol. He may be surprised to observe that eating three square meals a day can remove much of his craving for liquor.

The numerous difficulties a patient has experienced through his inability to control drinking, the general condemnation of society, and the disdain of his family, all contribute toward a depreciation of his self esteem. It is difficult to rebuild self esteem by reassurance, but an effort must be made, both in the waking state and hypnosis, to demonstrate to the patient that he has many residual assets which he can expand. Because alcoholics become negligent about their appearance, it is essential to rebuild their interest in how they look. Appearing neat and well-groomed always has a bolstering effect upon the person. Alcoholic women may be directed towards taking care of their complexions and hair by going to a beauty parlor. Whatever interest the patient shows in hobbies or external recreations should be encouraged. He must be reminded that he is not a hopeless case and that he has many good qualities which he has neglected. His guilt may be appeased by showing him that he is not solely responsible for his alcoholic craving. It will be possible to substitute for it something much more constructive. The physician will help him make a proper substitution. In discussing his work situation, a battery of vocational tests may disclose that the patient's interests and aptitudes are in a direction other than his existing work. He may be helped to develop along the lines indicated by his tests. The ultimate aim of these efforts is to get the patient to accept himself as a person with value and dignity.

Because the alcoholic is extremely hostile, some outlet should be provided for his aggressive tendencies. Joining a Y. M. C. A. or athletic club, engaging in competitive games and sports, in swimming, archery or boxing may be of value here. As release is provided for the patient's aggression, he will become much less tense, and the character of his dreams will change from fighting destructiveness to more peaceful actions.

Teaching the alcoholic to handle frustration will require considerable effort. The patient must be brought around to a realization that everyone has frustrated feelings, and that an important job in life is to exercise control. Because of what has happened to him, he may be informed, he is apt to misinterpret any disappointment as a sign of his own personal failure. It is mandatory that he build up a tolerance of frustration, even though he has to extend willful effort in this direction.

Since frustration is usually accompanied by gastric distress, it may stimulate a desire for drink. The patient may therefore be advised to carry with him, at all times, a piece of chocolate or candy. Whenever he feels frustrated, or, under any circumstances, where a craving for drink develops, he can partake of this nourishment. Hot coffee, cocoa and malted milk are also good for the same purpose and can act as substitutes for alcohol. As the patient gains more respect for himself, it will be possible for him to tolerate greater and greater amounts of frustration.

At some stage in therapy, the patient must be encouraged to stop drinking. The physician does not condemn him for alcoholic indulgence; but because liquor has a destructive effect, he must try to control its intake. The close relationship with the physician, the increased self esteem that comes from positive achievements, the correction of difficulties in his life situation, and the heightened ability to handle frustration, all help to reduce his thirst. Substitutes for the alcoholic craving also help to convince him that drink need not be an integral necessity in his life.

When the propitious time arrives, an explanation may be given the patient of how alcohol is poisonous to him because he has built up an allergy for it. It must be stressed that physiologically he is different from other persons, and for this reason he is unable to tolerate drink. Many alcoholics regard their inability to drink as a sign of weakness. An organic reason for their intolerance usually has a soothing influence on them. The patient may be told that because of his allergic condition, alcohol is as much a poison to him in the long run as cyanide. While he has needed alcohol to appease his tension, he will find that he can utilize other methods now and can, therefore, reduce the amount of his alcoholic intake. Gradually he will want to give alcohol up entirely.

The patient must abandon the prevailing idea, so current among alcoholics, that eventually he will get to a point where he can drink like anyone else. He must be assured that one drink is equivalent to a thousand, and that because of his allergic indisposition to drink, he must make up his mind to forsake alcohol completely. One way to do this is to live his life and make resolutions for only twenty-four hours in advance. There are a number of excellent scientific books on alcoholism that the patient may be encouraged to read, which will help him to achieve abstinence.[7-9]

Should the patient be unable to stop drinking, hypnosis is often quite effective as a support. No more than a light trance is required in which strong suggestions are given him emphasizing the destructive effects of alcohol, the distaste that he will have for all forms of drink, his ability to control his craving, and the need to substitute food, hobbies, sports and social activities for liquor. If nothing seems capable of controlling alcoholic indulgence, conditioned reflex therapy may be started, utilizing hypnosis or emetine hydrochloride.

An important phase of therapy is encouraging the patient to make social contacts and to affiliate himself with groups. If a branch of "Alcoholics Anonymous" exists in the community, the patient will find that he can make many friends there, and that he can involve himself in numerous constructive activities that will engage his energies and consolidate the gains he has made in therapy.

REFERENCES

[1] VOEGTLIN, W. L.: Treatment of alcoholism by establishing a conditioned reflex. Am. J. M. Sc. *199:* 802 (June) 1940.

[2] ——, LEMERE, F., BROZ, W. R., AND O'HOLLAREN, PAUL: Conditioned reflex therapy of alcoholic addiction: V. Follow-up report of 1042 cases. Am. J. M. Sc. *203:* 525 (April) 1942.

[3] TILLOTSON, K. J., AND FLEMING, R.: Personality and sociologic factors in the prognosis and treatment of chronic alcoholism. New England J. Med. *217:* 611 (October) 1937.

[4] LEMERE, F., AND VOEGTLIN, W. L.: Conditioned reflex therapy of alcoholic addiction: II. Specificity of conditioning against chronic alcoholism. California & West. Med. *52:* 268 (December) 1940.

[5] VOEGTLIN, W. L., LEMERE, F., BROZ, W. R., AND O'HOLLAREN, PAUL: Conditioned reflex therapy of chronic alcoholism: IV. A preliminary report on the value of reinforcement. Quart. J. Studies on Alcohol *11:* 505 (December) 1941.

[6] ——, ——, AND ——: Conditioned reflex therapy of alcoholic addiction: III. An evaluation of present results in light of previous experience with this method. Quart. J. Studies on Alcohol *1:* 501 (December) 1940.

[7] PEABODY, R. A.: The Common Sense of Drinking. New York, Little, Brown & Co., 1935.

[8] STRECKER, E. A., AND CHAMBERS, F. T.: Alcohol—One Man's Meat. New York, Macmillan, 1939.

[9] SELIGER R. V., AND CRANFORD, V.: Alcoholics are sick people. Nat'l Com. on Alc. Hyg., Inc.

XVIII

HYPNOSIS IN PSYCHOSIS

HYPNOSIS has, for obvious reasons, a limited utility in the psychoses. It may, however, occasionally be employed as an adjunct to other treatment procedures.

A psychosis represents a total collapse of the resources of the ego when the individual is no longer capable of adjusting to external pressures and internal demands. It follows failure of the customary defenses of the person to handle anxiety and to restore psychobiologic equilibrium. A combination of adverse constitutional and environmental factors renders the ego of the psychotic person incapable of adapting him on a realistic level of integration when he is exposed to conditions of extreme stress.

The psychosis is characterized by a retreat from normal relationships with people with regression to defenses characteristic of a more primitive stage of psychic development. There is an impairment of repressive functions with emergence of unconscious fears, conflicts and strivings. A diminished ability exists to test reality and to differentiate fact from fantasy. The psychotic reaction is not a purposeless one, but represents a form of adjustment. The hallucinations, delusions and other symptoms are not actually as chaotic as they seem. They follow definite laws governed by a prelogical type of thinking.

The shattered repressive function of the ego produces filtering into awareness of impulses whose gratification on a conscious level has been considered dangerous or repulsive. Hostile and erotic strivings, an exaggerated interest in oral and excretory activities, are apt to express themselves in a relatively undisguised manner. Impaired reality testing produces an inability to function to the demands of everyday life. Ideas and fantasies may be projected outward in the form of delusions and hallucinations. Shattered integrative capacities cause a disorganization of cognative, conative and affective elements of the personality.

There is also a return to archaic forms of thinking, behaving and pleasure striving reminiscent of infantile stages of development. For example, a profound state of helplessness with strong dependency impulses may develop that resembles the early attitude of the child toward the parent. Feelings of omnipotence and delusions of grandeur may occur which are similar to the bloated notions of self importance and narcissism experienced in childhood. Masochistic expiatory technics to gain love and approval, and coercive domineering reactions to force things from people are definitely regressive in nature. There may even be a return to a stage of development prior to the complete differentiation of the ego, a period before the individual distinguished himself from his environment and from others around him. Depersonalization, inability to recognize parts of the body, and delusions of nihilism are symptoms which belong in this category.

In the treatment of a psychosis the chief aim is to bring the ego back to a realistic level of integration, even though one has to restore habitual neurotic character traits that have maintained the person in a sort of functional relationship with life. For instance, the individual, responding to a feeling of inner paralysis and helplessness, may have mastered his anxiety on the basis of a strong dependency drive. However, the death of the person on whom he has depended may suddenly confront him with feelings of isolation and despair so profound that his integrative capacities will be shattered, with a resulting psychosis. In therapy an attempt can be made to restore equilibrium by providing the patient with a compensatory dependency relationship. Active guidance, manipulation of the environment, and other psychobiologic therapies may be useful in achieving this goal. Where the hold on reality is minimal, hospitalization, sedation and shock therapy may be required to bring the ego back to a more realistic stature. A most important element in the treatment program is establishing a relationship with the patient of an accepting nature, tolerating any psychotic projections he may display.

Hypnosis can sometimes be utilized to consolidate the interpersonal relationship once contact has been established with the patient. Trance induction is not as difficult as might be imagined provided the patient's attention can be maintained. Sedatives are helpful in getting the patient to relax to a point where he is accessible. As the patient gains confidence in the physician, he will become more susceptible to suggestions. Hypnoanalytic probing should at first be assiduously avoided, since the emotions released cannot be handled by an already overburdened ego. Treatment efforts during an acute psychosis are in line with repressing rather than expressing the unconscious content. Where the ego has been sufficiently strengthened to repress anxiety, and where reality testing is restored, the cautious use of a hypnoanalytic approach may then be attempted.

Manic-Depressive Psychosis

With all the studies that have been done on manic-depressive psychosis it is still impossible to say whether the disease is an entity in itself or whether it is a symptom complex that is the result of a variety of causes including organic factors. The outstanding feature of the disease is emotional lability, with mood variations of an extreme nature ranging from stuporous depression to frenzied destructive elation. Cognative and conative elements of the personality as well as the vegetative functions participate and are probably influenced by the prevailing mood.

In depressed phases there is a general retardation of ideational and motor activities. There is a loss of confidence with feelings of helplessness, worthlessness, contemptibility and lowered self esteem. There is a retardation of the physiologic processes with diminished salivary secretions and gastrointestinal activity. Associated are anorexia, constipation, and insomnia. Impotency or frigidity are also frequent. In severe depression the retardation of motor and ideational processes may become so extreme as to approach stupor.

The manic phases of the illness are associated with elation, and with an acceleration of psychomotor functions leading to flight of ideas, distractability and motor excitement. Assertiveness and self confidence are definitely increased here, and, in the wake of his ecstatic mood, the patient may exaggerate his capacities and accomplishments to the point of grandiosity. In the most extreme cases the manic attack resembles a delirium.

Fisher and Marrow[1] have experimentally produced many of the symptoms of manic-depressive psychosis by inducing in normal subjects, during the hypnotic state, emotions of depression and elation. They have thus added to the evidence that whatever symptoms appear in the disease, these are the consequence of the associated emotional change.

Whether the disease is of organic, constitutional or psychogenic origin is not definitely known. Vegetative disturbances are often present,[2-5] but whether they are the cause or the result of the illness is difficult to say. Most evidence points to the latter. Hereditary and constitutional factors are also definite in manic-depressive psychosis.[6-8] However, heredity alone is probably insufficient to produce the disorder, and in some cases a hereditary influence may not be present.[7]

Many authorities believe that manic-depressive psychosis develops on the soil of a peculiar type of personality structure. Strong parental fixations, emotional infantility, narcissism and a tendency toward marked mood swings are frequently listed as prepsychotic personality traits. Many individuals who develop hypomanic and manic reactions show, during the period when they are free from psychosis, a marked optimism, outgoingness, buoyancy and an inclination towards unsustained brief enthusiasms. Those predisposed to depression often are dependent, submissive people who are easily discouraged, fear disapproval, depreciate themselves and feel hopeless.

Whether the prepsychotic personality is related to hereditary and constitutional factors, or whether it is produced by specific environmental experiences, is to many authorities controversial. It is possible that prepsychotic personality traits are reactions of the ego to the same stresses and conflicts that produce the manic-depressive attack, and that they are, to a certain extent, defensive devices aiding in the adjustment of the individual to his various fears and needs.

There is probably some association between manic-depressive psychosis and schizophrenia, but the nature of this association is vague. Some schizophrenic patients show manic-depressive symptoms while a number of manic-depressive disorders are difficult to differentiate from schizophrenic reactions. Errors in diagnosis are thus often made.

To understand the mechanism of manic-depressive psychosis it is essential to review the genetic development of the child. Following birth the infant is completely helpless and at the mercy of the parent for every type of service. Tension related to hunger, cold, wetness and pain are alleviated by the mother with whom the child feels a peculiar unity, as if she were a part of himself. As his ego develops, and as he perceives that she is separate from himself, he associates her presence with the alleviation of tension and pain. Her absence then is apt to stimulate what is probably a primordial form of anxiety. To avoid this unpleasant emotion he strives to keep her at his side at all times. The screaming tantrum is one of his earliest technics. Later on, as the boundaries of his ego expand, and as his perceptual organs develop, he becomes conditioned to respond more adaptively in order to win the love and approval of his mother in the attempt to offset possible abandonment. He even absorbs her prohibitions and demands, and he conditions his behavior to avoid her disapproval. These prohibitions act as the nucleus of the conscience or superego which determine many of his future reaction tendencies.

In a later phase of development the child's motor system matures sufficiently so that he is capable of dealing more aggressively with his environment. Aggression and various other coercive technics appear, and the child, instead of complying passively, has a striving for power and mastery, and seeks to force his parents to yield to his will. Overconfidence and an inflated sense of his own importance develop. The driving motive of life is to coerce people to give him coveted bounties.

In children who develop normally, this stage proceeds to a more mature stage of personality growth characterized by independence and self sufficiency. Some children, however, perhaps because of certain constitutional defects, or because of excessively traumatic environmental influences during infancy, particularly rejection and overprotection, never reach this phase and cling to technics of adjustment characteristic of infancy. Such children may develop character structures of compulsive dependency with strivings to gain security by clinging to people in a parasitic way, utilizing ingratiation, aggression, submission, perfectionism, masochistic self punishment and other technics in line with this objective.

In manic-depressive conditions the basic character structure is often of a helpless and dependent, or of a domineering power-driven nature. However, not all dependent or power-driven persons develop manic-depressive reactions when their compulsive character strivings fail. The manic-depressive syndrome appears to represent an actual return to helplessness such as existed during infantile phases of development. The reparative measures that the individual employs to gain security, namely, complete passivity or coercive rage, are identical to those he used as a child. Hereditary and constitutional factors are probably decisive in molding an ego organization that regresses to the point of utilizing such infantile technics.

The individual who is predisposed to manic-depressive psychosis reacts to important situations of insecurity with the feeling that he is a helpless child at the mercy of a rejecting world. In many cases the precipitating factor appears to be a real or fancied blow to the person in the form of loss of money, position, work, self esteem, a love partner, friend or relative. These deprivations are symbolic of loss of love or loss of support which in turn are representative of abandonment by the parent. In endogenous depressions there is no demonstrable precipitating factor, and a subtle internal change of an endocrine nature, or a minor physical illness, may create the insecurity that generates the manic-depressive attack, bringing into play the primitive parental invoking mechanism.

The depressive attack thus represents the falling back to the protecting agencies of infancy, the parents, with re-establishment of old dependency ties. The machinery of depression is a regression to a type of behavior and attitude similar to that of a child who is dependent for his security on the good graces of a superior person, namely, the mother. The reaction may be looked upon as a psychologic campaign to restore the patient to a position where he is loved by a mother symbol. The latter may be an actual person, male or female, or may be a fantasied inner image of the mother. The ultimate goal is the reconciliation with a maternal object. Fantasies of suckling, of incorporating the mother cannibalistically, and other oral elaborations may appear.

Along with reparative efforts to recover security by restoring the lost parent, the patient develops symptoms which represent the abysmal lonesomeness and isolation that he feels. There may be fantasies of being an infant, of starving, of being tortured, or of being dead, which signify his conviction of nothingness. Psychologically he reacts as if his ego has been removed by the withdrawal of the parent. Mourning, self punishment, self denial and fasting are, in part, forms of penitence used to bring the parent back to the patient's side. At the same time a tremendous amount of hostility is released in rage at the parent for the desertion. Because expression of hostility presumably further compromises the patient with the parent, he is apt to repress his rage and direct it inwardly, accusing himself of the indignities he really feels toward the parent. The self depreciation, blame and contempt one finds so often in this condition are explicable on this basis. Hostility may discharge itself also through autonomic channels with the development of psychosomatic symptoms.

The manic attack appears to be a form of flight from conflict, the overactivity representing an escape from pressing inner problems. The person behaves as if he has achieved coveted goals in life and has eliminated injuries and threats to himself. Mania then becomes a triumphant victory over all the forces that oppose the individual, with resulting joy and exaltation. Having achieved outstanding success in his own eyes, the manic feels himself worthy of praise and love.

There are many reactions of the manic phase that correspond to the period of development in the individual where he strives to coerce the parents to yield to his whims. In vanquishing authority the manic individual manages to subdue his own superego, liberating repressed conflicts and desires. It is as if the flood gates of his unconscious no longer exist. There results a tremendous upsurge of unconscious hostility and sexuality with drainage of these impulses in ideation and action. The elation corresponds to the release of inner impulses. The grandiosity and expansiveness represent a liberation of the self from reality restraints.

The treatment of manic-depressive psychosis depends upon the phase and the severity of the illness. Hypnotic therapy is obviously impossible during manic stages because of the distractability of the patient. Sedatives may be helpful in milder cases in rendering the patient able to concentrate on suggestions. Where a trance can be induced, suggestions of a calm relaxing nature may be made. Following the acute phase of the illness, psychobiologic treatment, and, in selected cases, a modified analytic approach may be possible.

Hypomanic and manic patients are often extremely difficult to manage at home. They will seek to involve the physician in all of their fantastic plans. They will make demands of him which, when unfulfilled, will release great hostility or aggression. They will try to overwhelm and dominate those around them, and they may become uncontrollable when their wishes are not acceded to. During this period an effort must be made to calm the patient. Assignment of productive outlets for his energy may be attempted. Unfortunately, resistance is usually great, and hospitalization may be required for sedation, hydrotherapy, and, where indicated, shock therapy and prolonged narcosis.

One of the chief reasons for hospitalizing the manic patient is to protect him from involving himself and other people in projects which issue out of his overconfidence. Because he is inclined to be erotic, he must be protected from sexual indiscretions and from a hasty marriage, which he may contract on the crest of an ecstatic wave. Another reason for early hospitalization is that some manic cases will go into a state of delirium when they are not treated intensively at the start. These delirious attacks may be fatal due to exhaustion, dehydration and hypochloremia.

Psychotherapy is also very difficult in depressed patients because their demands for help and love are insatiable. Consequently, no matter how painstaking the physician may be in supplying their demands, they will respond with rage and aggression, often accusing the physician of incompetence or

ill-will. The patient should be told that the physician understands and sympathizes with his suffering. Such measures as
active guidance, sympathy and externalization of interests
may be attempted. As in schizophrenic patients, the basis of
treatment is a warm relationship between the patient and the
physician. The relationship that the patient establishes with
the physician will, however, be extremely vulnerable, because
of the existing infantile ego. Much patience and tolerance is
needed and an attempt must be made to share with the
patient his fears and misgivings.

This attempt is more easily said than done, because the
treatment of depressed patients must be carried out in the
medium of their distrustful nature. Distrust springs from the
fusion of hate with love. Hostile feelings generate guilt which
may be so disabling that the person will want to discontinue
treatments. The slightest frustration during treatment, such
as the unavoidable changing or cancelling of an appointment,
may be equivalent to rejection and will mobilize a tremendous amount of anxiety. Under the surface there is always
fear of abandonment, and the patient will tend to misinterpret casual actions. He has a tendency to seek reassurance,
but he resents its being called psychotherapy.

The aim in treatment is to develop and to reinforce all
positive elements in the relationship. This will involve much
work since the deep attitudes of the patient are so ambivalent that he will feel rejected spontaneously, no matter what
the physician does. It is best to let the positive relationship
take root without attempting to analyze its sources.

One of the ways of maintaining the relationship on a positive level is by reassuring the patient constantly, by avoiding
differences in opinion, by trying to see his point of view and
sympathizing with it. It is essential to convey to the patient
the idea that he is liked and that the physician is his friend in
spite of anything that happens. An attitude of belittling,
harshness, ridicule or irritation must be avoided. Treatment

is bound to be prolonged, and is always punctuated with relapses corresponding to the cyclic phases of the disorder.

Hypnosis can aid some of the milder depressions. The trance state is used primarily as a means of inducing relaxation and as a vehicle for persuasion in the attempt to bolster self esteem. A number of depressed patients appear to thrive under hypnotic therapy probably because it appeals to their dependency need.

Mild depressions may be treated at home under supervision of a psychiatrically minded attendant or nurse, or, better still, the patient should be admitted to a rest home. Isolation from parents and friends, bed rest and constant care by a motherly attendant may prove very beneficial. Massage and hydrotherapy should not be neglected except in agitated patients who may be acutely upset by such treatment. Because of anorexia efforts should be made to bolster the diet with high caloric and high vitamin intake in the form of small but frequent feedings. In severe cases of malnutrition a few units of insulin before meals may be helpful. If sedatives are needed, phenobarbital one-quarter of a grain at 3 P.M., 7 P.M. and 10 P.M. may suffice in allaying tension, and also in producing sleep at nighttime. In extreme insomnia, three grains of seconal or one dram of paraldehyde may be necessary. Rest is important and a midday nap or rest period can be prescribed. Where it is essential for the depressed patient to continue work, dexedrine or benzedrine sulphate, five to ten milligrams after arising and before lunch may be helpful as a stimulant. Where these efforts fail to control the depression, electric shock therapy should be used.

Where the depression is more than mild, hospitalization is advisable. Suicidal attempts and depression occur in almost one-third of cases, and deaths from suicide are many times that of the general population. The patient's complete loss of interest in himself makes mandatory the establishment of definite daily routines such as a hospital can best supply.

Electric shock therapy is the treatment of choice and often dramatically arouses the patient from the depths of his depression.

Psychotherapy is usually ineffective during extremely depressed phases. The only thing that can be done is to keep up the patient's morale. He should not be forced to engage in activities that he resists because this may merely convince him of his helplessness and of his inability to do anything constructive. Where there is little suicidal risk, he should be encouraged to continue his work, if he feels at all capable of managing it, since inactivity merely directs his thinking on his own misery. In all cases active work should be started with the patient's family and environment. This is necessary since the family of the patient often chides him for "not snapping out of it," and constantly reminds him that he must make up his mind to get well. The family must be instructed that recovery is more than a matter of will power, and they must be urged to avoid a nagging and critical attitude.

The material elicited during the periods of active psychosis, both as to mental content and as to the character of the relationship with the physician, may yield important clues to the inner conflicts of the patient. Notes may be made for later reference, but all interpretations during the active period must be suspended. Only during a remission can interpretive work be helpful. Many patients spontaneously express a desire to know more about their illness. Here a modified analytic approach may be used. The majority of patients, however, show an unwillingness to go into their difficulties and resist analytic psychotherapy. Having recovered they are convinced they are well, and they desire no further contact with the physician. Without the "wish" to get well little can be accomplished in the way of deep psychotherapy.

Once the patient has emerged from his depression, either spontaneously, as a result of shock therapy or through psychotherapy, an attempt may be made to work with his character strivings, analyzing the relationship to the physician actively in an effort to make the patient more assertive and self sufficient. Here hypnosis can facilitate the analytic process. Whether or not psychotherapy helps prevent the onset of an endogenous manic-depressive reaction is difficult to say, since one cannot entirely validate a cure or illness where a tendency to spontaneous recovery exists, as in this illness. Development to a point where the individual is capable of tolerating frustration, and where he is able to achieve greater self sufficiency and independence, will probably require a period of years during which a number of relapses are to be expected.

Involutional Melancholia

Involutional melancholia appears most frequently in women in their late forties and less frequently in men in their late fifties. It is characterized by a decreased functional activity of the endocrine and reproductive organs, and by metabolic and vegetative changes throughout the body. Early symptoms are those of uneasiness, worry, fatigue, insomnia and feelings of inadequacy. There is a withdrawal of interest from the environment and a concentration on the self and the body activities. This may proceed to an extreme depression which is usually of an agitated nature, although in some cases hypomotility may occur. There is a great loss of security and a tremendous devaluation of the self, its capacities and functions. The agitation often takes the form of hand wringing, moaning, groaning, pinching and picking of the skin. There are delusions of sin, nihilism, unreality and disease, and a misery so acute that the patient may attempt to escape it through suicide. In some patients the psychosis takes the form of a paranoid reaction which is indistinguishable from a paranoid condition or a paranoid schizophrenia.

The exact role of the climacteric in this illness is indefinite. Normally, the menopause is associated with a deranged ovarian function, a diminished secretion of estrogens, and a compensatory increase in gonadotropins as the result of pituitary hypersecretion. Vasomotor changes in the menopause are apparently due to this endocrine imbalance. There is probably a corresponding endocrine change in most aging males.

In many females and in some males, middle age is a period of psychologic and physical stress. Endocrine changes probably reinforce the feeling that one has passed the creative stage of life and is headed for a period of lessened capacity. Chills, flushes, sweating, insomnia, vertigo, headaches, fatigability, lassitude, depression, difficulties in concentration, numbness, frigidity, impotency and mood changes occur.

Only in a fraction of cases, however, do signs of an involutional psychosis develop. What factors are responsible for the precipitation of a psychosis is not clear. The consensus is that the prepsychotic personality is the basic thing, and that rigidity and an inability to develop adequate compensations for the stress that is inevitable to the involutional period produces a breakdown. Evidence is accumulating that involutional melancholia is probably not due to the menopause itself. Some women go through the menopause without difficulty only to succumb to involutional psychosis some years later. In examining patients one may find that it was not the menopause or menopausal disturbance, but rather the patient's outlook on the menopause that was pathologic.

The prepsychotic personality in the individual predisposed to involutional melancholia often shows, in contrast to the prepsychotic personality of the manic-depressive, a rigid inelasticity with few mood swings.[9-10] The person is extremely inhibited with a strong moral sense, and manifests compulsive and obsessive features such as scrupulousness, meticulousness, overconscientiousness and tendencies toward self discipline. Interests are definitely circumscribed and the person is inclined to be worrisome, sensitive, apprehensive and fretful. There are inclinations toward submissiveness and subordination, although, in some cases, sadism and aggression are the dominating characteristics. Often the patient has had a borderline or an actual compulsion neurosis prior to the onset of his illness.

The rigid character structure of the individual is bound to create an extreme problem for him when he is pitted against the various stresses, psychic and physical, of the involutional years. Among the blows to the ego are those that involve diminishing physical powers, earning capacity, health, vitality, sexual potency and ability to gain love and influence. Recognition that one has passed the zenith of life, and a sense of failure developing from a realization that one's early hopes and wishes are not to be realized, contributes to insecurity. In women there is the fear of not winning the love of a man, or of losing the love of her husband because of her age. The fear of loss of attractiveness, of productiveness, of pleasure from sexual activity, may create the illusion of being dead in so far as one's future is concerned.

The dynamics of the depressive reaction are similar to those in manic-depressive psychosis. Nihilistic delusions symbolize the conviction that one's ego has dissolved and that nothingness exists. The world, as Schilder[11] pointed out, becomes an object of nutrition or the transformation products of nutrition, as feces and products of putrefaction. Masochistic self punishment is rooted in guilt feelings originating out of the conviction that the individual has, through his own actions, done something prohibited that may result in the withdrawal of love or punishment on the part of the parent or introjected parent as embodied in the superego. Genetically this reaction is based on the fact that an acknowledgment of guilt, and condign punishment, brings forgiveness. This establishes a mechanism of remorse and penitence as a means of restoring the child to the good graces of the mother. Later on when the person feels insecure he may unconsciously believe that he has done something wrong, and, on the basis of his guilt, he may seek to expiate his crime through remorse, pleas for forgiveness, fasting, self denial and other masochistic devices. There is a compulsion to confess and to punish oneself in order to anticipate punishment.

In the agitated depressions, aggression is directed against the self as an expiatory mechanism. In the paranoid reaction, a projection mechanism occurs with an externalization of hostility. This is a defensive attempt on the part of the ego to rid itself of the destructive effects of hostility. The projected hostility may become structuralized as an obstinate paranoid state permitting the ego to function without undue anxiety.

The prognosis of involutional melancholia is considerably less hopeful than of manic-depressive psychosis. Cases without schizophrenic-like symptoms offer the best prognosis. Where relative stability has been reached on the basis of a paranoid reaction, the prognosis is guarded.

In the treatment of involutional melancholia the matter of endocrine therapy comes in for consideration. Both good results[12–15] and poor results[16–17] have been reported following treatment with estrogenic hormones in females, and with testosterone in males.[18–21] As a general rule, endocrine therapy is indicated where there are such evidences of endocrine insufficiency as vasomotor instability, flushes, sweats, headaches and tension. In certain cases an estrogenic deficiency, as determined by accurate tests, seems to be coincident with the psychosis. Here substitution therapy produces dramatic results. In other cases tests may show an estrogenic deficiency, but injection of estrogen has little effect. In most patients, however, the psychosis is a product of more complicated factors than endocrine substances.

Milder cases of involutional melancholia may be cared for at home, or better still in a nursing home under the constant supervision of a nurse or attendant. At all times it is essential to keep in mind the great risk of suicide, and to make plans to forestall any suicidal attempt. In some cases treatment may best be started by complete bed rest for a few weeks. Attention must be paid to the patient's diet and to his insomnia. Many patients refuse to eat and tonics prove of little avail. Forced feedings may have to be utilized to avoid emaciation. Insulin and barbiturates in small doses are often helpful.

In disturbed, agitated, acutely paranoid, and suicidally inclined patients hospitalization is mandatory. Some type of sedative therapy is advisable, at least at first, and in occasional cases prolonged narcosis therapy appears to have a real value. Continuous baths and wet packs may reduce the need for sedatives. However, massage is contraindicated. Occupational therapy may be of some help in diverting the interest of the patient from himself.

By far the most effective therapy in involutional melancholia is shock treatment. Electric shock therapy has a definite advantage over other types of shock and is to be preferred from the standpoint of safety. The results of shock therapy are often dramatic, and experience has shown that physical contraindications to shock treatment need not be too stringent.

Involutional melancholics are largely inaccessible to psychotherapy. All psychic probing in an analytic sense is to be avoided, and efforts must be directed at increasing repression rather than stimulating and interpreting the material that emerges from the unconscious. Persuasion and reassurance sometimes have the effect of tiding a patient over a crisis. Many patients confide that they have been immeasurably cheered by the physician who reassured them during their acute disorder, even though they were unable at the time to acknowledge the beneficial effect.

In mild cases of involutional melancholia, hypnosis can have a beneficial influence. Hypnosis should be used to induce relaxation and to reinforce reassurance and persuasive suggestions. It is essential to adjust the individual to his life situation and to the limited capacities induced by his advancing years. If hypnosis cannot be induced, psychotherapeutic talks can be conducted on a waking level. If possible the patient should be diverted from concentrating on his various symptoms, and his attention should be directed to daily activities, hobbies, recreations and occupational therapy.

Psychotherapy is particularly indicated following shock therapy, and the patient, at this time, may be quite accessible to hypnosis. The patient should be shown that advancing years inevitably bring with them convictions that one's views are considered old fashioned and intolerable, along with feelings that one may be unable to gain praiseworthy recognition. There are numerous other blows to self esteem at this time of life. Some persons attempt to compensate for this by becoming markedly egotistical or bigoted in their opinions, by clinging to their convictions stubbornly against logic, hoping thereby to regain their self respect. Others react by depression, hopelessness, inferiority feelings, hostility and rage directed at the world at large. One must always recognize the limitations inherent in the process of aging. He should also realize that many creative capacities are unimpaired and some actually increased.

It is important for him to appreciate that as a person grows older, he does have modified physical and working powers. If he is so constituted that he considers an inability to compete physically with younger and stronger persons a blow to his self evaluation, the results can be catastrophic. He will then become sullen and defiant, or perhaps he will evolve expansive notions regarding his own capacities, projecting his inability to function perfectly on the basis that he is misunderstood by others or menaced by a hostile world. He will then become more and more unable to withstand frustration, and he will be victimized by his own emotion of rage. He may even withdraw from social contacts and encrust him-

self in a bitter vituperative shell, isolating himself from relations with others.

The patient must be shown that some people attempt to
adjust to the problem of advancing years by a vicarious display of aggressiveness and energy, resenting any curtailment
of activities. There is in this a frenzied attempt to regain lost
youth by proving to the world that one is still physically
virile and should therefore not in any way be considered
aged. The most essential need in the patient is to tolerate
certain frailties within himself. If the person continues to
refuse to recognize self limitations, he may continue to operate under exorbitant expectations of what he must accomplish in life. The realization that the most active period in
his life is past, that he does not have as strong sexual feelings as he used to have, may arouse considerable anxiety.
It is thus necessary to appraise honestly one's impulses and
demands in relation to expected goals in life. It may be difficult at first to admit weaknesses in oneself; but the gradual
understanding that later years bring with them mellowness
and measures of contentment that cannot be approached in
the impetuosities of the early decades can lead to self tolerance and acceptance. It is essential to remember that in this
self acceptance there is no element of "giving-up," that reasonable physical activity is still essential to health, and that
mental activity can continue in a vital manner. It is urgent
also to increase one's social contacts and interests so as not to
be upset with the spectre of being "left alone."

Hypnosis in Schizophrenia

What actually constitutes the schizophrenic state is a
matter of dispute. There are some authorities who believe
that the regressive process that develops in schizophrenia is
essentially an organic condition. There are others who present considerable evidence of a hereditary and constitutional
factor in schizophrenia. On the other hand, there are certain

authorities who, while admitting that organic factors may exist in schizophrenia, believe that the essential cause lies in inimical experiences and frustrations suffered during infancy, at a period before the self has become completely differentiated. These environmental difficulties lead to an ego structure so weak that it crumbles in the face of external stress or internal conflict. Whereas the average individual is capable of handling anxiety with characterologic and neurotic defenses, the ego of the schizophrenic person finds security only by a regression to an infantile period.

A schizophrenic tendency is an extremely common thing and often goes unnoticed. Rorschach tests among large groups of people frequently show schizophrenic-like reactions. It is possible that many individuals who are capable of functioning in a relatively protected environment without the development of a schizophrenic state, may, when subjected to extraordinary stress, show schizophrenic-like symptoms or actual schizophrenia. This was born out during the last war when soldiers who, prior to induction, had shown no evidence of schizophrenia, developed schizophrenic states of an acute nature consequent to the hardships of war. When removed from the battlefield or when released from the army, many of these persons went back to their previous levels of integration and were capable of functioning, seemingly without any psychotic manifestations.

In some instances, neurotic defenses prevent the individual from experiencing more anxiety, and consequently make it possible for him to get along without a further breakdown. In other instances, the neurotic tendencies and defenses seem incapable of protecting the ego, which begins to shatter and to demonstrate regressive tendencies that are so characteristic of schizophrenia. The breaking point of the individual depends entirely upon his ego strength.

Persons with a schizophrenic tendency, who have a minimal ego strength, often intuitively protect themselves by functioning in an extremely protected atmosphere, circumscribing their activities, and limiting their relationships with people. Somehow they realize that a more intimate type of relationship, or the tackling of life on a more aggressive level, may result in a breakdown. In spite of this, some schizoid persons seem incapable of repressing threatening fundamental needs and impulses, the fulfillment of which involve them in situations which result in their collapse. For instance, a person who utilizes apathy and detachment as a defense in his relationships with people may, during adolescence or early adult life, be so carried away by sexual desires that he will seek to express his sexual needs. In trying to relate himself intimately with others, he will exhibit anxiety that issues out of fear of injury or destruction. Defenses against anxiety may be so completely inadequate, that the ultimate result is a schizophrenic condition. On the other hand, had the person circumscribed his activities, and had he maintained himself in an essentially detached state, it is quite possible that he might have avoided a breakdown.

The matter of prepsychotic personality in schizophrenia is one that requires considerable clarification. A so-called "schizoid personality" frequently precedes the development of the outright schizophrenic psychosis. Analysis shows that the schizoid personality is actually a reaction to the same stresses that later result in schizophrenia proper. Such traits as shyness, seclusiveness and apathy are manifestations of early defensive tendencies of the individual which serve a protective function, detaching the person from active contact with others in an effort to avoid anxiety and ego injury. Where the schizoid individual is incapable of holding back the strength of his inner drives, or where in spite of his tendencies to insulate himself from contact with others, he finds he is actually unable to do so, a schizophrenic psychosis may be the outcome.

Important in the considered therapy of the schizophrenic

individual is the possibility that he is actually constituted differently from the average person. A constitutional weakness of basic ego ingredients, it is assumed, makes it difficult for the individual to adjust adaptively to average frustrations and conflicts. The person then develops a "schizophrenic tendency" of ego shattering under the impact of extreme anxiety. An active schizophrenic breakdown may occur either because external stress is so severe or internal conflict so overwhelming as to destroy the adaptive resources. The degree of stress the individual is capable of tolerating depends entirely upon the existing strength of his ego. There are many persons, as has been mentioned, who are capable of adjusting to ordinary stress, but who, in the face of extraordinary environmental strain, will develop a schizophreniclike disorder. The example has been cited of the many soldiers who seemed to be well-adjusted in civilian life, exhibiting no demonstrable difficulties, but who collapsed under the rigors of wartime army discipline, showing acute schizophrenic symptoms from which they recovered in a quiet and protected environment. On the other hand, there are other persons whose ego structures are so weak that they will suffer a schizophrenic collapse as a result of tension, anxiety, and rage generated in everyday relationships with people.

While the regression which is characteristic of schizophrenia appears to be a defensive device to adjust the person, it actually makes a realistic adjustment impossible. In regression, the person withdraws into himself and attempts to recreate a world such as existed in his childhood. His attitudes, mannerisms and behavior tendencies reflect defenses and attitudes similar to those of an earlier phase. The regression that exists in schizophrenia is not an actual back-tracking of a developmental process; rather, it is a new and unique situation in the life history of the individual that draws upon defenses that existed in the past. In this new form of behavior, there is a partial reproduction of conditions that existed at a time when the person felt himself to be most secure.

The depth of regression varies and may be interrupted at any level at which stability can be maintained. In some instances, the individual seems to be able to stabilize himself through a childish dependent relationship with a maternal object. The withdrawal into himself does not go to an extreme. In other instances, regression proceeds to a point where there are actual disturbances in self awareness, with a loss of ego boundaries. Here, there is a reproduction of a primitive stage of ego growth with archaic types of thinking and behavior.

One of the first evidences of regression is in the emotional sphere. The individual becomes colder, more aloof, more apathetic, than the average person. He does not seem to feel the same nuances of emotion; he does not show the same resilience in his rapport with a group. This emotional blunting may be the initial sign of the schizophrenic process. It is often the forerunner of more severe symptoms. As a result of his apathy, there is an impairment in the emotional life with a splitting of affective and cognitive processes. In more severe forms, there is lack of congruity between emotions and thought content. The apathy that the patient feels and expresses is in part due to an insulation from other people. In part, it is a result of the fact that reality functions have come to mean less and less to him, and he tends to respond more and more to his internal emotional life. In the more pernicious types of schizophrenia, where reality has been abandoned, incongruous emotions come to the surface and the emotional life is extremely disorganized.

Another early symptom of schizophrenia is reflected in language disturbances. There is generally a decrease in linguistic fluency and an impaired ability to compare, abstract and generalize. There is loss of apperceptive capacity, a weakness of associative links, an interference with judgment and a tendency to deal with the concrete rather than with the abstract. The schizophrenic person tends to think in inconsistent terms which leads to an acceptance of contradictory ideas. A confusion of fantasy with fact, a subordination of knowing to wishing, and an inability to differentiate things emotionally identified, are produced by an increasing unreality sense. A withdrawal from objects and an attachment to words and ideas is common. The individual is mostly preoccupied with himself, indulging in day-dreaming and in inner speculations. Fantasies give him more satisfaction than realistic experiences. As the withdrawal continues, words and thoughts become omnipotent; ideas of bodily influence are more manifest; relationships with people are less important; and finally, word symbols become the objects themselves. Later on fragmentation may occur in the field of mental activity. There develops a peculiar repetitiousness with the use of personal idioms and neologisms.

Disturbances in behavior are also common in schizophrenia. The withdrawal from reality causes the individual to come more and more under the influence of his unconscious impulses and conflicts. The individual operates, in his associations with the world, more on the basis of inner wishes and fantasies than on the basis of judgment and intellectual reasoning. Bizarre activities of a random nature appear from time to time. The person may get himself involved in difficulties by engaging in behavior of a seemingly senseless nature. As the distortion of reality continues with further regression of the ego, changes in attitude and behavior become even more extreme. Stereotypy, negativism, automatic obedience and automatic movements may develop, and there will be an increased inability to coordinate behavior with social demands. The individual may become totally unable to mediate his internal needs or to take advantage of environmental opportunities to fulfill basic impulses.

As reality testing becomes further impaired there develops an actual substitution of fantasy for reality. A projection of inner ideational processes to the external world is inevitable, and ideas of reference and of influence, delusions and hallucinations are consequent. The individual becomes less and less capable of judging what is realistic as contrasted with what originates within himself, and the boundaries of the ego become more and more diffuse.

Regression shatters the repressive function of the ego. The individual's mind becomes flooded with unconscious material, with repressed sexual and hostile impulses, and with various primitive symbolizations. In early schizophrenic states, before the ego is totally overwhelmed by unconscious material, the individual, while in contact with reality, has the capacity of entering into the realm of unconscious fantasy much more facilely than the average person. Being in closer association with his unconscious, he is able to portray in literary and art productions bizarre symbols of his unconscious life.

Another symptom of ego regression is a diminution in the integrative functions of the ego. The individual seems unable to fuse his cognitive, emotional, and behavioristic functions in pursuit of his fundamental needs. His life becomes quite discordant, with a dissociation of moods, thought content, and behavior.

The regressive process usually ceases when the individual is capable of maintaining himself on some level of stability. In simple schizophrenic states, there may be no further regression than that involving the emotional life. Apathy, disinterest, and a general detachment from people will exist; but there will be no disturbance in the reality testing function. The individual may thus be able to integrate himself fairly well with life, although he will eschew close interpersonal relationships. In the paranoid reaction, the person may find it possible to utilize projection as a technic to rid himself of his disturbing emotions. As a consequence, he may be able to externalize his deepest conflicts, and in this way allay anxiety sufficiently to prevent a shattering of his ego. In the catatonic reaction, the individual does not seem capable of maintaining stability except on an extremely primitive level of integration. There may be a return to early phases of development. Indeed, in certain forms of catatonia, the regressive state is associated with infantile muscular control and vocalization. The breathing function, for example, may come to have a magical significance, forceful breathing being associated with hostile murder fantasies in which the person believes that he kills with his breath. Or controlled breathing may fill him with a sense of power, withholding his breath seeming to keep his parents alive. Regression may actually proceed to a stage prior to the formation of the ego with the inability to differentiate himself from the environment. There may be depersonalization, misidentification, and finally, collapse into a stupor which psychologically resembles death. During this stage, the patient may actually be living an active fantasy life, engaged in a struggle between the forces of good and evil, with jumbled notions of death, redemption and rebirth. In the hebephrenic state, there is an extreme shattering of ego functions, although the regression may not be as deep as in catatonia. The individual may find it possible to function in his relationships with life, although there may be a marked impairment in affect, and a distortion of the reality sense with fantastic delusions and hallucinations.

The treatment of schizophrenia depends upon the stage of the disease, the depth of regression, the grasp on reality that remains, the desire of the patient for therapy, and his ability to establish some sort of relationship with the physician. The first object in therapy is to bring the patient from his inner regressed state to a more realistic level of integration. Once this is achieved, the second stage in therapy may be attempted, which is to determine the cause of the patient's anxiety that has forced the ego to shatter in schizophrenic illness.

Where the patient's psychosis has been precipitated by overwhelming external traumatic situations, simple environmental manipulation may suffice to bring the patient back to his prepsychotic level of adaptation. For example, a man inducted into the Armed Forces may develop an acute schizophrenic reaction as a result of an inability to adjust himself to the demands and disciplines of army life. The personality resources of the individual, while adequate to permit a satisfactory functioning in civilian life, are not now sufficient to cope with the added burdens imposed on them. In such a case the discharge of the man from the Army, and his return to his previous civilian capacities, may achieve a complete cure of the psychosis.

Most schizophrenic reactions, however, are associated with such great weakness of the ego that the person is unable to withstand even average stresses. Ordinary processes of living and mixing with people may be more than the person can mediate. Environmental manipulation does not suffice to restore the patient to reality here, because he senses menace everywhere around him even in the most obviously congenial atmosphere.

Fears rooted in past inimical conditionings and damaging conflicts generate anxiety continuously and prevent the ego from emerging from its regressed level of integration. The patient erects a wall around him to protect himself from further hurt, and it is this wall of detachment and isolation that interferes so drastically with any attempted therapy.

The key to the treatment of schizophrenia lies in the ability to establish some sort of contact with the patient. Most schizophrenics fear relationships with people desperately, and they erect all kinds of obstacles to any interpersonal threat. The withdrawal from reality, and the archaic type of thinking and symbolism, enhance the individual's isolation from people, since there is no common means of communication. Yet beneath the surface the patient yearns with all his might for a friendly and loving relationship. He wards it off, however, because he has been injured by past interpersonal contacts. He does not wish to encounter further rebuffs. His apathy, his detachment, and his expressed hostility and aggression are means of protecting him from his desire for a closer union with people. Establishing a contact with the patient is in line with two objectives: first, to reintegrate the patient in his relationships with people to where he can obtain at least partial gratification of personal needs without fear of abandonment or injury; and second, to bring him back to the realistic world by proving to him that reality can be a source of pleasure rather than of pain.

The technic of developing a contact varies with the patient. A great deal of activity is essential. In very sick patients whose productions are seemingly irrelevant and incoherent, a careful analysis of the productions will disclose a language that is very meaningful to the patient. The ability to show the patient that his words and gestures are understood sometimes secures a transference that is the first chink in the defensive armor. Sullivan[22] has emphasized the need of understanding the patient's language and gestures as a means of solidifying the interpersonal relationship. In order to do this it may be necessary to talk to the patient on his own regressed level. Tidd[23] has practiced this to a point of using childish utterances. Grotjahn[24] was able to establish an astonishing transference with a hallucinated patient by attempting to hallucinate with her. In several hallucinating schizophrenic patients, I was able to gain their confidence by listening attentively to the voices they imagined were present in the room, expressing at the same time an interest in their interpretations of these messages. The fact that I had entered their own world made them much more amenable to appeals for them to re-enter mine. Rosen[25] interprets the utterances of the patient in terms of their symbolic meaning, and he has been able to develop a remarkable relationship with his patients with marked success in their treatment.

In mute patients therapy may consist of nothing more than

sitting with the patient without prodding him to express himself. The very fact that the physician refrains from probing his trends, and avoids discussing the causes of his breakdown, but accepts him as he is, causes the patient to regard the physician as a less threatening force than other people. In many cases therapy may consist of working with the patient at occupational projects, playing cards, checkers or chess with him. Sometimes a more positive approach is made to the patient by giving him milk, candy and cake. For a long time it may seem that these gratuities are the only reason that the patient desires to see the physician. In querying the patient after his recovery, however, one becomes convinced that the patient actually had a desire for closeness and was testing the physician constantly.

Any relationship that the patient is able to establish with the physician is at first bound to be extremely unstable. The schizophrenic individual feels very vulnerable and helpless within himself. His level of frustration tolerance is inordinately low. He is distrustful, suspicious and inclined to misinterpret the motives of the physician in accordance with his inner fears and prejudices. He feels incapable of coping with life, and he resents the intentions of the physician to return him to reality which holds for him unbounded terrors. He fears injury and frustration from people, and it may be months, sometimes years, before he is willing to accept the physician as a friend. Even then he will sense rejection and neglect in the most random attitude of the physician. Anxiety with a temporary return to regression will interrupt therapy repeatedly, and it must be handled by a consistently reassuring and friendly attitude. Violent hostile reactions may punctuate treatment from time to time, especially when the patient senses that his liking for the physician is forcing him to leave the relative security of his retreat from reality.

Fromm-Reichman[26] has commented on the unpredictable nature of the schizophrenic's relationship to the physician.

A sympathetic, understanding and skillful handling by the physician of the relationship is far more important than any intellectual comprehension of the patient's illness. She ascribes difficulties in therapy to the fact that the physician is unable to understand the primitive logic and magical reasoning which governs schizophrenic thinking.

Unless the physician analyzes his own reactions repeatedly, his own sense of frustration may arouse aggression that will interfere with treatment, because it is manifestly impossible to treat any psychotic person where there is no genuine liking for him. If the physician looks upon the patient as essentially a child or an infant, he will better be able to understand the latter's vagaries and behavior. Cold logic fails miserably in explaining the reactions of the schizophrene. Despite his age, the patient seeks a childish relationship to the physician, and he desires unlimited warmth, understanding, protection, and help. He seeks mothering rather than a give and take relationship between two equals.

Therapy in schizophrenia must, therefore, be oriented around the fact that the ego of the patient is extremely immature. As a result the individual is as helpless as an infant in his dealings with life. He requires the aid of a stronger person upon whom he can depend. Like an infant, furthermore, his emotional reactions with people are unstable and ambivalent. He is easily frustrated, and he feels rejection for insufficient reasons. He is unreasonable and demanding. His concept of reality is wholly unreliable. He often confuses inner mental processes with outside reality. He may believe that the person on whom he depends is omniscient and will supply his every demand, expressed or unexpressed. He will react with hostility if he is not given what he believes he deserves. Alone, his ego is so weak that he is unable to tolerate the impact of the world. He needs unqualified help and support.

Because of this it is usually advisable to enlist the aid of a relative or friend, preferably a motherly person who can take upon herself the responsibility for the patient. Federn[27] stresses that no schizophrene be left to his own resources. He should at all times be surrounded by an atmosphere of love and warmth. His stability and his strength grow as a result of positive identifications with loved ones. If he is at all able to develop to self sufficiency, his independence will grow best in the soil of this positive identification. The hope is to bring him to a point where his own ego can function satisfactorily without the aid of a parental figure. In many cases the latter stage of self sufficiency is never attained, and all one can do is adapt the individual to reasonable social functioning, attached to some kindly person.

The need to surround the patient with a favorable atmosphere necessitates work with his family or with people with whom he lives. This is essential to relieve the burden on the patient induced by demands and responsibilities he is incapable of fulfilling. Often the inertia and apathy of the patient stirs up resentment in his parents or siblings, and when the patient is aware of their hostility, he may retreat further from reality. Considerable work with the patient's relatives may be required before they are sufficiently aware of the dynamics of the patient's reactions to be willing to aid the physician in the treatment project.

The chief emphasis in treatment must be on the creation of a human relationship with the patient that has pleasure values for him. Only by this means will he relinquish the safety and gratification of regression, and, utilizing the relationship with the physician as a bridge, return to reality. The handling of treatment, however, is one that requires considerable tact. No matter how detached the patient is, he is extremely sensitive to everything the physician says or does. An avoidance of things that evoke anxiety is essential. This is often a very difficult task because the most casual remark may stir up powerful emotions in the patient.

The patient may choose to remain silent throughout the treatment hour and he will appreciate the physician's refusal to force him to talk. It is expedient with such a mute patient to point out occasionally that he perhaps refrains from talking because he believes that the physician is interfering with him, or because he is afraid of what he might say. The patient may feel more at ease on this account, and he may finally break through his silence.

In most cases the patient at first will feel alone, helpless and misunderstood. He resents the intrusion of the physician into his private life, and he will believe that the physician, like everyone else, is unable to understand him. The initial task is to show the patient that his impulses and wishes are respected, and that he is not required to comply with dictatorial commands. Usually in all of his previous interviews he has been bombarded with questions about his breakdown, and, even when he has responded to these questions in a more or less frank manner, he has sensed disapproval. The fact that the physician accepts him as he is, eventually builds up his own self respect and strengthens his desire to return to reality.

Constantly, during treatment, the patient will react by detachment or withdrawal, or he may subject the physician to a testing period during which he is recalcitrant and hostile. His purpose is to determine whether the physician is the kind of person who can be trusted, or whether he is like all other people in his experience, who make unfair demands or react to his hostility with counterhostility. The patient may believe that what the physician demands of him is to be "good." This "goodness" means to the patient that he must comply with standards that all other people impose on him. At first he will act as if the physician expects him to abide by these standards, threatening him with rejection or aggression if he resists. The testing period may be a trying one for the physician, since it may continue for many months during which the patient constantly rejects the physician's friendship. When the patient realizes that the doctor does not expect him to do certain things, that he actually sides with him against his family, he will begin to re-evaluate the doctor in a new light.

The beginning of a feeling of closeness may precipitate panic, and the patient may try to run away from therapy, or he will exhibit aggression toward the physician. The ability to see the patient through this stage finally may succeed in breaking down his reserve and in establishing for the first time an identification with a person based upon love. There exists within every schizophrene a psychic tug of war between the spontaneous forces of mental health that drive him to seek relationships with people in order to express his basic needs, and the security of his regressed state that harbors him from the imagined dangers of a hostile world. The physician's attitudes will determine which of these impulses will triumph.

The method of handling the treatment hour is an important one. It is best not to cross examine the patient because he may interpret this as censure. He must be convinced that the physician does not want to invade his private world, but rather that he seeks to help him. This does not mean assuming a cloying sweetness because the patient will be able to see through this. At all times it must be expected that the patient's attitudes will be ambivalent. He may profess little interest in the interview, yet resent its termination at the designated time. He may attempt to defy or to provoke the physician, or he may refuse to cooperate. If the physician becomes ill and cannot keep an appointment, the patient may react with rage and refuse to continue treatments. If the physician is unavoidably late for an appointment the same thing can occur. The patient may resent the physician's taking any vacation or assigning another person than himself to care for him. In all instances where the customary routine has to be interrupted, it is best to prepare the patient far in advance, and also to enlist the help of those members of his family with whom he has an attachment. If the patient becomes hostile toward the physician every attempt must be made to understand in which way he believes the physician has failed him. Should he persist with hostility and desire to see some other doctor, his wishes should be respected, because it is futile to do any work with a patient while he is governed by feelings of resentment.

Once a positive relationship has been established, it is necessary to use it in order to strengthen the ego of the patient. Nothing must jeopardize the relationship. For example, the patient must never be led to feel that his delusions are ridiculous. His feelings and attitudes must be respected at all times. It is unnecessary to reinforce these attitudes by agreeing with them; but they should be accepted as something the patient believes sincerely, even though there might possibly be another explanation than the one he imagines. All probing for dynamic material must assiduously be avoided. This is one of the most frequent errors in the handling of psychotic patients. It is also an error to cross examine the patient regarding previous mental upsets.

Because the aim is to increase repression, because the ego is already too weak and permits the filtering through of disturbing unconscious material, such technics as free association should be discouraged. Rather, the patient should be enjoined to talk about everyday reality happenings. In general, the past had best be avoided and the patient may be told he should regard it as a bad dream or something that is best forgotten. Under no circumstances should the positive relationship to the physician be analyzed. Where the patient exhibits inhibitions or phobias these too should be respected since they probably have protective values. All resistances he uses to repress psychotic material should be reinforced, although the symbolisms he employs may sometimes be interpreted to him. Unlike neurosis, analysis of resistances should be refrained from to avoid the release of the unconscious content which will upset the patient more. When the patient himself brings up delusional material or symptoms and spontaneously sees the connection with traumatizing circumstances in his past, an effort may be made to explain in everyday terms how these manifestations originated. The rule never to dissolve resistance does not apply to resistances to getting well, or to integrating himself more closely with the physician and with reality. When these exist they should be analyzed and removed if possible. Guilt feelings should be met by reassurance, and hostilities should be analyzed and dealt with in a manner that does not put responsibility or blame on the patient.

One of the ways in which a positive relationship with the physician may be used is to try to show the patient that his thoughts and ideas often appear to be realistic, but that it is necessary always to differentiate between what seems to be real and what actually is real. In the patient's own case he may confuse the two feelings even though there is no question of doubt in his mind that the two states are identical. An excellent sign of restoration of ego strength is the ability of the patient to recognize the irrational nature of his associations and ideas while he was in a psychotic state.

The matter of institutionalization is an important one. Sometimes it is essential for the safety of the patient and the protection of his relatives to hospitalize him. Occasionally it may be advisable to admit the patient into an institution even when he manages to get along well on the outside.

Shock therapy is administered best in the protective atmosphere of a hospital, and such treatment may dramatically bring the patient to a more realistic level of integration. Whatever the psychologic effect of shock, regressed patients are often enabled to establish an adequate contact with reality. This can materially shorten the period of therapy. Along with shock treatments, psychotherapy is essential. All the general rules in the handling of schizophrenic patients are applicable to patients in a state of remission as a result of shock therapy. If possible the physician who administers psychotherapy should be the one who carries out shock treatments. A very close relationship to the physician is often established during the administration of shock therapy.

On the other hand there are certain disadvantages to hospitalization. The most insidious feature of institutionalization is that the patient's tendencies to regress will be reinforced enormously by any lack of stimulation in the hospital. As one of a large group of patients the individual may lose his identity. He becomes dilapidated in his appearance and oblivious to customary habit routines. There may be little in his environment to encourage his latent desires for growth and development. This unfortunate feature is due, to a large extent, to the overcrowding of institutions, and to the lack of enlightenment and education on the part of the personnel. The motives governing an employee's choice in working in an institution may not be those helpful to the patient in restoring him as an active unit of society.

That hospitalization can prove itself to be a stimulating rather than a regressing influence is illustrated by treatment of psychotic patients in institutions with an enlightened administration and well-trained personnel. Selected occupational therapy and craftsmanship carefully applied to the patient's interests and aptitudes can help prevent the abandonment of reality. Exercises, games, entertainment, dancing, music, social affairs and group discussions can also be of estimable benefit. The physical aspects of treatment should not be neglected. Correction of remedial physical defects, the use of glandular therapy where indicated, the employment of hydrotherapy or sedatives may be helpful. Many of the benefits derived from such therapies are psychologic, convincing the patient that he is not considered hopeless, in this way building up a feeling of confidence in the physician and in himself. It is probable that the so-called Aschner treatment for schizophrenia with its stress on detoxification, stimulation, exercise, baths, sweats, venesection, catharsis, emesis and hormone therapy was really psychotherapeutic in effect.

Hypnosis may be employed as an adjunct in the treatment of schizophrenia and, if adroitly used, is of value in a certain number of cases. A great deal of misinformation exists regarding the possible harmful effect of hypnosis on schizophrenics and schizoid individuals. If hypnosis is used as a means of inducing a pleasurable relaxed state, and if analytic probing is avoided, the effects can be most beneficial. Difficulties do arise if the patient is urged to recall traumatic incidents in his past, or if he is given posthypnotic suggestions to open up to people and to do those things that he finds terrifying. Such suggestions will destroy the relationship with the physician, the patient resenting being exposed to danger.

In most cases difficulties will be encountered at first in inducing hypnosis, because of the regression of the patient and his retreat from reality. A prolonged contact with the patient will be necessary before he expresses a desire for a more intimate relationship. In my experience schizophrenics have a strong motivation to be hypnotized, possibly because they seek a dependent type of relationship. Once the patient's confidence is obtained, and when he is able to establish rapport with the physician, hypnosis may be as easy to induce as in neurotic conditions. Because the word "hypnotism" has so many fearful connotations, it is best not to mention this, but merely to stress the fact that "relaxing exercises" can be very beneficial. Sleep suggestions are given to the patient, and if he turns out to be a good subject he should be brought to as deep a trance as possible.

As a general rule the use of hypnosis should be supportive in the form of reassurance, relaxation and gentle persuasion. Analytic probing must be eschewed, at least until the patient's ego is sufficiently strong to stand the powerful emotions liberated by unconscious conflicts. One must veer away from traumatic material even though the patient's conflicts become transparent to the physician as revealed by hypnotic productions. If a painful subject is introduced prematurely in the trance, the patient may suddenly shift from a relatively normal type of speech and behavior to an incoherent, neologistic, symbolic type of expressiveness. This is due to the return of his regressive defenses. It is essential to avoid interpretation of the material elicited during hypnosis. Strong commands should also be avoided, since they will arouse in the patient the feeling that the physician demands unreasonable things of him, or seeks to subjugate or to enslave him. The positive relationship with the physician should not be analyzed or discussed.

The chief use of hypnosis, then, is to solidify the relationship with the physician by making the trance a comfortable and pleasurable experience. This is illustrated by the treatment of a hebephrenic schizophrenic who was so terrified of people that ten years prior to his hospitalization he had confined himself in his room, avoiding all friends, and finally refusing to see even his parents and siblings. In the hospital he detached himself, sitting in a corner of the ward with his eyes fixed on the floor. Whenever any patient or attendant approached him, he walked away. Despite the entreaties of his family he refused to leave the hospital, since he was able to seclude himself better on the ward than at home.

During interviews the patient refused to bring his head up because of his "blushing sickness," and because of his fear of looking anyone in the eyes. He was encouraged to continue doing this, and it was suggested that so long as he felt more comfortable away from people he had best continue removing himself from other patients on the ward. Nevertheless, he was reminded that he was probably very lonely and that were he not so afraid he might perhaps like some companionship.

During ward rounds the patient was always cautiously approached and politely asked whether he might be spoken to. If he refused to reply, this refusal was respected. If he nodded his head, a few casual remarks were made to him. After two months of this type of contact, he was asked whether he would like to borrow one of my books. He refused to reply. Apparently he pondered over this because one day he spontaneously asked in an irritated manner where the book was that I had promised him. I brought several books to him. After he had finished them, I invited him to pick his own volume from my library. He refused to leave the ward at first, but after a week of urging he consented to accompany me to my office. He picked out a book and I invited him to discuss it with me later. In the course of these conversations it turned out that his most engaging interest during the period prior to his breakdown was music. Whenever he could afford it, he attended symphony concerts, and he bought books and phonograph records to appease this musical interest. At home alone in his room he had listened to symphonies on the radio. He particularly like Beethoven's *Sixth Symphony*.

During our conversations about music the patient admitted that he felt rather tense and afraid. With his consent, sleeping instructions were given him as he sat in his chair, and he immediately went into a somnambulistic trance. During the trance state it was suggested to him that he would hear the music of a symphony orchestra playing Beethoven's *Sixth Symphony*. He would experience, he was told, ecstatic pleasure as he listened to this music, pleasure which was greater than anything he hitherto had enjoyed. It was furthermore suggested that he would remember this experience when he woke up. These suggestions were repeated in later sessions. The patient looked forward to the sessions with great eagerness, and, as indicated by his spontaneous dreams as well as his behavior, his attitude changed from regarding me as a frustrating and terrifying person to one who was interested in him. He became more capable of standing up for his own rights and soon was able to obtain a ground parole and to engage in work that brought him into contact with others. His entire concept of reality changed, and there was little doubt that the pleasurable emotions he had experienced during the hypnotic state convinced him that a contact with another person could have pleasure values.

While many patients retain a fairly good grasp on reality and tend to return to their customary occupations, and even to tolerable relationships with other people on the basis of the close attachment that they establish with the physician, it may be necessary to do further work with the patient to prevent a relapse. Some of the patient's problems may be rooted in the fact that he harbors bloated ambitions of what he should accomplish in life. His grandiose expectations may have resulted in constant frustration. Under such circumstances it is essential to modify the patient's goals through the careful use of the transference. It may be possible, for instance, to convince him that it is better to devote one's life to the attainment of happiness in the immediate present than to strive for things in the unknown future. Other character disturbances may exist that make relationships with people fraught with anxiety. An active manipulation of the patient's environment through consultation with his family will make it possible for him to function more comfortably. Attempts should also be made to introduce him gradually into social contacts with other people. Hypnosis may be useful in facilitating these objectives.

In spite of such corrective measures, it is possible that hostility, tension and anxiety may constantly be generated by unconscious inner conflict. The patient's ego may again become unable to absorb and to deal adaptively with emotional stress. The danger of another schizophrenic collapse may therefore be imminent. Under these circumstances the cautious use of an analytic approach is indicated, and hypnosis may also be of some value here.[28] It is best not to attempt analysis until the patient, himself, evinces an interest in understanding his own problems. Schizophrenic persons are remarkably intuitive and can grasp the dynamics of their disorder better than most neurotics. This is probably because they live closer to their unconscious, and the ego barriers to deep impulses and fears are not so strong. It is for this reason that one must proceed very carefully in analyzing the patient's deepest impulses.

The realization of unconscious guilt, hostility and erotism through analysis has a dual effect on the psychic apparatus. On the one hand it floods the ego with destructive emotion; on the other, by forcing a more realistic adaptation, it serves to liberate the psyche from incessant conflict. In this way a dynamic probing is a two-edged sword; the ego has to be traumatized by the liberated emotions before it is able to mobilize defenses less destructive to the person than regression. The ego, however, may still be so weak that it shatters under the impact of emotion before it can adapt itself in a more normal manner. This is always the danger in psychotic and prepsychotic conditions. All interpretations must, therefore, be very cautiously applied. Analytic technics should be abandoned temporarily if excitment or great hostility develop. Only when the patient is positively attached to the physician is he able to bear the suffering brought out by a realization of his unconscious trends.

REFERENCES

[1] FISHER, V. E., AND MARROW, A. J.: Experimental study of moods. Char. & Pers. *2:* 201–208, 1934.

[2] McFARLAND, R. A., AND GOLDSTEIN, H.: The biochemistry of manic-depressive psychosis. Am. J. Psychiat. *96:* 49, 1939.

[3] LOCKWOOD, M. R.: A note on the relationship between the blood cholesterol and hyperglycaemic index in manic-depressive psychosis. J. Ment. Sc. *78:* 901–907, 1932.

[4] Strongin, E. I., and Hinsie, L. E.: Parotic gland secretions in manic-depressive patients. Am. J. Psychiat. *94:* 1459–1466, 1938.

[5] Baird, P. C., Jr.: Biochemical component of the manic-depressive psychosis. J. Nerv. & Ment. Dis. *99:* 359, 1944.

[6] Kallmann, F. J.: The operation of genetic factors in the pathogenesis of mental disorders. New York State J. Med. *41:* 1354, 1941.

[7] Rosanoff, A. J., Handy, L. M., and Plesset, I. R.: The etiology of manic-depressive syndromes with special reference to their occurrence in twins. Am. J. Psychiat. *19:* 725–762, 1935.

[8] Pollock, H. M., and Malzberg, B.: Hereditary and environmental factors in the causation of manic-depressive psychoses and dementia praecox. Am. J. Psychiat. *96:* 1227–1244, 1940.

[9] Titley, W.: Prepsychotic personality of patients with involutional melancholia. Arch. Neurol. & Psychiat. *36:* 19, 1936.

[10] Courtney, J. W.: "Involutional" as applied to involutional melancholia. Boston M. & S. J. *174:* 416, 1916.

[11] Schilder, P.: Introduction to a Psychoanalytic Psychiatry. New York, Nerv. & Ment. Dis. Publ. Co., 1928 p. 137.

[12] Werner, A. A., Johns, G. A., Hoctor, E. F., Ault, C. C., Kohler, L. H'' and Weis, M. W.: Involutional melancholia; probable etiology and treatment. J. A. M. A. *103:* 13 (July 7) 1934.

[13] ——, Kohler, L. H., Ault, C. C., and Hoctor, E. F.: Involutional melancholia; probable etiology and treatment. Arch. Neurol. & Psychiat. *35:* 1076 (May) 1936.

[14] Ault, C. C., Hoctor, E. F., and Werner, A. A.: J. A. M. A. *109:* 1786, (November 27) 1937.

[15] ——, ——, and ——: Involutional melancholia. Am. J. Psychiat. *97:* 691–694, 1940.

[16] Notkin, J., Dennes, B., and Huddart, V.: Folliculin menformon (theelin) treatment of involutional melancholia. Psychiat. Quart. *14:* 158 (January) 1940.

[17] Wittson, C. L.: Involutional melancholia. Psychiat. Quart. *14:* 167 (January) 1940.

[18] Hamilton, J. B.: Treatment of sexual under-development with synthetic male hormone substance. Endocrinology *21:* 649 (September) 1937.

[19] Schmitz, G.: Erfahrugen mit dem neuén syntehtischen Testeshormonpräparat "Perandren." Deutsche Med. Wchnschr. *63:* 230 (February 5) 1937.

[20] Sevringhaus, E. L.: Endocrine Therapy in General Practice. Chicago, The Year Book Publishers, Inc., 1938.

[21] Barahal, H. S.: Testosterone in male involutional melancholia. Psychiat. Quart. *12:* 743 (October) 1938.

[22] Sullivan, H. S.: The modified psychoanalytic treatment of schizophrenia. Am. J. Psychiat. *11:* no. 3, 1931.

[23] Tidd, C. W. A note on the treatment of schizophrenia. Bull. Menninger Clin. *2:* 91, 1938.

[24] GROTJOHN, M.: Some features common to psychotherapy of psychotic patients and children. Psychiatry *1:* 318, 1938.

[25] ROSEN, J. M.: The treatment of schizophrenic psychosis by direct analytic therapy. Psychiat. Quart. *21:* 3–37, 117–119, 1947.

[26] FROMM-REICHMANN, F.: Transference problems in schizophrenia. Psychoanal. Quart. *8:* 412, 1939.

[27] FEDERN, P.: Psychoanalysis of psychoses. Psychiat. Quart. *17:* 3–18, 470–487, 1943.

[28] WOLBERG, L. R.: Hypnoanalysis. New York, Grune & Stratton, 1945.

XIX

HYPNOSIS IN MISCELLANEOUS CONDITIONS

A VARIETY of habit disturbances and symptoms are amenable to hypnotic therapy. However, the extent to which they can be influenced, and the permanency of the improvement, will vary with the existing dynamics.

Such problems as overeating, insomnia, excessive smoking, nail-biting, drug addictions, enuresis, "stage fright" and stuttering, though appearing as isolated symptoms, are merely surface disturbances of much deeper emotional processes which affect vast areas of the individual's functioning. The patient may actually be unaware of the significance of his symptom in terms of broader personality implications. He will, therefore, resist any interference with his customary patterns of living, even though these are manifestly neurotic, and, without question, underlie his difficulties.

In treating any complaint by means of symptom removal, and by the various psychobiologic therapies, an effort must always be made to create in the patient a motivation to explore the sources of his problem. Unless some fundamental change develops in the patient's life pattern through a real alteration in the personality structure, amelioration or removal of a symptom may prove ineffective or temporary.

Unfortunately, the patient himself will impose limitations on the extent to which he will be influenced. He may be satisfied with himself and with the type of relatedness he has with people. He may regard his symptom or complaint as a foreign body, whose removal, he imagines, will open up for him new paths of health and achievement. He may superficially acknowledge the existence of deeper problems and acquiesce to their exploration, but his attempts will be hol-low and lack sincerity. Nevertheless, the physician must continue to bring to the patient's attention the existence of difficulties which will need further inquiry, if not now, then at some future date when there is a stronger incentive for more intensive work.

OVERWEIGHT

Overweight is exclusively the product of an intake of food in excess of the dietary requirements. It can be overcome by reversing the balance so that the caloric output of the body is greater than the intake. This may be done in several ways: first, by accelerating metabolism through exercise and endocrine substances, like thyroid; second, by restricting the diet so that more energy is expended than consumed; third, by deadening the appetite through the use of substances like benzedrine sulfate.

Since abstemiousness is anathema to the average overweight person, he is prone to depend upon measures other than dieting when he becomes concerned with his excess poundage. These devices are, of course, quite effective in reducing weight. However, they do not correct the basic cause of obesity which is the compulsion to overeat. Unless weight reduction is accompanied by a re-education of the palate so that the individual is content with a diminished quantity of less fattening foods, weight gain is inevitable.

The person who habitually overeats does so either to alleviate tension or to derive a vicarious gratification that comes from gorging himself to the point of satiety. Individuals who have been pampered or rejected in childhood, and who have suffered great insecurity or harsh illness in the first years of life, are most apt to overvalue oral activities. Stuffing the stomach with food materials becomes associated with a feeling of profound peace and contentment. Analysis of fantasies and dreams indicate that in eating the person strives to achieve a regressive type of security which is equivalent to being breast fed by a bountiful mother. Over-eating thus becomes a tension relieving mechanism as well as a most important source of pleasure fulfillment. The personality structure that provokes the overeating tendency also motivates the individual toward dependency on a stronger person who acts as a mother substitute. The death or absence of the latter individual creates depression, and stimulates the desire to overeat as a compensatory mecha-nism. The psychology of the obese person resembles that of the alcoholic. Both involve pathologic oral activities.

It would seem urgent to treat the basic personality dif-ficulty before any permanent improvement in the craving for oral gratification could be expected. Unfortunately, an alteration in the character organization of patients with this type of problem is an extremely ambitious undertaking. Even when the patient is motivated toward change, therapy is bound to be prolonged.

Consequently, at the start, a directive supportive technic may be expedient. Appropriate reducing diets are prescribed, and the patient is enjoined to weigh herself (or himself) daily and to tabulate, for the doctor's information, every item of food that she takes. Trance induction along authoritarian lines has a remarkable effect on the patient's ability to fol-low her diet. The trance facilitates a close relationship to the physician, satisfying the dependency drive, and causing a diminution of the oral craving. Strong suggestions to follow the diet rigorously, along with suggestions that the appetite will be under control and that feelings of gastric emptiness will disappear, serve to remove the urge to overeat. Where a very deep trance is obtained, it may be possible to condi-tion the patient so that she converts an urge to eat into work or social activities.

Under hypnosis, utilizing a persuasive approach, an attempt is made to create a strong incentive to follow the diet by stress-ing increased health, beauty, and better social and business opportunities. The dangers of continued obesity are brought to the patient's attention. She is then given detailed instructions about her diet: the types of food to avoid, the preparation of foodstuffs, the need for supplementary vitamins, the importance of mastication, the need to be continent on dining away from home or when attending social functions, and advisable forms of exercise.[1] Suggestions are repeated to the effect that the will to observe the diet will increase, while the urge to eat will diminish.

Should the person slip on any occasion in the strict observance of her diet, the physician must not become impatient. He should rather utilize this opportunity to point out the fact that overeating occurs as a direct result of certain emotional problems which may require coincidental correction. The circumstances underlying the break in the diet may be reviewed with the patient in an attempt to bring her to an understanding of attitudinal and interpersonal difficulties. Once the patient evinces an interest in inquiring more deeply into her existing problems, a re-educational or analytic approach will insure the greatest success in curing both the obese condition, and the much more fundamental personality difficulty.

INSOMNIA

Hypnosis is one of the most effective therapies for insomnia. It is the treatment of choice in acute conditions of sleeplessness which do not respond to drug therapy.[2] Here hypnosis is induced, and the patient is given strong suggestions to the effect that he will henceforth sleep soundly because he will feel able to face, with a different attitude, those situations which worry him. Often no more than one hypnotic session, which is carried to as great a depth as possible, suffices to relieve insomnia. Should the patient complain that his sleep is interrupted by disturbing dreams, he may be given suggestions, in the trance, to the effect that his sleep will be dreamless.

The treatment of chronic insomnia is much more difficult.

Patients with this condition have established a habit of sleeplessness which is extremely obdurate. Often they rely on sedatives to which they become addicted. Sedation is less and less effective with the passage of time, and the patient attempts to make up for this by an increased dosage.

The usual causes of chronic insomnia are worry over an adverse environmental situation, over-fatiguability, excitement, a generalized state of neurotic tension, obsessional fears and anxiety dreams. In treating the insomnia, it is essential to understand its source, since hypnotic suggestions are best directed at correcting the condition which creates the sleeplessness. The nature of the patient's problem will undoubtedly become obvious to the physician after several sessions.

Where the insomnia is merely a minor symptom of an extensive neurosis, and where the patient has the motivation to work through his deeper problems, treatment must be directed at the neurosis itself. Insomnia will diminish or disappear when the tension and anxiety associated with the neurotic condition are brought under control.

In the event a short-term approach is necessary, a direct attack on the symptom of sleeplessness may be indicated. Hypnosis is valuable here, but many resistances arise in the course of treatment. Because the word "sleep" has become a bugaboo with the patient, and because he has convinced himself that he is unable to sleep, the induction process must be carried out avoiding the use of the term "sleep." Instead the words "tired," "relaxed," and "drowsy" are used.

Once the patient has achieved as deep a trance as can be produced, he is informed that one of the most persistent causes of insomnia is worry about the harmful consequences of not sleeping. Studies have shown that merely lying in bed and relaxing is sufficient to take care of the waste products that are to be dissipated in sleep. If he does not sleep, no real harm will befall him. Of course he can drive himself to distraction worrying about not sleeping. Worry actually causes him more difficulty than his insomnia. What he must tell himself each evening before retiring is this: "If you happen to fall asleep, so much the better; if not, it will not matter." This well-known aphorism may sound trite, but it will help him enormously.

The patient must be enjoined to establish a proper routine in restoring his sleeping habit. Some exercise during the day is advisable to produce slight muscle fatigue. A hot drink of milk or cocoa and a hot bath are also helpful. The patient must retire at the same time each night for best results. Upon retiring he must make his mind as passive as possible. Following this he is to give himself breathing and relaxing exercises which are patterned after the technic of hypnosis with sleep suggestions as outlined in Chapter V. This technic is taught the patient while he is in a trance, and he is awakened and asked to put himself into "a relaxed drowsy state" in order to ascertain that he understands the procedure. As soon as the patient demonstrates his ability to utilize this form of self-hypnosis, it is suggested, while he is in a hypnotic state, that he will retire at a designated hour, that he will make his mind passive, and that he will put himself to sleep in five minutes or less by employing the technic he has just used. He will sleep soundly during the night and awake in the morning fully refreshed. In Volume Two, under "Hypnosis with Symptom Removal," will be found an illuminating transcription of the therapy of a patient with insomnia.

In the event the patient is accustomed to sleeping drugs, these should not be removed at the start. Suggestions are made to the effect that he will find it unnecessary to employ sleeping medications, and that he will gradually abandon them.

Persuasive suggestions, such as described in Volume Two, are often valuable, and those suggestions which are particularly applicable to the problems of the patient are given him both in waking and hypnotic states.

Needless to say, existing environmental and neurotic difficulties must be treated by appropriate methods to forestall a relapse of insomnia.

NAIL-BITING

Nail-biting is an extremely common habit, prevalent particularly in childhood and adolescence. In a series of three thousand school children, Wechsler[3] discovered that the incidence of nail-biting rose from 35.7 per cent at the age of 8, to 42 per cent at the age of 14.

Nail-biting serves as an outlet for tension. It may involve a vicarious form of masturbatory or sexual gratification along with self punishment, the two being fused in a masochistic manner.

The treatment of nail-biting may occur on a symptomatic level, or on the level of treating the deeper dynamic cause. Unfortunately most nail-biters have little motivation for real psychotherapy, and seek treatment merely because of embarrassment about their habit. They are usually unaware of the intense unconscious meaning of their symptom, and are often puzzled by the persistence of their urge to chew their finger tips.

Hypnosis with strong authoritarian suggestions to stop the practice of nail-biting is successful in many cases. In the trance the patient is told that henceforth he will experience a strong distaste whenever he brings his fingers to his mouth. It will be as if they taste bitter. Conditioning nausea to the biting of the nails may also suffice to control the habit.

Success is most marked where daily hypnotic sessions are utilized until the nails regenerate and the finger tips heal. Reinforcement of suggestions is advisable once every two weeks. Where practical difficulties interfere with daily visits at the start, the parent, mate or a friend may reinforce therapy by making suggestions during sleep. In the event this technic is to be practiced, the patient may be instructed in the trance that the person chosen as an ally will help him master his problem.

Leshan[4] has reported a most interesting experiment which demonstrates the efficacy of suggestions made during sleep in the treatment of nail-biting. Forty nail-biters in a boys' summer camp were divided into two groups. The first group of 20 boys was exposed during sleep for fifty-four nights in succession to the sentence repeated fifty times each night: "My fingernails taste terribly bitter." The other group of boys served as a control. At the end of this period, eight boys in the first group had given up nail-biting, while none of the control group had abandoned the habit.

This type of therapy does not alter coincident neurotic or character disorders which may be at the root of the nail-biting, and for this reason effort must always be made to motivate the patient to accept therapy aimed at his basic problems.

Excessive Smoking

A somewhat similar approach may be utilized in excessive smoking. Chain smokers have established a pernicious habit of alleviating tension by puffing on a cigarette. They are usually unable to break this habit through their own effort, and any attempt to do so mobilizes an enormous amount of anxiety. In treating the chain smoker, a persuasive approach may be utilized. Under hypnosis he is informed about the harmful effect of nicotine on his system. He is asked to verbalize a desire to control his smoking urge. Following this he is given strong suggestions to the effect that his craving for tobacco in any form will disappear, and that he will even develop a dislike for smoking. He will find that his powers of self control will increase progressively until he can give up smoking entirely should he so desire. Chewing gum or hard candy may be substituted temporarily for cigarettes in the event his tension mounts; however, he will learn to control and to dissipate tension as soon as it arises. The patient should also be told that if tension continues to bother him to the point of distraction, he had best get psychotherapeutic help to determine and eradicate its source.

ENURESIS

A urologic examination is essential in all cases of enuresis to rule out an organic factor. Assuming that the patient is not mentally defective or of borderline intelligence, the presence of enuresis probably indicates improper habit training, emotional immaturity, or conflicts related to sexuality or aggression. Frequently enuresis has positive values for the individual as a masturbatory equivalent. In some instances it represents a form of aggression against the parents or against the world in general. Often it signifies an appeal for dependence on the basis of being a childish, passive, helpless person. In this context enuresis symbolizes for the boy castration and the achieving of femininity. In girls it often connotes aggressive masculinity and functioning with a penis.

Strong emotional stress sometimes produces enuresis in persons who are ordinarily continent. This was brought out during the war when certain soldiers subjected to the rigors of induction or warfare displayed the regressive symptom of bed-wetting. Most soldiers who showed this symptom had a history of early bed-wetting, or of periodic attacks of this disorder prior to induction.

The treatment of such acute conditions consists of trance induction and the use of a persuasive approach. The patient is instructed regarding the immaturity of his reaction, and he is shown that bed-wetting serves a function of pleading for love or for mercy on the basis of his helplessness. He virtually tries to make himself a baby to avoid responsibility or to get out of a difficult situation. The dangers of passivity are emphasized and the patient is brought to a point where he verbalizes a desire to be a grown person. The need for adjusting himself to an irremediable distressing life situation is emphasized and active suggestions may be made in this direction. Should no change occur with this approach, a more authoritarian attitude may be necessary, pressure being applied to the patient "to give up being a baby," to "face his duties like a man," and "to be like the other fellows."

In chronic enuretic states a modified analytic approach is the best type of therapy from the standpoint of altering disturbed personality patterns. The origins of the bed-wetting disturbance are explored, and the unconscious fantasies associated with it are clarified to motivate the patient to accept a more adaptive attitude toward life. It may be expedient to combine this re-educational approach with a reconditioning process. In the event an analytic technic cannot be utilized, symptom removal through reconditioning may be employed.

In reconditioning the enuretic person, he is trained to enter as deep a trance state as possible. In the trance an attempt is made to teach him self mastery by showing him that he is able to produce various phenomena, like paralysis, muscle spasm, etc., and that he can shift or remove these by self suggestions. Fantasies related to the most horrible thing and the best thing that can happen to a person are obtained for purposes of reinforcing the conditioning process later on. The patient is then requested to experience a sensation of slight bladder pressure such as occurs immediately prior to urination. As soon as he feels this sensation, he is told that it will inspire a dream or will make his hand rise to his face, which action will cause him to open his eyes. Even though no dream or hand levitation occurs, his eyes will open nevertheless. The moment his eyes open, he will realize that he must go to the bathroom. Going to the bathroom will be associated with a feeling similar to that accompanying the fantasy of the best thing that could happen to a person. Refusing to go will be associated with the feeling inspired by the fantasy of the worst thing that can happen to a person. These suggestions are repeated a number of times.

The next stage in therapy is teaching the patient to control sensations which arise in his bladder, retaining his urine without needing to awaken until morning. Suggestions to this effect are given the patient as soon as he establishes a habit of going to the bathroom. The positive relationship with the physician may be utilized as a reinforcing agent in reconditioning, praise and reassurance being given the patient upon following suggestions successfully.

These technics are described in detail in Volume Two under "Hypnosis and Symptom Removal," where there will be found the complete transcribed record of the treatment of a patient with enuresis.

"Stage Fright"

The symptom of stage fright is a manifestation of anxiety which develops when the individual has to perform, express or assert himself before a group. It is associated with an undermined self esteem, and with expectations of hostility, disapproval or actual attack on the part of other persons who witness the performance.

Stage fright may be a diffuse symptom appearing under any circumstance in which the individual has to express himself. It may occur here irrespective of the nature of the audience. Strong perfectionistic traits complicate the picture and the individual makes inordinate demands of himself, being terrified of failure. In most instances, however, stage fright occurs when the person fears exposure to authoritative persons or to those he believes are superior to himself. Whenever he feels superior or contemptuous of persons around him, he is able to assert himself without fear. Strong competitive drives are often present, which, upon analysis, are frequently related genetically to defeat in a sibling rivalry situation.

Where stage fright is a symptom of a deep or pernicious character disorder, treatment on a symptomatic level is usually unsatisfactory. Therapy here is prolonged and involves an alteration in the dynamic components of the personality. A nondirective and analytic approach is useful, but results may not be satisfactory even with these methods, particularly when a schizoid element is present. The entire effort in therapy is toward rebuilding self esteem through liberation of the individual from unconscious conflicts and fears, and from pervasive passive and masochistic impulses. This effort is aided by expanding self confidence through positive achievement and gratifying interpersonal relationships.

Where the Rorschach test and the response of the patient to the initial interviews indicate a basically well-integrated personality, it may be possible to utilize a persuasive hypnotic approach. Here emphasis is placed on the fact that the patient's reaction is unrealistic, that because of early unfortunate conditionings, he fears assertiveness and anticipates failure in performance. He is encouraged to seek out opportunities where he can express himself. Suggestions are made to the effect that his self confidence will return soon and that he will want to be more assertive. Performance fears will diminish and he will grow stronger and stronger. Persuasive arguments, such as contained in Volume Two, may be utilized to bolster the patient's determination to conquer his timidity. In addition, self hypnosis is also useful.

Various devices can be practiced by the patient to overcome his fear of people. Where there is a tendency to avoid meeting others, the individual is encouraged under hypnosis to counteract this by actually going out of his way to come into contact with individuals or groups. When he meets people he is to resist the impulse to look at the ground or to direct his gaze away from people. In self hypnosis the patient may visualize himself meeting and talking to authoritative people, or actually addressing groups. He may give himself suggestions that he will be able to do this in real life. When talking to people, he must dwell on the conversation rather than on himself. Whenever he starts thinking about himself, he must shift his train of thought back to the conversation, since thinking about himself will bring on self consciousness. He must never expect or anticipate ridicule. Rather he must cultivate the attitude that he will be accepted by people if he accepts himself.

Should fear of people and stage fright be caused by an anticipation of criticism, it is essential for the person to cultivate the philosophy that if the criticism is proper, he will profit by it. If it is improper, he will not brood over it, but rather will be critical of those who have made this unjust decision. If one approaches people with the idea that he likes them, and is agreeable in his attitudes, he will find them responding to him in kind.

When the patient expects to make a speech or to present a talk, he must prepare himself for this thoroughly. Knowledge that he has mastered his subject in advance is of utmost help. It is best to have made the speech or to have read the paper to oneself several times in advance. At the time of the meeting, and before he has been called on to perform, he should attempt to socialize with others. Talking to people helps dissipate his tension. The attitude he must take is that his colleagues are his friends and that he has something to contribute to the group. Immediately prior to his introduction, at the time when a sense of panic strikes him, he can divert energy by tapping his foot, or opening and shutting his fist, in such a manner that these movements will not be noticed. Since excitement causes shortness of breath, he must inhale deeply. A thorough oxygenation of his lungs will tide him over the first few minutes which are the most crucial minutes of his performance. It is urgent that he memorize the first few lines of his talk or paper so that he can recite them during the initial period of panic. As he finds himself able to talk without shortness of breath, his confidence in himself will be restored. He must deliberately cultivate an appearance of confidence, since this will stimulate his assertiveness. One way of doing this is to speak slowly and precisely. Should any doubts arise as to his ability to perform, they must be checked immediately and attention again focused on what he is saying. In the event he has failed to perform well, he must try again.

These persuasive measures naturally deal in a topical way with the individual's problem. They do not tackle the central causative difficulty. They are, nevertheless, useful in certain personality types, particularly compulsive characters. They must always be utilized with the idea of shifting the approach to an analytic one as soon as the patient is motivated toward exploring his relationships with others.

A treatment program such as outlined further under "Speech Disorders" is also helpful where stage fright accompanies talking to a group.

DRUG ADDICTION

The principal drugs to which an individual may become habituated are opium and its derivatives, particularly morphine and heroine, cocaine, cannabis, barbiturates and benzedrine. Drug addiction occurs under the same conditions and involves somewhat similar personality problems as alcoholism. In the main there are two types of addicts: first, the individual who suffers from a psychoneurosis and who attempts to subdue tension and anxiety with drugs; second, a particular type of character problem similar to the "essential alcoholic" who lives chiefly for the "lift" and moments of ecstasy and euphoria induced by the drug action. After addiction has developed, a physical dependency on the drug develops, conditioned by a physiologic tissue change, which creates a yearning for the drug apart from the psychologic need.

The treatment of narcotic addicts is best achieved in an institution where withdrawal symptoms can be handled and where the person is kept under close supervision to prevent him from obtaining drugs. The treatment plan should be organized so that total abstinence is achieved within ten days. Supplementary barbiturate sedation, a high caloric diet with vitamins, hydrotherapy, massage and glucose infusions are most easily administered in an institution. Hospitalization is best planned for a period of at least six months, during which period psychotherapy should be utilized, since, unless the sources of conflict are removed and the basic attitudes toward life altered, a relapse of the addiction is almost inevitable.

Hypnosis is often effective in helping the patient through the rigors of the withdrawal period. A deep trance during which reassuring, persuasive suggestions are given the patient help ameliorate his suffering. The patient usually feels helpless during this phase of therapy and he is remarkably susceptible to a warm "mothering" approach. Relaxing suggestions aid him also in overcoming insomnia. Following total withdrawal of the drug, hypnotherapy is advisable along lines described for the treatment of the alcoholic. The patient cannot be considered cured until all craving for drugs has disappeared, and until he is able to resist taking them even though they are available.

The treatment of the barbiturate addict is also difficult and will require institutionalization except where the individual has stabilized his intake and does not require excessive amounts of the drug. Barbiturates in large doses are destructive to brain tissue. Withdrawal of the drug must be gradual to avoid convulsions or the precipitation of a psychosis. As in the treatment of narcotic addiction, abstinence must be complete before a cure is possible. Hypnotherapy is helpful and also follows closely the technic for the treatment of alcoholic addiction.

Hypnosis is often requested by persons who depend on barbiturates to overcome insomnia. Where the habituation has gone on for a period of many months or years, hypnosis will not in itself be able to produce sleep. Substitution of bromides or chloral for the barbiturates may be instituted as a temporary measure. Hypnotherapy for the treatment of insomnia, which has been outlined elsewhere in this chapter, is employed in conjunction with an exploration of existing conflicts and interpersonal problems.

The treatment of cannabis and benzedrine addictions may be carried out along the same lines as the hypnotic treatment of alcoholism.

Speech Disorders

Functional speech problems, which are sometimes arbitrarily called "stuttering," are the product of incoordination of various parts of the speech apparatus wherein the speech rhythm becomes inhibited or interrupted. Associated are vasomotor disturbances, spasm and incoordination of muscle groups involving other parts of the body. The speech difficulty is initiated and exaggerated by certain social situations, the individual being capable of articulating better under some circumstances than others. This is confirmed by the fact that the person is usually able to sing, and to talk without difficulty to himself and to animals.

Investigation discloses that the problem in talking stems partly from an undefined constitutional factor that renders the speech apparatus vulnerable to homeostatic imbalance, and partly from a personality disorder which involves the individual's incapacity to assert himself, to express his needs in relationship with others. The inhibitory mechanism is often inspired by a fear of hostile speech outbursts, with blocking of articulation to avoid rejection or counterhostility.

There is a fear here of the killing power of words. Speaking is regarded as an act through which the person believes he may reveal himself. It also becomes a means of proving himself, and his self uncertainties and feelings of ineptitude are reflected by wavering speech. Talking becomes charged with values which interfere with its functional utility as a means of self expression and of social contact.

The origin of speech disorders is believed to lie in damage to the individual's security feelings in the first months of life when the mouth and oral apparatus were the chief organs through which the individual established his contacts with the world. The most frequent provocative factor is inadequate mothering as reflected in deficient feeding, sucking and sensory stimulations. Early insecurity makes the individual vulnerable to deprivations around the period of toilet training and socialization. Hostility and pathologic interest in anal activities are intensified as a result. Sometimes the experiences the child encounters are so disturbing to him that he develops a character structure of a compulsive nature, with dependency strivings and sado-masochistic impulses.

On this sensitized soil the speech difficulty germinates into being, usually as the result of some precipitating factor. This may be a fearful incident, or may involve panic at being called upon to perform or to assert himself before adults or at school. Repetition of speech hesitation or speech disturbance under similar circumstances establishes a pattern of fear of speech failure. This intensifies the symptom. Once the speech disorder is established and the individual senses his expressive ineffectuality, and feels the ridicule and concern of those around him, talking becomes associated with anxiety and phobias develop to avoid situations in which he is most likely to stutter. He also elaborates a number of defenses in the form of hesitations, distracting rhythmic physical movements, preliminary sounds as helpers, and substitute synonyms for difficult words. The speech difficulty becomes exaggerated as he realizes his own helplessness in controlling it. Withdrawal from people is engendered by a fear of failure in talking. Self esteem is progressively impaired and outbursts of social defiance and aggression may occur. Stuttering is most pronounced where the individual believes himself to be in an inferior position. Hence it is especially marked in the presence of authoritative persons, and is least noticeable where the individual feels relatively superior.

The treatment of stuttering should proceed on two different levels: correction of the improper speech habit, and the handling of the deeper emotional problem which originally initiated and now sustains the difficulty. A guidance approach both in the waking and hypnotic states is of help in achieving the first objective. The second goal is obtained through a persuasive, re-educational, and, where indicated, a modified analytic approach. Hypnosis is useful here also. Therapy involves correction of patent difficulties in the environment that stir up the person's insecurity, and a dealing with disturbing inner conflicts. Since the character disturbance in stutterers is extensive, therapy is bound to be difficult, prolonged, and, in many cases, unsuccessful in so far as alteration of the personality disorder is concerned. The most that can be expected here is a symptomatic speech correction.

My experience with speech difficulties has convinced me that some forms of speech training may do as much harm as they do good. They are valuable only as a means of building up confidence in the individual's powers to articulate. Unfortunately, they may psychologically have the opposite effect, since they emphasize will power and control, and concentrate the stutterer's attention on the mechanics of his speech rather than upon what he says. Instead of becoming less conscious about his speech difficulty, he becomes more involved with it, thus intensifying his problem. This is not to say that proper exercises in diaphragmatic breathing, phonetics and articulation are of no value in certain patients.

Sometimes a symptomatic recovery may take place in mild cases with these methods. However, in severe cases, they are relatively ineffectual, and, especially where the person makes a voluntary effort to put his stuttering to a halt, the severity of his speech problem may increase. There is one method, known as the "chewing method,"[5] which has advantages over others since it diverts attention from the speech mechanism. Rhythmics and eukinetics are also useful. Training methods, when utilized, should be employed by a therapist experienced in speech methods.

There are certain evasions and defenses that the stutterer may learn in order to tide him over situations where he must talk. Drawling, speaking in a rhythmic manner or in a sing-song tone, utilizing distracting sounds like "ah" or a sigh prior to articulation, employing a gesture or engaging in some motor act like pacing or rubbing a watch chain, purposeful pauses, and a variety of other tricks may be taught the stutterer by the speech teacher. These are entirely palliative and must be considered escapes rather than therapeutic devices.

The only rational therapy involves a rebuilding of confidence of the individual in himself and in his capacity to establish a verbal contact with people. Toward this end therapy may be divided into a number of stages.

The first stage consists of convincing the patient that because of his experiences and disappointments he has come to overemphasize the speech function. To him it constitutes an insignia of aggrandizement and defamation. His self esteem has become linked with how he performs in his speech. Because of this he concentrates his attention on the way he talks more than on what he says. It is essential to remember that while his speech problem is important in his mind, it is probably not regarded with the same emphasis by others. It is essential for him to realize that he will overcome his stuttering more easily when he stops running away from acknowledging it. He must face the situation and even admit his speech problem to others. When he does this he will be more at ease and his speech will improve.

A talk such as the following is helpful: "There is nothing disgraceful about stuttering. Avoiding social situations because of fear of ridicule merely serves to exaggerate the sense of defeat. It is necessary to regard stuttering in the same light as any other physical problem. It you stop being ashamed of it, and do not concern yourself with embarrassing others, people will notice your speech less and less. As you become more unconcerned about *how* you talk, you will concentrate on *what* you say. Keep concentrating on what you say and pay no attention to how it sounds. Fear and embarrassment exaggerate your speech difficulty, so make yourself act calm and you will feel calm."

The last precept may be illustrated to the patient in hypnosis. A trance state is induced utilizing sleep suggestions, and atonicity is produced involving the various muscle groups. Suggestions are also made to the effect that muscles of the face, mouth and throat will become relaxed. Slow, deep breathing exercises are given the patient and he is asked to visualize the most calm, peaceful scene that he can bring to his mind. He is then informed that in his calm and relaxed state he will describe the scene as he sees it with ease and without stuttering. As a general rule, patients respond to these suggestions by talking in a perfectly normal manner. The occasion is utilized to point out to the patient that his speech now shows no evidence of stuttering because he is calm and relaxed.

A suggestion is next made to the effect that the patient visualize himself with people that he knows and likes. The calm relaxed feeling will continue. As soon as he indicates that he has visualized this scene by a signal like hand levitation, he is told that his calm relaxed state will enable him to talk easily to the people in his fantasy. He is asked to imagine himself talking to them, and urged to tell the physician about his imaginary conversation.

Should the patient carry out this suggestion successfully, he is again reminded that he was able to talk without stuttering because of his calm, relaxed feeling. The next fantasy involves his being with people whom he admires and respects, but of whom he is in awe. He will visualize himself talking to them, but instead of being upset and fearful as he talks, he will be calm and unafraid. He will find that he can talk without any difficulty. He is then asked to report on what he has said.

The fantasies brought to his mind following this involve his going to parties, addressing small groups and then large groups, in each instance with the same calm, relaxed feeling, a feeling as if he is as good as anyone in the group, as if he is totally unafraid. When the patient reports a successful performance in each of these instances, he is informed simply that the purpose of the demonstrations was to show him that when he is calm and relaxed, he can speak unhesitatingly. He is then told that being calm and relaxed with people is enormously important for him, and that he will soon become more assertive and self confident and will be able to feel calm and relaxed in any social group. He will be able to speak with greater freedom and will be able to meet life with more assuredness.

The next stage of therapy consists of demonstrating to the patient how he becomes upset and loses his sense of calm in certain situations. There will be no lack of material, since the patient will bring to the physician's attention many instances in which his stuttering became exaggerated. Examining his emotional reactions to these situations as well as his dreams will give the physician clues as to the dynamic elements involved in the patient's speech condition. These may be pointed out to the patient at levels that approximate his existing capacity to absorb insight. The aim is to show the

patient that his speech difficulty appears when he loses his
sense of calm and relaxation, and to demonstrate to him why
his emotional instability develops.

Should the patient be deeply hypnotizable, an experimental conflict may be induced which recapitulates his
important conflicts and fears, and the patient will learn in a
dramatic way how his speech breaks down under certain conditions. Later on this technic may be utilized for purposes of
desensitization to enable the patient to master life situations
of a most disturbing nature.

A persuasive approach may be combined with re-education.
In a trance, suggestions are given the patient to the effect
that as he understands himself better and sees how his speech
is influenced by his emotional reactions, he will want to correct those difficulties that upset his stability. He will adopt a
more tolerant attitude toward himself and toward other
people. He will analyze and do something about any remediable disturbing elements in his environment. Should environmental difficulties be irremediable, he will adjust himself to
them. He will accept his limitations and expand his assets
within reason. Since inner resentment aggravates his stuttering, he will better his relations with others to prevent anger
from piling up. He will stand up for his rights, but he will
also give in to reasonable demands. It is extremely important
that he assert himself as much as he can, and that he externalize his interests preferably in social channels.

The patient is encouraged to cultivate a calm, unemotional
tone of voice. He may practice this with a friend or with
members of his family. One half hour each day devoted to
reading aloud from a book, jotting down those words that are
difficult to pronounce is helpful. He may then practice enun-
ciating words several times during the day. Some persons find
it helpful to talk for a short time daily in front of a mirror
watching their facial movements as they utter sounds. Other
individuals find such autosuggestions as the following useful:

"I am able to talk and to pronounce each word. I shall be able to do this better and better, under all conditions. I will make myself calm and unemotional when I am with people. I will concentrate on what I say rather than how I say it. Under no circumstances will I get discouraged. If my speech gets bad on any occasion, I will do better next time."

Two important adjuncts in speech therapy are self hypnosis and group therapy. Persuasive autosuggestions in a self-induced trance reinforce the patient's expanding self confidence and assertiveness. Group therapy, in which the patient comes into contact with other persons suffering from speech problems, removes his sense of isolation. The fact that his companions experience the same trepidations as himself helps him to re-evaluate his reaction. An opportunity is provided him to speak and to recite in a permissive setting. The identification with the group, along with the growing confidence in his ability to express himself, have a most positive effect on his speech performance.

As the patient begins to experience improvement in his interpersonal relationships, his speech problem will plague him less and less. Utilizing the speech group as a bridge, he will be able to integrate himself with other groups and to consider himself on an equal plane with its constituent members.

The patient must be prepared for an occasional relapse of his stuttering. He must not regard this as a failure; rather he must look upon the experience as something that will teach him more about his interpersonal problems. A thorough understanding of these will give him the best opportunity to overcome his neurotic attitudes and to better his speech.

ORGANIC DISEASES

Organic disease is always complicated by emotional factors. The extent of the emotional element is dependent upon the significance to the patient of his illness. Treating the emotional factor raises the resistance of the patient and may result in more prompt healing.

Some people respond to their illness with a fearful secretive attitude, attempting to conceal its existence from others as well as from themselves. They regard it here as a contemptible thing that will result in ridicule. Power-driven and perfectionist people are particularly prone to respond to illness in this way. Weakness of any sort is equated with being a pitiable, mutilated person, who is unable to achieve an idealized stature. Self contempt in possessing limitations imposed by the illness, and fear of being injured and taken advantage of by surrounding people, produce a need to deny one's disability.

Obsessive personalities react to physical illness with tremendous tension and anxiety. This is because the illness symbolizes to the individual death or castration. The emotional response may be so extreme that it far outweighs the physical illness itself.

Individuals who are basically dependent are prone to utilize a physical illness for its secondary gain to justify their collapse on society. The abandonment of purposeful aggressive striving may create tremendous difficulties for the person and he will respond anxiously to the passivity that his illness imposes on him. Homosexual strivings, and dreams of mutilation and castration, accompany his reaction and symbolize his desire for and fear of passivity.

Persons who are more or less detached and who function through their own independent efforts resenting encroachment on the part of others may react to physical illness with a similar reaction. They may interpret the illness as a threat to their detachment, since it, of necessity, makes them dependent on others both physically and financially.

Psychotherapy is usually unnecessary in acute physical illness unless the resulting anxiety precipitates a psychoneurosis or psychosis. Treatment here is directed toward the underlying personality problem, dealing with the physical illness solely as the precipitating factor.

Chronic disease, on the other hand, and particularly disease which is associated with partial disability, will require a different kind of psychiatric handling. Where the person is suffering from a nonfatal illness, and where there is a possibility of a residual disability, as in coronary disease, apoplexy, arthritis, tuberculosis and various orthopedic and neurologic disorders, an effort must be made to get the patient to accept his illness. A desensitization technic may be utilized, encouraging the patient to discuss his illness and to ventilate his fears concerning it. The need to recognize that his illness does not make him different from others, that all people have problems, some of which are more serious than his own, that it is not disgraceful to be sick, may be repeated in waking and hypnotic states.

Persuasive talks may be given the patient to the effect that the most important thing in his achievement of health is to admit and to accept the limitations imposed on him by his illness. This need not cause him to retire in defeat. He will still be able to gain sufficient recognition and success if he operates within the framework of his handicap. It is most important for his self respect that he continue to utilize his remaining capacities and aptitudes, expanding them in a realistic and reasonable way. Many people suffering from a physical handicap have been able to compensate for a disability in one area by becoming proficient in another.

In patients who tend to regard their disability as justifying a completely passive attitude toward life, an effort must be made to stimulate activity and productiveness. The dangers of passivity and dependency, in terms of what these do to self respect, are emphasized. The person is encouraged to become as self assertive and independent as his handicap will allow.

Where it is important for the patient to relax and to give up competitive efforts, persuasive therapy may be combined with a reassuring, guidance approach aimed at externalizing his interests along lines that will be engaging but not too stimulating. The cultivation of a different philosophy toward life directed at enjoying leisure, and looking with disdain on fierce ambitious striving, will help the patient to accept this new role.

In the course of therapy, it may be necessary to modify the patient's attitudes toward life and people by working with his character problems along re-educational and analytic lines. A period of preparation may suffice to motivate the patient toward accepting a deeper approach to his basic personality difficulties.

In incurable, progressive, and fatal ailments, therapy involves the elimination of pain and acceptance of the progressive nature of the illness. Hypnotherapy is useful here, too, and often reduces pain and suffering. A trance, in which the patient is told that he will pay less and less attention to his suffering, and that his pain will disappear, frequently results in reduction or elimination of analgesic drugs. Persuasive hypnotic suggestions to face his remaining years with calmness and courage may be very reassuring to the patient. The patient may be told that while his life span is limited, he may extend it and enjoy his remaining years by the proper mental attitude. A guidance approach helps reduce the disturbing effect of environmental factors, and permits the patient to divert his interests toward outlets of an enjoyable nature. Where the patient is so disposed, he may be encouraged to cultivate religious interests in which he may find much solace.

Hypnosis in Dentistry, Obstetrics and Surgery

The use of hypnosis in dental, obstetrical and surgical procedures is limited by the fact that only one-quarter of subjects inducted into a trance are capable of achieving a sufficiently deep hypnotic state to make these procedures possible. Chemical anesthetics, on the other hand, are fool-proof and applicable to the majority of people. Where, for any reason, chemical anesthesia is contraindicated, hypnotic anes-thesia may be attempted. It may also be used where the patient is known to be a good hypnotic subject.

In the majority of cases four or five induction sessions will be required before an operation is possible. Once the patient has been trained to achieve anesthesia, a posthypnotic sug-gestion may be given him to the effect that he will, at a given signal, immediately enter a trance and display a total insensi-tivity to pain.

The anesthesia under hypnosis is profound, and, except for major surgical procedures, is as effective as chemical anesthesia. Obvious advantages are the ease of administra-tion, the immediate removal of anesthesia when desired, and the absence of postoperative reactions to the anesthetic. Of advantage also is the fact that posthypnotic suggestions may be given to the patient directed at postoperative pain. Where a major surgical operation is required, the hypnotic anes-thesia will make only a small amount of chemical anesthetic necessary.

In dental surgery, anesthesia, once it has been produced in the patient, can be invoked after a few minutes. It may be localized in any part of the mouth. It is possible, Stein[6] claims, to control salivation and to reduce bleeding. Advan-tages include the fact that fear and nervousness can be re-moved by suggestion. The patient may be placed in any position, and gags, mouth props and retentive devices need not be utilized. Stein points out that it is possible to produce anesthesia for postoperative pain, and that there is an absence of nausea and sickness which occur in other dental anesthetics.

Wookey[7] emphasizes that hypnosis is, in addition to an anesthetic, a therapeutic agent. It removes preoperative fear and dread, and promotes more rapid healing and the arrest of hemorrhage. It also acts as a psychologic aid in helping people get used to dentures. Wookey believes that the period of training required to induce hypnotic anesthesia is justified by virtue of the fact that, once achieved, it can be obtained almost immediately for years thereafter.

In obstetrics, hypnosis may be used during childbirth and for various obstetrical procedures. The patient is trained to enter a trance state during her pregnancy, and skin anesthesia is produced to demonstrate to her that a removal of pain is possible on suggestion. In the last month of pregnancy, suggestions are given her to the effect that at a given signal she will sleep deeply and will feel no pain in her delivery. Where the patient responds positively to these suggestions, a total absence of pain results and postpartum discomfort is minimal.

REFERENCES

[1] WOLBERG, L. R.: The Psychology of Eating. New York, Robert M. McBride & Co., 1936. (Reprinted as: Weight Control Through Proper Diet. New York, World Pub. Co., 1942.) pp. 192–219.

[2] KRAINES, S. H.: The Therapy of the Neuroses and Psychoses. Philadelphia, Lea & Febiger, 1943.

[3] WECHSLER, D.: The incidence and significance of fingernail biting in children. Psychoanal. Rev. 18: 201–209, 1931.

[4] LESHAN, L.: The breaking of a habit by suggestion during sleep. J. Abnorm. & Social Psychol. 37: 406–408, 1942.

[5] FROESCHELS, E.: Pathology and therapy of stuttering. The Nervous Child 2: 158–160, 1943.

[6] STEIN, M. R.: Anaesthesia by mental dissociation. Dental Items of Interest 52: 941–947, 1930.

[7] WOOKEY, E. E.: Uses and limitations of hypnosis in dental treatment. Brit. Dent. J. 65: 562–568, 1938.

XX

DANGERS, LIMITATIONS AND FAILURES
OF HYPNOSIS

FROM a medical standpoint the question of whether it is possible to influence a subject to perform a crime in a trance is purely academic. It is assumed, even if such a situation were possible, that the therapeutic objective as well as the moral code of the physician would preclude such use of the hypnotic state.

It is quite unlikely, however, that any person could be induced to do anything in a trance or posthypnotically as a result of suggestion, that he would not do with adequate persuasion in the waking state. In a small number of cases, it is conceivable that a subject may be influenced toward antisocial and even self-injurious acts which are contrary to his personal wishes and to his moral nature. In the waking state such persons could undoubtedly also be persuaded with proper arguments to engage in activities opposed to their best interests and to their customary moral stature.

People in the trance state easily sense when they are being used for experimental purposes. They will play a role with great sincerity, and, where they have faith in the hypnotist's integrity, will expose themselves to presumably dangerous situations. There is, nevertheless, a limit to how far they will go.

While doing experimental work with hypnosis, I suggested to a somnambulistic subject in a trance that he would open his eyes and conspire with me in a crime. I informed him that two lumps of sugar in a bowl, which I marked with a pencil, contained a deadly poison. He was to select them and place them in the cup of tea served to a doctor friend whom I expected shortly. This doctor was an evil fellow who had perfected a virus with which he planned to kill a number of people. It was best to get him out of the way before it was too late. I asked the subject if he would cooperate with me in getting rid of the man. While no one would find out that the man had been killed, the subject would, if it were ever known, be hailed as a benefactor. The subject readily agreed to cooperate with me. On signal the supposed victim entered the room and the three of us started a conversation. The subject, it was noted, was very irritated with the doctor and made biting sarcastic remarks about people who put on a front. I suggested that we have tea, and the subject volunteered to make it. I noticed that he carefully put the marked lumps into the victim's tea and passed the cup to him. The doctor drank the tea, without effect of course. I then called the subject to one side and mentioned there was probably some mistake, that we had not given the doctor a large enough dose of cyanide. Thereupon I gave him two capsules from a box marked "Potassium cyanide" and asked him to put these in the next cup of tea. He immediately awoke from the trance. So long as he was playing a role, he was willing to follow suggestions. He knew very well that the lumps of sugar were not really cyanide. However, the possibility that there might be cyanide in the capsules brought him out of the trance.

Experimental work with artificially induced dissociated states, in which a suggested criminal personality alternated or operated in conjunction with the usual personality, has convinced me that the patient, even though he is a potential criminal, is capable of inhibiting any impulses he conceives to be wrong. However, the fact that criminally inclined persons may, under the protective alibi of a trance, seize the occasion to act out their criminal drives, is one reason why hypnotic practice should be made illegal among unqualified lay practitioners.

In competent hands hypnosis has no harmful effects, but where it is utilized to evoke nonsensical and dramatic phenomena by showmen and parlor pranksters, and where symptom removal is attempted without some understanding of the dynamics of the patient's illness, neurotic persons may be influenced adversely. The neurotic individual already has serious problems in interpersonal relationships. He mistrusts people and constantly doubts their motives. When he is exposed to an injudiciously applied trance, he may become acutely upset, and his mistrust and resentment will become exaggerated.

Hypnosis has been associated with crystal balls and Frankensteinian monsters for so long that it has a definite dramatic appeal. By and large the field of hypnosis has been dominated by untrained lay hypnotists and charlatans. The latter, abetted by popular magazines and the radio, have tended to dramatize the most spectacular aspects of hypnosis. As a consequence an aura of quackery permeates the practice of hypnotherapy.

The medical profession cannot hold itself entirely blameless for the situation; for they have never delineated which of the aspects of hypnosis belong exclusively in the province of medicine. Urgently needed are laws forbidding the use of hypnosis for entertainment purposes, and limiting its therapeutic employment to trained and licensed practitioners.

Even when employed by persons skilled in its use, occasional complications arise. Posthypnotic nausea, dizziness and headaches which last for a short time are common. Spontaneous trance states sometimes develop, the individual experiencing dissociated bodily sensations with no apparent provocation. One of my experimental subjects, in whom a dual artificial personality had been induced, utilized this personality to justify bouts of drinking. Spontaneous trance states and hysterical phenomena may be controlled by firm suggestions in hypnosis to the effect that these conditions cease to exist. In so far as permanent alteration of personality, falsification of reality, elaboration of escape mechanisms, compulsive reactions to immoral suggestions, and hypersuggestibility resulting from the continued use of hypnosis are concerned, Erickson[1] has shown these to be very much exaggerated.

Another question is how dependent on the therapist the patient becomes who has had his symptoms removed by authoritative suggestion. Theoretically one would assume that dependency and an interminable attachment would result. In actual practice the patient becomes no more dependent than with any other kind of therapy. Whether or not the patient will become dependent seems to reside in his needs rather than in the technics used. People who have a need for a dependency relationship will become dependent upon a therapist—often to the latter's dismay—who utilizes a nondirective, passive approach exclusively.

The individual's basic character structure determines his attitude toward hypnosis. The compulsively dependent person does not need hypnosis to bring out his dependency. He will react to hypnosis as he does to any other interpersonal relationship. There is no evidence that hypnosis infantalizes a person, weakens his will, or renders the person any more dependent than any other therapeutic technic. I have induced trances in patients and volunteer subjects virtually hundreds of times, and not in a single instance has any patient become overly dependent on me or has become addicted to the trance state. There is no justification for the fear that a hypnotic subject will remain under the influence of the operator who will be able to wield a Svengali-like power over him.

The danger to the operator is also minimal. Rarely, unstable and hysterical persons are apt to claim a sexual assault on the basis of projected wish fulfillment. While such accusations are extremely uncommon, the possibility must be kept in mind, and where a patient displays strong sexual fantasies, these must be explained to the patient in terms of deeper motivational patterns. The notion that hypnosis in the mind of every subject is a symbolic sexual phenomenon is not borne out by facts. Indeed it is extremely uncommon for the patient to conceive of it in this light, unless he regards all close contacts in terms of sex. There is no real danger that the person will act out sexual fantasies in a properly conducted hypnotic session.

Limitations of the patient's ability to respond to harmful suggestions apply also to suggestions which are therapeutically useful. The dramatic effect of hypnosis on the psychic, somatic and visceral functions may lead the novice to overvalue its suggestive influence. One reason for the cyclic disappointment with hypnosis in the past has been the fact that with all its vaunted powers it can fail to remove many neurotic symptoms by suggestion.

Maladaptive as it may seem, a neurosis constitutes for the individual an equilibrium in the face of overwhelming anxiety. The patient, sensing that his neurosis interferes with effective reality functioning, comes into therapy with a dual motivation. He desires to escape from his restricting neurotic symptoms; yet he seeks to maintain his neurosis to protect him from anxiety. These motivations structure the character of all of his interpersonal relationships and will condition how he reacts to the therapeutic relationship.

Any attempt to produce changes in the individual which do not fit into the framework of his motivational system will be resisted. The individual who is not properly motivated will, when put into a trance and enjoined to give up a symptom, or to change his attitudes toward his illness, or to adopt a different philosophy of life, or to act in a more congenial manner with people, or to recognize his important unconscious conflicts, fails to respond.

There is nothing miraculous about the trance state. It has many values; but it does have limitations in terms of the individual's existing motivations and his capacities for change. Therapeutic failures occur with hypnosis as with any other form of therapy.

One of my most spectacular failures with hypnosis was with a physician who asked me to hypnotize him so that he could pass his State Board examinations. He had recently completed an internship in a Midwest hospital, and had returned to New York to establish a practice, which was being set up with the financial aid of his parents. By scrimping and scraping they had put their son through medical school, had supported him during his internship, and now they were about to realize their ambition of having him at home as a successful medical practitioner.

Although he realized that he would have to take his State Boards, he could find no time to study for them while interning; and, after leaving the hospital, he discovered that whenever he opened a book, his mind went blank. As time passed by, he became more and more panicky, and now that the examinations were only several days away, he had become so agitated that he could scarcely contain himself. He begged me to hypnotize him and remove by suggestion his mental block. He was quite certain that powerful pressures put upon him while he was in a trance would enable him to recall his medical studies and to complete his examinations successfully.

Under ordinary circumstances I would have refused to take this assignment; but because he was so disturbed, and because there was so little time, I consented to try to put him into a suitable frame of mind for the examination. He cooperated eagerly and entered a deep trance, during which I regressed him to the period of his life while he was at medical school. He recalled many details of his studies, of which he had, in the waking state, only a faint recollection. For instance, he was brought back to his anatomic dissection laboratory, and he painstakingly went through the motions of dissecting out the radial nerve, explaining its course and distribution. In a similar way he recalled many details of his other studies. I suggested that when he presented himself for examination he would recall as much as was necessary for him to remember. On the evening before, he would retire early and sleep soundly during the night. He would awaken refreshed with a clear mind, with sufficient vigor and self confidence to apply himself adroitly to the task of completing this examination.

On the evening before the examination he telephoned me and asked if it might not be advisable for him to spend the night at a hotel instead of at his parents' house, because he would be able to sleep better there and thus be in a better frame of mind. I agreed that this was probably advisable.

In the late afternoon, I received another telephone call from the man, and he informed me in a calm and even droll manner that never in his life before had he slept so soundly. As a matter of fact he had just gotten up, having slept through the examinations. There was no point now, he insisted, in taking the remainder of the tests. He volunteered to come to my office to talk things over.

When he reported, he seemed to be in excellent spirits. There were no signs of tension or anxiety, and he even adopted a humorous attitude towards the incident. He considered it peculiar, however, that he had slept so long since he rarely spent more than eight or nine hours in bed. In talking, he confided that there now was no reason why he could not go back west to visit a young lady in whom he had become interested while interning. His parents had opposed his marrying the girl, and because he felt he owed them a debt, he had given up his plan to settle in his girl's home town.

He was obviously torn between love for the girl and loyalty to his parents, and his inability to study seemed due to this conflict. He was unable to get himself to yield to the desires of his parents, nor did he wish to incur their disapproval or rebuke. Inhibition in thinking was a symptom which had for its purpose a frustration of the plans his parents had made to have him practice in New York. Guilt feelings, however, created anxiety and caused him to seek a desperate measure in hypnosis to break down his inhibition. So strong was his guilt that hypnosis was successful. When, during the trance, he realized that he might be able to remember enough to pass the examination, his conflict again became dominant and eventually it triumphed over my suggestions. His prolonged sleep was a means of escaping from the possibility of becoming licensed in New York. He had obtained implied permission from me to sleep when I agreed to his plan to spend the night at a hotel. When these facts were brought to his attention, he laughed heartily and declared that no longer was he going to deceive himself. He would tell his parents that they no longer had a claim on him, and, as soon as he was financially capable of so doing, would repay them for what they had expended towards his education.

Several years have gone by since this incident, and the man has established himself in practice in the Midwest. He is married to the young woman in question, and the situation with his parents has resolved itself more or less successfully.

This case is an example of how hypnosis indiscriminately applied can fail to achieve certain goals. It is essential to understand what motivations lie behind the patient's desire for hypnotherapy. These may be so distorted as to militate against any satisfactory result.

For instance, a young man applied for hypnosis with a list of items he desired to have injected into his personality. The first was: "You will be masterful at all times, expecially with women"; the second, "You will always think clearly, speak effectively in a low, modulated tone"; the third, "You will go to bed at 1:00 A.M. and wake up at 7:00 A.M. fully refreshed"; the fourth, "You will be a success in life in spite of all obstacles." The man had failed to gain these objectives after an extended psychoanalysis, and he felt certain that hypnosis could succeed where psychoanalysis had failed.

Many people have the misconception that hypnosis is a form of magic which can inject aptitudes and correct defects in a miraculous way. A number of persons have visited me for

this purpose, from a seventy-five year old man who had become impotent, to a six year old mentally defective child who
had never learned to talk, but whose mother had heard from
her family physician that a cure was possible if hypnosis
could be induced.

Failures in hypnosis can be subdivided into two types;
those that involve failure of induction and those that involve
failure to achieve a set therapeutic goal.

Induction failures are, with a good technic, fortunately
rare. They do occur, nevertheless, and are usually the product of a fear of submission on the part of the patient. In
instances where there is terror of interpersonal relationships,
and particularly a fear of yielding to an authority conceived
of as destructive or dangerous, resistances may develop
which prevent the attainment of a hypnotic state. The personality of the hypnotist and his experience may be determining factors here, and by adroit handling resistances to
induction may be successfully circumvented.

An example of how a patient can fight against hypnosis
while desiring it is illustrated by a man who asked to be hypnotized in order to learn how to control his homosexual drive.
During the process of induction he clenched his teeth and his
fists, and almost physically tried to fight off sleep suggestions.
As hypnosis proceeded, he panted violently, precipitously
arose from his chair and shrieked, "I can't, I can't let myself
go." He then confided that he had experienced an orgasm,
and that he seemed to want to yield himself to a higher power
who would be able to possess him completely. He had wedged
hypnosis into the framework of his neurosis, and had responded to the suggestions that I gave him as if I were virtually a lover whom he could not resist. Desiring both to yield
to and to resist suggestions, he experienced panic when he
realized he was actually entering a trance state.

A proper motivation to be hypnotizable is essential before
induction is possible. This motivation seems to exist universally, but sometimes, especially in emotional problems, may

not be present. It is usually impossible to hypnotize a subject if he wills otherwise; he must either desire to obey the orders of the hypnotist and enter a trance state, or he must have the feeling that in spite of his own will he is unable to resist the hypnotist's commands. An unconscious motivation to be hypnotizable may be stronger than the conscious desire to resist hypnosis. There are a number of persons who fight against entering a trance state, yet they are unable to stay awake once the induction process has begun.

Failures in induction may be reduced to a minimum where the physician is cognizant of the factors that militate against the patient's wanting to be hypnotized. If, by his manner and attitude, the physician can inspire trust; if he can dissipate the patient's misconceptions regarding hypnosis; if he can mobilize the patient's healthy impulses to get well and convince him that through the medium of hypnosis he may be able to achieve health, or to satisfy certain ambitions and objectives, it may be possible to overcome the fear of hypnosis.

A proper induction technic is also indispensable. There are innumerable hypnotic technics, some of which are successful with one type of individual, and others with another. A technic which inspires confidence, which makes the subject feel that he will gain a great deal from hypnosis and lose very little, that permits him to focus his attention exclusively on one stimulus, or a limited number of stimuli which repeat themselves monotonously and rhythmically, is most successful.

Among the more common resistances to trance induction are a desire to defy the authority that is vested in the hypnotist, a fear of losing one's will power or independence, a wish to prove oneself superior to and stronger than the hypnotist, or a conviction that one will fail in the task of hypnosis. These resistances are manifestations of personality problems which must be treated as symptoms.

Where the nature of the resistance is known, it may, in

some cases, be worked through. For instance, where a patient spontaneously admits that he has a fear of yielding up his independence, the physician may assure him that no suggestions will be given him without first gaining his consent. The hypnotic state may then be conducted in such a way that the patient vetoes or accepts the suggestions given to him in accordance with his own free will. Where the patient is defiant of the physician's authority, ventilation of his feelings toward the latter may sometimes make him susceptible to trance induction.

The ability to modify the hypnotic technic to coincide with the patient's character structure calls for an infinite amount of patience and ingenuity. It is sometimes possible to utilize the patient's resistances themselves as a means of increasing trance depth. Most often, however, this involves complications that may be disastrous to the therapeutic objective. It is usually essential to enlist active cooperation and participation and to abandon trance induction where it is obvious that the patient is resistive to the procedure.

An example of how an attempt to break through resistances without analyzing them may create difficulties can be illustrated by a patient who was referred to me after two years of unsuccessful psychotherapy. The patient was a compulsive individual who had built up a rigid detached system in which he maintained bloated arrogant notions of his own abilities and a defiant attitude toward any type of encroachment. Psychotherapy had constituted a threat to his neurotic structure, and he defended himself by a supercilious and hostile attitude toward the psychiatrist which interfered with all attempts to establish a type of transference which might have brought about beneficial results.

As he had proceeded with his therapy, he had become more and more frustrated, and finally he insisted that his analyst hypnotize him, claiming that only through hypnosis would he be able to get to the bottom of his difficulty. The psychiatrist sent him to a number of hypnotists who attempted hypnosis unsuccessfully, the patient resisting the induction process, yet experiencing intense frustration and disappointment because he could not be hypnotized.

The psychiatrist enjoined me to attempt hypnosis with him, believing that were induction successful, it might be possible to get around his detached attitude. When the patient appeared for the initial visit, the first words he said to me were, "I'll bet you can't hypnotize me." He then smiled in an arrogant manner and remarked that four hypnotists who were considered skilled in their profession had failed; he had challenged each of them to put him into a trance, stating that he had made a bet with himself that nobody would be able to do this. I inquired why he thought I might be successful when others had failed, and he replied that he was not sure that I would be successful, but that he had heard about sodium amytal as a catalyst to hypnosis. If I were to give him three capsules of the drug, his resistance might be removed. I had on my desktop blue placebo capsules consisting of sodium bicarbonate. The patient pointed to the capsules and said, "Those are sodium amytal capsules, aren't they? Could I take them now?" I agreed that a powerful sedative often facilitated hypnosis and that the capsules on my desk might possibly put him into a state where he could not resist hypnosis.

To my surprise, shortly after he had imbibed the tablets, he began to complain of feeling drowsy. I then started trance induction and succeeded in putting him into a deep hypnotic state. When he awoke, he was very elated, but almost immediately thereafter he had an anxiety attack with severe heart palpitations, inability to breathe, and a feeling as if the walls were closing in on him. Apparently what had happened was that he had cajoled himself into believing that he could be hypnotized through the agency of the blue capsules, and he had permitted himself to relax his vigilance to a point where he could enter a trance state. The feeling that he had yielded his defenses even temporarily was enough to create panic.

The psychiatrist reported to me that the anxiety attack lasted the greater part of one week. He believed the experience to have been valuable for the patient, because it permitted him the opportunity of bringing to the patient's attention for the first time how anxiety was associated with closeness in his relationships with people. Even though the induction of hypnosis was probably justified on the aforegoing basis, the case illustrates how an abrupt breaking through of an individual's defenses can produce severe anxiety.

Assuming that hypnosis can be induced successfully, therapeutic failures can occur under the same conditions and for precisely the same reasons as failures with any type of psychotherapy.

The most frequent reason for failure is an inadequate or distorted motivation for hypnosis. As has been mentioned before, hypnosis has so many occult associations that it is apt to attract persons who seek a magical essence of some sort that can inject qualities in them which they do not possess. Compulsion neurotics are particularly attracted to the hypnotic method for this reason; they want a magical formula, and often desire from hypnosis a means of controlling themselves as well as the universe.

In some instances a distorted motivation of this sort which is symbolically satisfied in hypnosis may put to an end, for a while at least, certain disturbing symptoms. To illustrate, a man came to see me with the request that I hypnotize him in order that he be able to learn the process of self hypnosis for the purpose of inducing skin anesthesia. He justified this peculiar request by alleging that if he were in an automobile accident, many miles away from a town, he might require surgical help. In such an emergency he wanted to be able to induce anesthesia so that he would feel no pain. It seemed

obvious to me that his motivation for hypnosis was a distorted one, and that it probably concealed a much deeper
motive of which he was not entirely aware.

Prior to inducing hypnosis I suggested that we discuss any
problems that he might have; but he refused to do so contend-
ing that since his sole interest was to learn self hypnosis,
there was no reason for going into his various difficulties, one
of which was a problem with his fiancée. As a matter of fact,
he confided, he had already gone through a period of psychotherapy with a qualified psychiatrist, and was certain that
he had gotten sufficient help out of treatments so that he now
required no further psychotherapeutic aid.

Hypnosis was easily induced and the patient rapidly learned
the technic of self hypnosis. In the course of training, through
the medium of dream induction and other hypnoanalytic
technics, it was possible to learn what was behind his request
for self hypnosis. Because of early inimical experiences, the
patient had developed a character structure with detachment
as a primary defense. He had been able to manage his life
successfully by maintaining a certain distance from people,
and by an aloofness which prevented him from getting himself involved too intimately with any person. On the surface
he gave the appearance of being a self-contained and self-
confident individual who was capable of a congenial relationship; but he noticed that when a friendship started developing he had to terminate the relationship of his own accord.

In the past few months he had become seriously involved
with a young woman, and for the first time in his life he had
begun to experience emotions of love. These disturbed him,
and he wanted to escape his feelings; but no matter what he
did, proximity with the young woman continued to bring out
emotions which he felt he could not handle. In desperation he
conceived of a plan whereby he might possibly be able to
function if he could bring himself to where he could control
and deaden his feelings. He then might perhaps master his

emotions to a point where he could continue his relationship with the young woman and yet not get so involved with her as to experience panic and his other usual reactions to closeness. These deliberations were not completely conscious. They reflected themselves symbolically in a desire to control skin sensations and to deaden them through will power reinforced by self hypnosis. He had rationalized his wish to abnegate all feeling by convincing himself that he desired solely to learn how to impose anesthesia on himself.

During a trance these facts were presented to the patient, and he was told that he might not be able to accept them in the waking state, but that when he felt sufficiently strong within himself to want to tackle the deeper problems of his relationships with people and his need for detachment, he would be able to proceed to where he could divest himself of any fears that prevented him from living realistically and productively.

Very little effect of this talk seemed to have registered, the patient having complete amnesia for it. He was apparently satisfied to have mastered the technic of hand anesthesia, and he practiced inducing anesthesia over various parts of his body. After five sessions he declared that he had gained all he desired from hypnosis.

Several months later he telephoned me and remarked that self hypnosis had made a new man out of him and that he no longer felt upset with his fiancée. However, it suddenly had occurred to him that he had wanted to learn self hypnosis because it would enable him to control his feelings as well as sensations. From his conversation it was apparent that he had utilized the insights that I had given him during the trance. He realized that he required further help for his problem and shortly thereafter he started psychotherapy with me.

Among other inadequate motivations for hypnosis is utilization of the trance as a means of submitting to an omniscient authority, in order to derive masochistic gratifications from this submission. Under this circumstance hypnotherapy usually ends in failure. Many passively homosexual individuals, who are frustrated in their homosexual interests, seek hypnosis both as a means of fighting against and finally yielding to powerful authority. Even though they may ostensibly desire hypnotherapy to aid in controlling homosexuality, their neurotic motivation, if not understood and analyzed, can completely block the achievement of a satisfactory therapeutic result. When a motivation of this kind is present, it is essential to work with it on a waking level in order to get the patient to a point where he can accept therapy on a different, more rational basis. When he refuses to do so, hypnotherapy may merely exaggerate rather than help his problem.

A further reason for therapeutic failure with hypnosis is that some persons seek from it a cure of a rapid nature, being impatient with the prolonged time period consumed by the traditional psychotherapies. Because hypnosis is such a dramatic phenomenon, it is easy to understand why most people are susceptible to the notion that hypnosis can bring about, in an incredibly short period of time, results that are not possible with any other treatment method.

While it is true that hypnosis can often shorten the therapeutic procedure, it is not true that it can break through habit patterns of an obdurate nature thus enabling the individual to function successfully in life without the formality of working through his deep conflicts and disturbances in interpersonal relationships which militate against a successful adaptation. The impatience of an individual to overcome his neurosis is quite understandable; however, time is the essence of those forms of psychotherapy that have as their objective the complete rehabilitation of the individual in his functional relationships to life and to people. Where the patient does not understand that therapy will take time, he is apt to expect the impossible of hypnosis, and, failing to gain his wishes, he may blame himself, adopting a completely hopeless attitude towards his illness. It is essential, too, that the physician understand that hypnotherapy may not in itself be able to rectify certain aspects of the personality. Such components as self confidence and assertiveness may require the putting into action in actual life experience the lessons learned in therapy. This may require a considerable period of time.

In order to understand more completely the reasons for therapeutic failure, it is essential to understand what we mean by a therapeutic success. Success in therapy implies that we have achieved a certain determined goal. As a matter of fact therapeutic failures, as well as therapeutic successes, can be spoken of only in the context of a delineated therapeutic goal. Once this goal is outlined, we can determine whether our results approximate this goal, and we are then able to classify our effort as either a success or a failure. We may decide that on the basis of inadequate time, or inadequate motivation, or of diminutive ego strength that we can achieve only a limited goal, as, for instance, the removal of a disabling symptom. From the standpoint of our delineated goal, then, we would say that our therapy is successful. However, we must admit that we have not really influenced the personality structure of the patient, nor altered his basic neurotic patterns. We must thus, from another point of view, consider our therapy a failure.

For instance, a neurotic patient comes to therapy with the chief complaint of being unable to sleep, and he looks to hypnotherapy to cure his insomnia. Through the medium of suggestion during the trance, we may be able to relieve or cure his symptom by direct attack. However, because the neurotic structure itself is not touched, the individual will continue to suffer from disturbances in relationships with people and from disabling neurotic manifestations. Can we then rightfully speak of the cure of the patient's insomnia as a therapeutic success? Where our goal has been merely to treat the symptom of insomnia, we may say that we have treated him successfully. However, where our goal is to re-habilitate him as a functioning unit in society, we must admit that our effort is to be classified as a failure.

Another example may clarify this point. A patient was sent to me some years ago for hypnotherapy in order to recapture memories that he had been unable to bring to the surface in several years of psychoanalysis. The analyst believed that through the medium of regression it would be possible to return the patient to a period in his life where he would be able to remember and to live through a traumatic experience which might account for his homosexuality. When I saw the patient it was apparent to me that he was markedly disabled in his relationships with people. He had been seeking a means of circumventing his anxiety and, through reading, had be-come convinced that were he able to uncover a secret in his past regarding some traumatic injury that had been inflicted upon him, it would explain and remove his fear of people, particularly of women. It was apparent to me that during his prolonged period of psychotherapy he had successfully evaded relating himself closely to the psychiatrist, and had spent most of his time attempting to enucleate elements in his past history which seemed to account for his difficulty. He had become progressively more and more frustrated as he discovered that memories and the recounting of early diffi-culties had very little ameliorative effect upon his anxiety and present interpersonal difficulties. He had become convinced that all the early incidents he had produced were merely cover memories and that deeply imbedded within himself there was a memory so traumatic and so devastating to his conscious mind that it had successfully evaded all attempts at probing. He therefore wanted help in hypnosis in order to get to the bottom of his difficulty.

It was possible to induce a fairly deep trance, and, through the medium of automatic writing in the regressed state, **the**

patient was able to recapture an experience in which he had
witnessed his parents having sexual relationships. He lived
through the frightening experience of encountering for the
first time the sight of the female genital organ which he conceived of as mutilated. This incident had aroused deep fears
of castration and a horror of observing female genital organs
for fear of being confronted with the possibility that he too
might become castrated.

The recapturing of this early traumatic event, his living
through the emotions related to this event, exhilarated him
temporarily. However, it did not alter in the least his customary character patterns, nor did it make it possible for him
to give up his fear of women.

The result was that he insisted that what he had recaptured
was valid, but that there was probably something even deeper
than this, which if enucleated would immediately remove his
anxiety. Here, while the goal of recapturing early memories
had succeeded, we had failed to produce any change in his
neurotic structure. From a therapeutic standpoint, this case
had to be classified as a failure, even though the failure was
not the fault of hypnosis, but rather the product of the generally mistaken notion that recapture of early traumatic
memories can bring relief to a character problem.

Another example of what I would consider a therapeutic
failure, but which, on the basis of the actual reasons for coming to therapy would ordinarily be classified as a therapeutic
success, is the case of a psychopathic personality who had
gotten into innumerable conflicts with the law, and who had
indulged in episodic bouts of intoxication during which he
signed worthless checks and involved himself in serious problems with authority. He came to me primarily with the desire
to have something done so that when he was in an alcoholic
state he would not be able to sign blank checks.

Although he professed a desire for a better life, it soon became obvious that the secondary gain element of his illness

was too important to enable him to desire to abandon his disturbed and irresponsible way of life. Therapy was started with the object of establishing a conditioned reflex which would prevent him from passing worthless checks. Another further objective was gradually to bring the patient to a realization of his own destructiveness in order to make it possible for him to wish for therapy on a deeper level. During a somnambulistic trance, a conditioned reflex was set up so that when he started signing a worthless check, a spastic paralysis prevented him from completing the action. This reflex was successful and with reinforcement the patient found that, even though drunk, he was not able to sign checks. Furthermore, during reinforcement, attempts were made to bring the patient to an understanding of his actual neurotic problems and acting-out tendencies. The latter effort failed, since sufficient motivation for change could not be brought about, and, while the patient was inhibited in his attempt to sign worthless checks, he continued to engage in bouts of alcoholic activity which he rationalized with extreme ingenuity.

The conditioned reflex was successful, but after several months reports came to me that he had passed several more worthless checks. Upon questioning under hypnosis, the patient confessed to having practiced signing his name with his left hand when he discovered that he was unable to use his right. A conditioning process then was set up which prevented him from signing checks with either hand. However, he soon found a way of circumventing this by getting one of his friends to forge his name. Therapy was then interpreted as a complete failure. This case illustrates the fact that working with a patient in whom the motivation for therapy is inadequate usually is unsuccessful.

A definition of an adequate goal in therapy must take into account the fact that what we strive for as an ideal is the complete rehabilitation of the person in his relationships with life. We seek to bring the individual to a point where he can derive pleasures from creature comforts of life, from food, sex, work, and relaxation. The capacity to satisfy these drives in conformity with the mores of the group, and the ability to find opportunities and to execute successfully fulfillment of needs in line with existing resources and environmental opportunities, is an important objective. The patient must achieve the capacity to relate himself productively and con-genially with other people. He must establish a relationship to authority so that he can assume a subordinate role without fear or rage, and, in certain situations, still be capable of assuming leadership. He must develop the ability to adapt himself to stress and to frustration without resorting to child-ish forms of defense or fantasy. This involves the ability to withstand a certain amount of deprivation without anxiety, when it is reasonable or necessary to group welfare, or when consequences of impulse fulfillment entail more than their worth in compensatory pain. There must be a healthy regard for the self as an individual, with a capacity to face the past and to isolate from the present anxieties related to childhood experiences. There must furthermore be a realization of limi-tations and an ability to fulfill oneself within the bounds of these limitations. Other objectives are self confidence, asser-tiveness, a sense of freedom, spontaneity and self tolerance.

These goals, as will be recognized, are extremely ambitious and, in many cases cannot be achieved. There are a number of reasons for this.

One of the chief causes of failure is the individual's lack of adequate motivation; he sees no need for working out his problem, is satisfied with an inadequate adjustment to life and to people, or is unwilling to work with the type of technic that would make it possible for him to achieve these goals. Another reason is the individual's possession of an ego struc-ture so weak that it is unable to tolerate anxieties which are incident to an understanding of his deeper problems and to the relating of himself to people in such a way that he can experience and live through these problems. This is the case in preschizoid, in very dependent or detached characters, in whom close relationships mobilize such intense anxiety that they are incapable of utilizing available strengths to work out a more adequate solution to their difficulties. A third reason is the derivation by the individual of so many secondary gains from his neurosis that these more than counteract the anxiety associated with the neurosis. A fourth reason is misdirected conduct of the therapeutic session itself, the therapist assuming an authoritarian approach, setting values for the patient and coercing or persuading him to adopt these values. While an authoritarian approach has certain advantages, particularly in brief psychotherapy where partial goals are to be achieved, it can block the achievement of the goal of complete rehabilitation.

The patient always comes to therapy with a problem for which he wants active help. He assumes that, as in other contacts with doctors, he merely has to present his problem to the physician and the latter will either remove his difficulty or tell him how he can get well. In this assumption lie the seeds of a great deal of misunderstanding, inasmuch as the acceptance of direction and suggestions from the therapist may block the patient's development. What we most desire as a goal is the bringing of the patient to a point where he can function through his own resources as a strong, capable, assertive person, making his own choices and decisions in his effort to lead a productive life. The patient has been unable to do this hitherto and many of his difficulties are the product of excessive demands upon authority, of dependencies and hostilities that are consequent to a feeling of self paralysis. Where the treatment session is so conducted that the therapist does the bulk of the therapeutic work, where he gives the patient suggestions, and where he assumes the attitude of the leader who extends moral judgments on the thoughts and actions of the patient, the latter is virtually infantalized, and never has the opportunity to work out an adequate acceptance of himself in line with values that he himself formulates. He continues to need reinforcement in the form of prohibitions or support, and he never liberates himself from the tyranny of authority.

The traditional conduct of the hypnotic session itself is such that it plays into the authoritarian demands that the patient may make on the therapist. When the patient comes to a physician for hypnosis he immediately adopts an attitude of passivity. He assumes that he will be put into a suggestible state, that directions will be given him, and that through some magic he will be able to function in ways that will bring him health or success. The very fact that suggestions are given to him, and that he enters into a relationship in which he is submissive immediately circumscribes the therapeutic goal.

Seemingly we are confronted with an insurmountable contradiction for, it will be said, the induction of hypnosis itself involves the passivity of the patient, and suggestions given the patient are similar to those in a child-parent relationship. How then is it possible for the patient to achieve the goal of complete rehabilitation in a medium where the hypnotist is the commanding authority?

These objections are valid and, in my opinion, the individual is never capable of liberating himself from authority, nor of achieving the utmost change in his character structure where the hypnotic situation is conducted in the traditional manner. Self growth and the ability to become an independent, assertive individual are most effectively achieved in a treatment experience in which the patient is capable of working out his problems through his own capacities and resources. The entire conduct of the hypnotic session, therefore, must be modified to a point where the patient no longer puts himself into a passive state and expects suggestions from the omniscient hypnotist which will direct him towards mental health.

Achievement of the ultimate goal in therapy, of complete personality rehabilitation, involves the abandonment on the part of the patient of the notion that he can depend exclusively on directions and suggestions from the therapist. Otherwise, therapeutic failures will be unavoidable.

The fact that the use of hypnosis in the traditional sense revivifies the child-parent relationship, and prevents the growing up of the patient, makes it mandatory to modify the induction technic itself as well as the conduct of the session under hypnosis. With the usual method of inducing hypnosis, the patient responds to suggestions that he feels are imposed upon him. He gradually becomes more and more drowsy and finally upon command sinks into a trance state. He then continues to follow suggestions that are given to him by the hypnotist, either because he desires to do so of his own free will or because he feels powerless to resist these suggestions. Under these circumstances, he conceives himself to be under the power of a stronger individual, and he complies because he feels that compliance is expected of him.

In order to remove the patient from this expectation, the essential modification of the induction process may be accomplished in several ways. One method is to couch suggestions in such a way that the patient himself feels that he is participating in the induction process. The technic of hand levitation which has been described is extremely helpful in this respect, and makes for many induction successes that would otherwise have ended in failure. Furthermore, it prepares the patient so that he himself, with proper direction, begins to assume the responsibility of participating in his own growth process. Gradually, as he learns the technic of entering the trance state, the direction for this is transfered to the patient. He is told that he himself will, when he so desires, upon giving himself a certain command, be able to enter a trance and will be capable of giving himself suggestions to achieve certain tests through his own efforts. What occurs is that the patient who first dreams upon suggestion, or writes automatically, or follows posthypnotic suggestions upon command, discovers that he, himself, can apply these technics to himself. The feeling on the part of the patient that he has the capacity to execute activities by himself and to work out his own problems has an enhancing effect on ego growth, and liberates him from the feeling that he needs the help of a stronger person.

While the conduct of the therapeutic session in this way, makes for a minimum of therapeutic failures where complete rehabilitation of personality is the goal, it must be remembered that there are many persons who are not amenable to therapy of this sort. There are those whose problems are so vast, whose ego structures are so weak, whose motivations are so inadequate, that they resent and refuse to participate in a treatment process where they themselves are expected to make decisions and to develop along the lines which they themselves dictate. Here it is essential to abandon the therapeutic goal of complete rehabilitation for one that is more inadequate, but which will make it possible for the individual to experience symptomatic relief in the face of a neurotic character structure.

The aim in therapy of this sort is more or less supportive. It tends to bring the ego to as stable a condition as possible through supplying needs that are lacking, or through giving the patient direction and suggestions that will enable him to live with his neurotic defenses as comfortably as possible.

An example of this is the immature personality who, having functioned through the medium of dependency all his life, responds to the death or departure of his host with depression and anxiety and comes to treatment in a state of collapse. Under these circumstances, the therapist, in inducing hypnosis, assumes the role of an authority who replaces the individual on whom the patient hitherto depended. The therapist deliberately enters into a neurotic type of relationship with the patient, supplying the needs that the patient wants fulfilled. In this situation, anxiety, tension and other symptoms are bound to vanish. It is important to remember that despite symptomatic relief the patient is essentially the same neurotic person he was before, and that he has merely entered into a new relationship that satisfies his neurotic needs. Where the therapeutic goal is the relief of symptoms, or the dissipation of anxiety, we may credit this type of result as a therapeutic success. However, we must not delude ourselves about the quality of the success, because the individual actually has not solved his basic problems.

There are some individuals who are susceptible to an authoritarian approach only. Here the traditional use of hypnosis, with authoritative commands to abandon symptoms, or enjoinders that anxieties will vanish, or persuasion to change attitudes towards life may bring success in the form of symptom relief.

Many successes have been reported with hypnosis in which the session has been conducted exclusively in an authoritarian manner. I, myself, have had some successes of this type. For instance, one of my experiences with hypnosis was a patient who had hysterical aphonia for a number of years, and who, in several treatment sessions with hypnosis, which were conducted along the lines of forcing her to talk, suddenly recovered her voice and has not shown a relapse of her aphonia over a period of five years. In another instance an alcoholic patient, who had failed to stop drinking with conditioned reflex therapy, shock therapy and psychotherapy, succeeded in giving up drinking following one hypnotic trance, and has remained dry for almost two years.

In most cases, however, authoritative commands to the patient to abandon symptoms will end in complete failure.

A modified technic in which the symptom is made to disappear through a ruse instead of by direct attack may sometimes succeed. For example, a man who was a cornet player by profession came to see me with the complaint that he had over a period of two years developed a spasm of his masseter muscles whenever he brought the mouthpiece of his instrument toward his mouth. A clenching of the jaws also occurred when he brought a utensil to his mouth while eating. The symbolic nature of the patient's symptoms seemed obvious, but the patient himself had absolutely no insight into its significance nor did he have any desire to probe its nature. His Rorschach test indicated an extremely coarcted person with rigid characterologic defenses and manifest ego weaknesses. He desired a cure within a period of three weeks, inasmuch as he had a contract to play in a band on the coast. Financial circumstances made it mandatory for him to work as soon as possible, and the job that was open to him afforded him an opportunity to earn a fairly substantial salary.

Under deep hypnosis an attempt was made to get the patient to play his cornet. This was unsuccessful. Spasm of the jaw muscles occurred even when strong injunctions were given to the patient that he allow his jaws to relax and that he shift his attention from the cornet. At the next session a new technic was tried. The patient was given the suggestion that whenever an object approached his mouth the spasm that previously occurred in his jaw would be transferred to his left foot. A conditioned response was set up so that automatically as soon as an object approached the patient's mouth, the muscles of his left foot contracted in substitution of those of his jaw. The object was to transfer spasm, with its symbolic values, to a less incapacitating part of the body. With this ruse it was possible for the patient to play his cornet under hypnosis, and while playing he was awakened. Upon awakening he joyously leaped up from the chair, but found that his left leg was in a cramp. However, as he spoke the cramp disappeared. Enthusiastically he lifted the cornet again to his mouth, and his foot again went into a cramp. He declared that the cramp bothered him, but not sufficiently to prevent him from playing the cornet. This conditioned reflex was reinforced during the period that he remained east. So far as I know to this day he is able to function at his work.

Individuals with inadequate motivation, or whose ego strength is doubtful, cannot be expected to achieve the goal of complete personality rehabilitation. Here adjustment to the existing neurosis with a utilization of available resources to the full, and minimization of liabilities, is all that can be expected. Hypnosis may be helpful in enabling the ego, weak as it is, to cope with existing pressures. However, relapses must be expected, because the individual does not with this type of therapy ever achieve a self stature that will permit him to handle the stresses of life in a mature and realistic way. This is why hypnotherapy which is used as a means of removing symptoms, or of persuading the individual to change his attitudes, is bound to bring only temporary success. So long as the hypnotist relies entirely upon the authoritarian powers with which the hypnotic situation automatically invests him, his therapeutic effectiveness will be no greater than cures achieved by miraculous healing.

Direct symptom removal or ruses to permit symptom removal are usually inadvisable, unless the significance of the symptoms is studied and some means of compensation provided. Where no other therapy than symptom removal can be used, the patient must be given some compensatory symptom that will have a significance to him symbolically similar though less incapacitating than the symptom which is to be removed. For example, where a patient possesses a paralysis of an arm which is associated with hostility toward a parent, and which represents an attempt to incapacitate him from yielding to his murderous impulses, an attempt to remove the paralysis may precipitate intense anxiety. However, where the function of the paralysis is understood, and where the patient is given suggestions such as that instead of his arm beoming paralyzed, one of his little fingers will be affected, and where this ruse is accepted by the patient, anxiety may be averted. In several instances I have seen patients who have been plunged into intense anxiety states, and in one instance into a psychotic condition, because of symptom removal by authoritative suggestion, when the symptom itself served the protective function of keeping anxiety in check.

In spite of these limitations, suggestive hypnosis has a place in the therapeutic armamentarium. It is essential always to realize that the objective is a partial one and does not permit the patient to function to the full measure of his capacities. Wherever possible attempts should be made to guide the patient to a proper motivation, and to promote a stabilization of his ego so that he can accept a more rational type of therapy.

REFERENCE

[1] ERICKSON, M. H.: An experimental investigation of the possible antisocial use of hypnosis. Psychiatry 2: 391-414, 1939.

INDEX

443